Realism

A Study in Human Structural Anatomy

Second Edition

Carol F. Edwards, RMT

Brenda A. Grosenick, RMT

Kasterstener Technical Director: Jonathan Hill

3D Images by: Darryl Lajeunesse, CD Media Studios Inc.

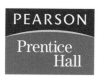

PEARSON

Prentice Hall

Upper Saddle River, New Jersey 07458

Grosenick, Brenda, A. [Date]
   Realism : a study in human structural anatomy / by Brenda A. Grosenick and Carol F. Edwards. -- 2nd ed.
     p. ; cm.
   Rev. ed. of: Realism / Darryl Lajeunesse, Carol Edwards, Brenda Grosenick. c2003.
   Includes bibliographical references and index.
   ISBN 0-13-812745-X
   1. Human anatomy--Atlases. 2. Anatomy, Artistic--Atlases. I. Edwards, Carol, [Date] II. Lajeunesse, Darryl,
[Date] Realism. III. Title.
   [DNLM: 1. Musculoskeletal System--anatomy & histology--Atlases. WE 17 G8765r 2009]
   QM25.L34 2009
   611.0022'3--dc22
                                                                              2008003314

Publisher: Julie Levin Alexander
Publisher's Assistant: Regina Bruno
Executive Editor: Mark Cohen
Associate Editor: Melissa Kerian
Editorial Assistant: Nicole Ragonese
Senior Marketing Manager: Harper Coles
Marketing Specialist: Michael Sirinides
Marketing Assistant: Lauren Castellano
Managing Editor: Patrick Walsh
Senior Operations Manager: Ilene Sanford
Operations Specialist: Pat Brown
Cover Art Director: Jayne Conte
Cover Design: Bruce Kenselaar
Full-Service Project Management: Kevin Bradley, GGS Book Services
Printer/Binder: Courier Printing, Kendallville IN
Cover Printer: Phoenix Color Corporation
Typeface: 10/12 Helvetica

Pearson Prentice Hall™ is a trademark of Pearson Education, Inc.
Pearson® is a registered trademark of Pearson plc
Prentice Hall® is a registered trademark of Pearson Education, Inc.

Pearson Education Ltd., London
Pearson Education Singapore, Pte. Ltd.
Pearson Education, Canada, Inc.
Pearson Education–Japan

Pearson Education Australia PTY, Limited
Pearson Education North Asia Ltd., Hong Kong
Pearson Educación de Mexico, S.A. de C.V.
Pearson Education Malaysia, Pte. Ltd.
Pearson Education, Upper Saddle River, New Jersey

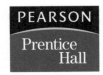

10 9 8 7 6 5 4 3
ISBN-13: 978-0-13-812745-9
ISBN-10: 0-13-812745-X

Dedication

Carol—To my children, Cassandra and Ryan. Your patience throughout has been steadfast and your supportive natures have been an incredible blessing. Your belief in me is what motivates me. To Melvyn "Rod" MacLeod. Your friendship and advice have been cornerstones providing companionship and insight.

Brenda—To my loving and supportive husband Darrin, with whom I cherish each and every day. To my beautiful children, Adam, Kaitlynn, Logan, and Leigha, who are always my inspiration. For all of you…my heart is filled with gratitude.

The Authors

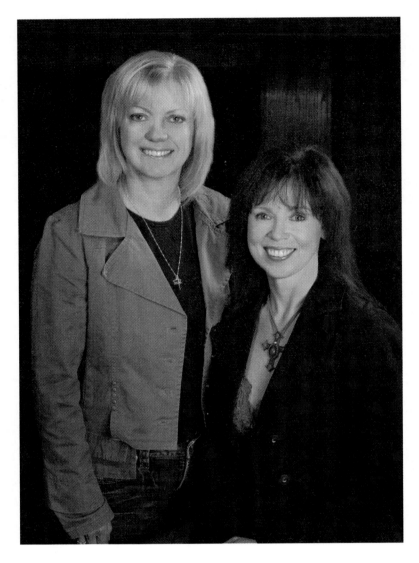

Carol F. Edwards, RMT   Brenda A. Grosenick, RMT

Photo by:
Dean Ward
Highview Photo
3434 50th Avenue
Red Deer, Alberta
T4N 3Y4
(403) 343-1808

Contents

The 3-dimensional, digitally enhanced models literally leap off the pages bringing God's awesome creation to light! All students of musculoskeletal anatomy will definitely benefit from the incredible clarity presented here. The fruition of the painstaking work is evident in the remarkable views not depicted in other anatomical texts. I certainly look forward to the accompanying CD that will advance learning in the twenty-first century.

— *Todd Newfield, DC*
   Red Deer, AB

The amount of detail in the models is unparalleled. Anyone who is a student of the human body should have this book in their collection. References are constantly needed during the character creation process in gaming and having a book with so much detail only helps to create a better product. In my field having such a good reference is invaluable.

— *Jesse Brophy, Senior Artist*
   Atari Interactive
   Silver Spring, MD

The visual impact of this graphic representation provides a great guide for anatomy professionals. It gives a 3D picture that provides a clear description of bony landmarks and muscle attachments.

— *Dr. Réal Gaboriault, Ph.D.*
   CTRC President (Canadian Touch Research Center)
   Montreal, QC

The book is truly "user friendly"—the visual display is appealing and you have managed to include the photos and descriptors in such a way that one does not get the sense that information is crammed onto a page—the succinct labeling with clear lines to the visuals makes finding the anatomical detail very easy. The use of OIAN (origin, insertion, action, and nerve) is helpful and provides valuable information in a succinct and predictable manner. I have used the book in my advanced health assessment course, and students have been able to Find any item they have searched for. The varied views truly provide the 360-degree visualization one needs to understand the core anatomy in its fullest.

— *Madeleine Buck*
   Assistant Director B.Sc.(N)
   School of Nursing
   McGill University

Human anatomy is an old science and one could probably argue that everything related to it has been said and done shortly after Leonardo da Vinci's time. Althouh this may be true in general, every once in a while something truly outstanding happens, which advances a field where no major advances are to be expected anymore. One such event is "Realism," which pushes the level of graphical detail available in human anatomy to unprecedented heights. Thousands of computer objects, representing the bones and muscles of the human body, were constructed in three dimensions. Image maps with very high resolution were painted onto the objects to give them very realistic color rendition and textures. The resulting anatomical objects are astounding in their appearance and will be extremely useful for teaching and research. Students and teachers alike will enjoy the book, which allows one to marvel at the beauty of the construction of the human body. In addition, I hope that this book will find an even wider audience of people who enjoy the computer artwork presented in this book and who might learn something about the organization of the human body by studying the following pages.

The truly important breakthrough presented here though is the fact that all objects were rendered in the computer. This will allow people with access to the files to manipulate them in three dimensions. Using computers, objects (e.g., muscles or bones) can be removed to look at the underlying structures and study them in detail. The computer model becomes a toolkit, which can be used and reused in many different settings. This certainly pushes the envelope of human anatomy modeling and can already be considered a new paradigm on how to store and present anatomical data. With the complete human genome now available from public databases, imaging is becoming more and more important as a tool, which allows the mapping and visualization of very complex data sets, for example, related to gene expression patterns and posttranslational protein modifications.

The data set presented in this book will be an important step on the way to understanding how the human body is organized and how it functions. In the future, three-dimensional displays, from stereo goggles to fully immersive virtual reality environments could be used to view and manipulate the anatomy data. Other data sets might be superimposed onto the anatomy to understand spatial and temporal phenomena in the human body. This will go far beyond the printed information presented here, which in itself is already absolutely outstanding in quality and depth of information. I certainly hope that the readers enjoy the book as much as I do and I hope that the authors can continue their important work and complete the model of the human body.

Calgary

— *Prof. Dr. Christoph W. Sensen*
  Professor of Biochemistry and Molecular Biology
  University of Calgary, AB

Acknowledgments

The undertaking of *Realism* has been sedulously nurtured and as a result, we humbly submit this credible portrayal to a venerable society of sages and a new generation of learners.

Throughout this incredible journey, our "portraiture of legacy," we have experienced personal blessings in our own growth and development of character. Among these blessings was the extraordinary revelation of how incredibly intricate and complex the human structure is. This awareness gifted us with an immense appreciation of the hard work and fervent dedication of previous authors and illustrators.

An endeavor of this magnitude would not be possible without the collective support of family, friends, and colleagues, who believed in our vision and our abilities. It would be remiss of us not to recognize their contribution to our "link in the chain." We wish to acknowledge and give heartfelt thanks to the following people, who have in various ways enriched our lives and enhanced our quest.

Ms. Jennifer Thomas, "The Keeper of All Things"—for her optimistic enthusiasm, unwavering faith and efficient administrative assistance.

Dr. David Dawson—for his delightful encouragement, inspirational discussions, invaluable input, and dependable wisdom

Dr. Real Gaboriault—for his voice of confidence and visionary spirit

Dr. Greg Gellert—for his sincere motivation, uplifting assurance of our abilities, much respected guidance, and eloquent percipience

Dr. Todd Newfield—for his belief in us, his perceptive regard of the vast efforts in achieving this goal, and his polished understanding of anatomy

Prof. Dr. Christoph Sensen—for reinforcing our purpose, corroborating our achievement, seeing beyond the present, and opening a new door of opportunity

Staff at University of Calgary Medical School cadaver lab—for providing us with the privilege of enhancing our knowledge of the human body

Honorable Victor Doerksen—for his sincere interest in our endeavors and informing us of available resources

Ms. Dianne Dawson—for her spirit of celebration and genuine admiration of our venture

Ms. Linda Oman—for helping to facilitate in the delivery of *Realism* with such vivacious passion

A.I.M./E & H staff—for their inexhaustible patience and outstanding dependability

A.I.M. students—for their eternal pursuit of knowledge and refreshing desire to explore it

Family and Friends—for their motivation, steadfast prayers, and for giving us the courage to seize the day

And as always,

Our Heavenly Father, creator of life—we give thanks for your love, direction, and ever present faithfulness.

From Brenda

George and Mary Smallbones—my parents. Thank you for inspiring me to believe in myself and for teaching me the importance of following my dreams with the faith to accomplish my goals. I will always draw strength from your love and support.

The late Rod W. McLeod, my father—"Hold fast McLeod." You taught me when facing a challenge to never give up; to persevere with stubborn tenacity…I think you would be proud.

Bob and Dianna Grosenick—my father- and mother-in-law. Thank you for loving me with open hearts and allowing me the privilege of being part of your lives. Bob, your humor and quick wit have summoned many a chuckle when most needed.

Meechan Fleury—Although the newest member to our family, you have already proven to be a loyal and strong-spirited addition

Kathy Faulk, Tammy Smith, and Lorrie Scherger, my sisters—you have gifted me with laughter, tears, hugs and many treasured memories. Each of you are astonishing women in your own rights and have each touched my life in a special way.

Arla Kaye—my sister, although we don't share childhood memories you have extended your heart and I thank you.

From Carol

Gordon and Gladys Green—my parents, your unconditional love is never wavering. You have allowed me countless opportunities to grow and expand my horizons and have always believed in me. Your life example has taught me the importance of a humble spirit.

Verna Bellerive and the late Karen Green—my sisters, thank you for the experiences that we have encountered together. You have afforded me a unique and humorous outlook on life and have played a most important role in the development of my character.

The rest of my extraordinary family (all of you, you know who you are)—you continually motivate me, and for that I am truly grateful.

The creation of this textbook has been a profound privilege. It has offered us the opportunity to serve those that have a desire to pursue a greater knowledge of the human body as it pertains to structural anatomy.

During our years of introducing the study of the human body to aspiring learners, we have searched for an encompassing teaching tool that realistically and accurately portrayed the complexities of the human structure.

Although there was several quality textbooks published with exceptional content, we were continually searching for *the* textbook. This exhaustive search for a compilation that presented *consistent* illustrations, displayed varied angles of imagery and exhibited a definitive collection of bones, muscles, tendons, ligaments, and nerves was challenging yet futile.

This paucity of conclusive documentation became our motivation to conceive a dream, to identify the deficiencies, to set our goals, to rise to the challenge and to realize the immense satisfaction of proffering an outstanding contribution to a community of past, present, and future scholars.

We began to envision a text that would bridge the gap between what was currently available and what we knew (*based on our experience and the valued input of our instructors and students*) would become a favored resource for educators and learners alike.

Of great importance to us were three issues:

1. That of depth perception (being able to facilitate the learners' visual comprehension of geometry and functionality)
2. That of maintaining integrity and consistency of an image when shown from different angles and perspectives
3. That of illustrating structures independently as well as amalgamating them to portray the synergy of structure and function

Of primary concern to us were two issues:

1. That of accuracy withstanding cogitation
2. That of uncompromised quality

We are confident that we have achieved and in some aspects exceeded our goals in the development of this work of art. The advent of our mapped and textured, three-dimensional models abolish ambiguity, thus eliminating the prevalent concern of continuity in numerous illustrated textbooks. Our hallmark has been our pursuit of excellence and pride, in the creation of *Realism* our first edition and its anticipated progenies.

Utilizing the Textbook

The authors would like to offer the following suggestions to equip the reader with a clearer understanding of how to better utilize the textbook:

n   The standard layouts traditionally employed (e.g., anterior, posterior) are utilized within the sections of this text and some are supplemented by our "unique viewpoints" termed "perspective, exploded, macro, and/or transparent."

n   Origins, insertions, actions, and nerves are depicted by the first letters of each word and are presented as follows: O. Origin, I. Insertion, A. Action, and N. Nerve.

n   When describing origins and insertions, the bone(s) or the specific bony landmark(s) that the muscle attaches to, will be listed first. The adjunct descriptive terms are documented thereafter.*

n   The color blue has been used to signify bursas and synovial sheaths. These structures are not labeled but are included for reference.

n   For each specific grouping in the **muscle group movements unit**, the primary muscles that move the joint are listed first and the synergistic muscles that assist them are listed last and in *italics*.

n   On each page that displays varied vantage points that are dedicated to "showcasing" a specific muscle, that muscle is only labeled once. When referencing the index to find a particular muscle displayed with O., I., A., and N., the bolded page number will direct you to the primary page.

n   There are five units; each is prefaced with a unit page that lists the sections, contents, and image numbers

n   The specific format set for general content within a unit is: a header displaying section, image number, identification, and distinctive views, if applicable. The unit number and category are listed at the bottom of the page,

E.g., *Section 6.10 Thorax, Perspective, (Macro)*—(header)
      Unit 1 Skeletal System—(footer).

n   When accessing the muscle sections, pay particular attention to the sequence of presentation. The arrangements have been carefully laid out to show the musculature in the order of placement on the human body. Macro views are displayed first to facilitate the relativity of surrounding structures. Next as individual muscles within that macro image are removed, from the *superficial layers down to the deepest layers*,* the reader can associate the residency of each definite muscle. At this point, accompanying the composition is a detailed description of attachments, actions, and innervations.

n   The nerves within Unit 5 have been color coded to provide visual impact and clearly distinguish the plexuses. A checkered pattern was used to denote the nerve roots.

* These are guiding principles applied whenever possible.

Skeletal System

Realism   *a study in human structural anatomy*

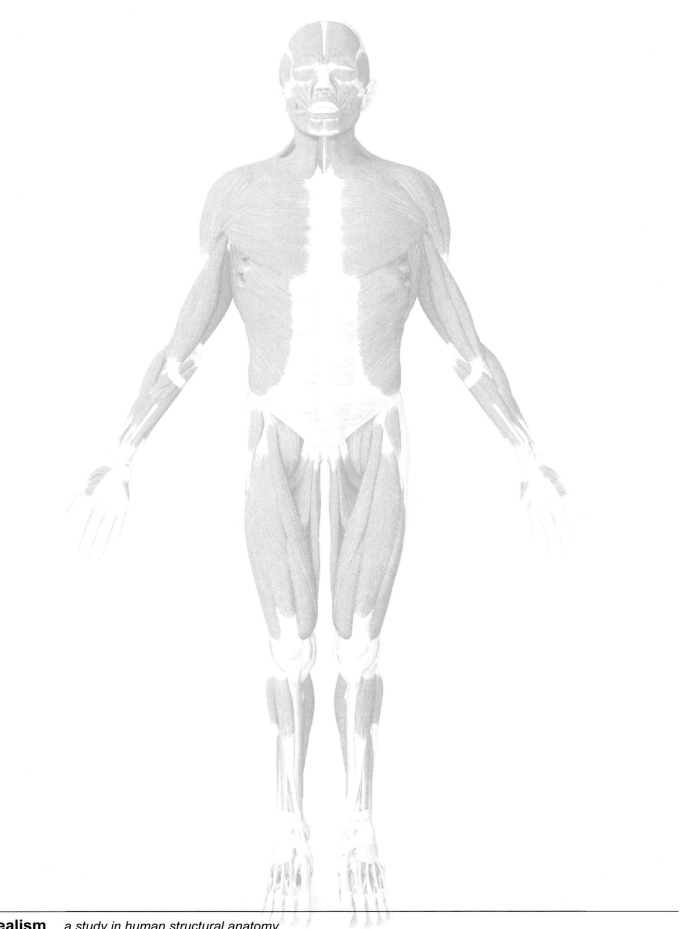

Realism   *a study in human structural anatomy*

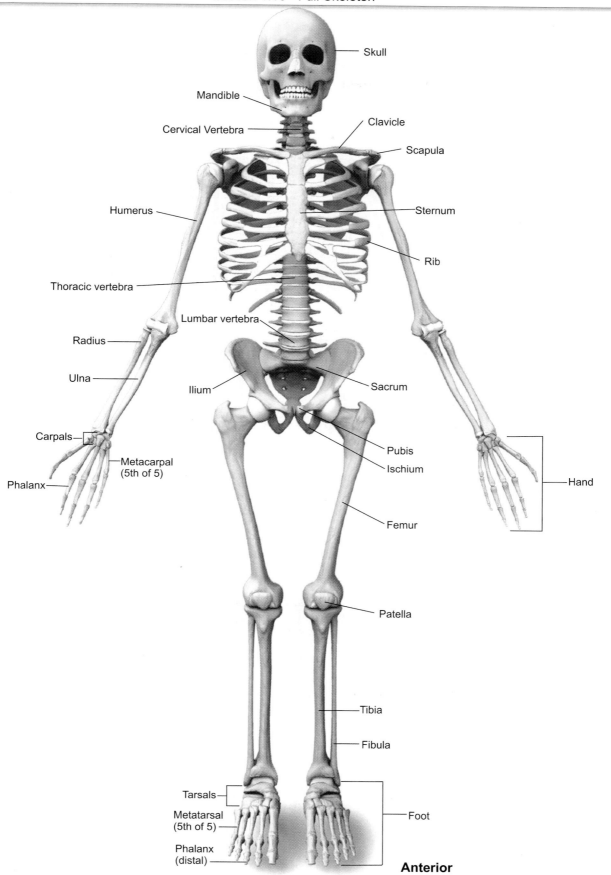

Skull

Mandible

Cervical Vertebra

Clavicle

Scapula

Humerus

Sternum

Rib

Thoracic vertebra

Lumbar vertebra

Radius

Ulna

Ilium

Sacrum

Carpals

Pubis

Ischium

Metacarpal
(5th of 5)

Phalanx

Hand

Femur

Patella

Tibia

Fibula

Tarsals

Metatarsal
(5th of 5)

Foot

Phalanx
(distal)

Anterior

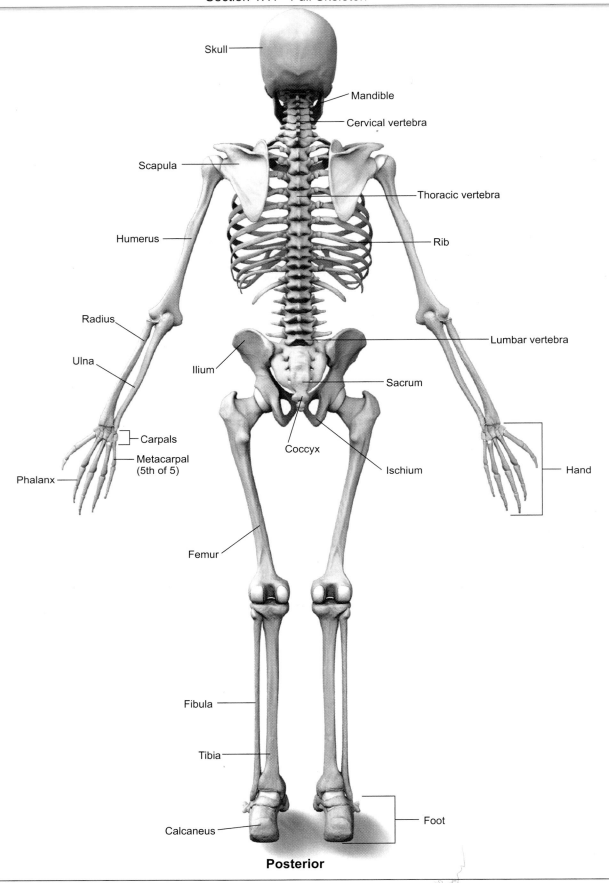

Skull

Mandible

Cervical vertebra

Scapula

Thoracic vertebra

Humerus

Rib

Radius

Lumbar vertebra

Ulna

Ilium

Sacrum

Carpals

Coccyx

Metacarpal
(5th of 5)

Ischium

Hand

Phalanx

Femur

Fibula

Tibia

Foot

Calcaneus

Posterior

Unit 1 Skeletal System

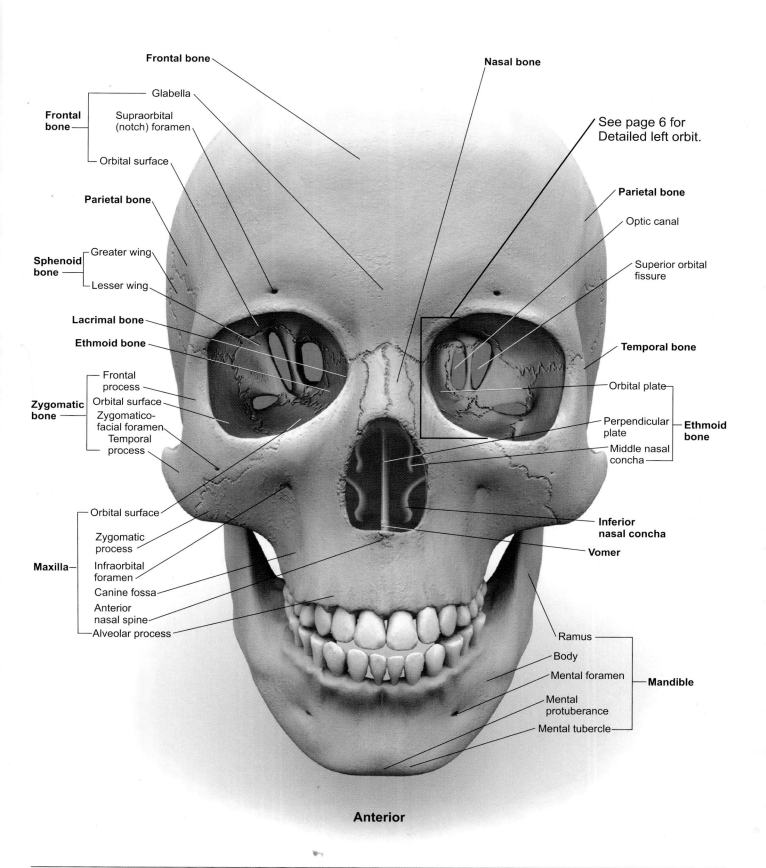

Frontal bone

Frontal bone

Glabella

Supraorbital
(notch) foramen

Orbital surface

Parietal bone

Sphenoid
bone

Greater wing

Lesser wing

Lacrimal bone

Ethmoid bone

Zygomatic
bone

Frontal
process

Orbital surface

Zygomatico-
facial foramen

Temporal
process

Maxilla

Orbital surface

Zygomatic
process

Infraorbital
foramen

Canine fossa

Anterior
nasal spine

Alveolar process

Nasal bone

See page 6 for
Detailed left orbit.

Parietal bone

Optic canal

Superior orbital
fissure

Temporal bone

Orbital plate

Perpendicular
plate

Middle nasal
concha

Ethmoid
bone

Inferior
nasal concha

Vomer

Ramus

Body

Mental foramen

Mental
protuberance

Mental tubercle

Mandible

Anterior

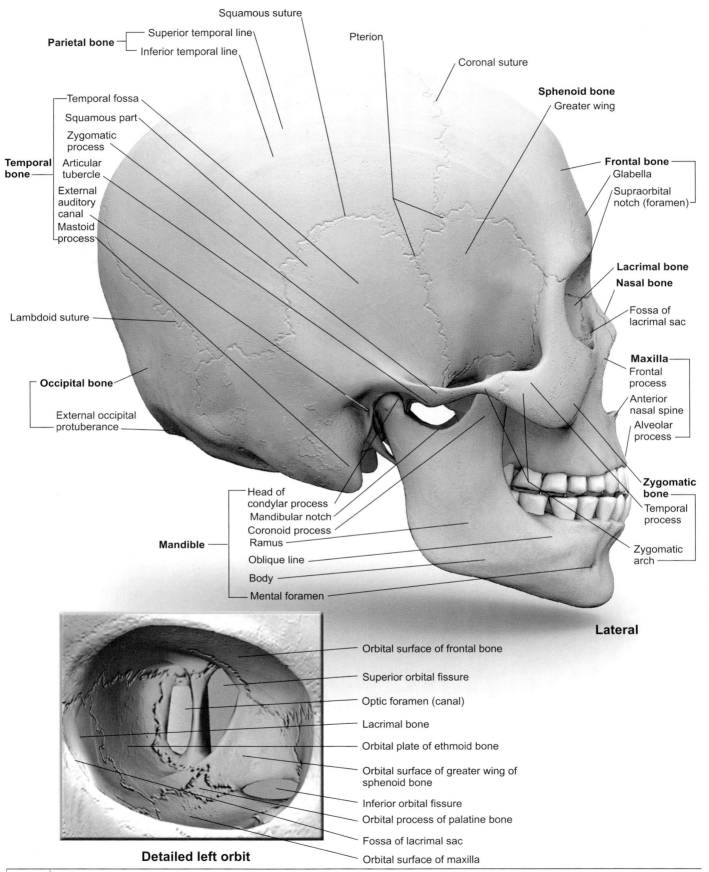

Parietal bone — Superior temporal line
Inferior temporal line
Squamous suture
Pterion
Coronal suture

Temporal fossa
Squamous part
Zygomatic process
Temporal bone — Articular tubercle
External auditory canal
Mastoid process

Sphenoid bone
Greater wing

Frontal bone
Glabella
Supraorbital notch (foramen)

Lacrimal bone
Nasal bone
Fossa of lacrimal sac

Lambdoid suture

Maxilla
Frontal process
Anterior nasal spine
Alveolar process

Occipital bone

External occipital protuberance

Zygomatic bone
Temporal process

Head of condylar process
Mandibular notch
Coronoid process
Mandible — Ramus
Oblique line
Body
Mental foramen

Zygomatic arch

Lateral

Orbital surface of frontal bone

Superior orbital fissure

Optic foramen (canal)

Lacrimal bone

Orbital plate of ethmoid bone

Orbital surface of greater wing of sphenoid bone

Inferior orbital fissure

Orbital process of palatine bone

Fossa of lacrimal sac

Orbital surface of maxilla

Detailed left orbit

Unit 1 Skeletal System

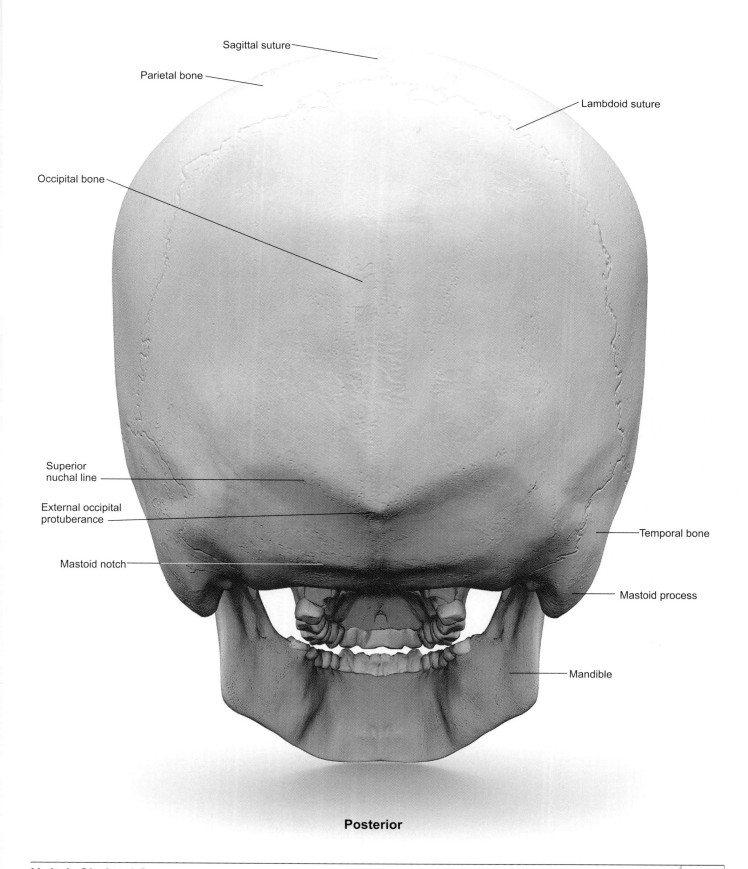

Sagittal suture

Parietal bone

Lambdoid suture

Occipital bone

Superior
nuchal line

External occipital
protuberance

Mastoid notch

Temporal bone

Mastoid process

Mandible

Posterior

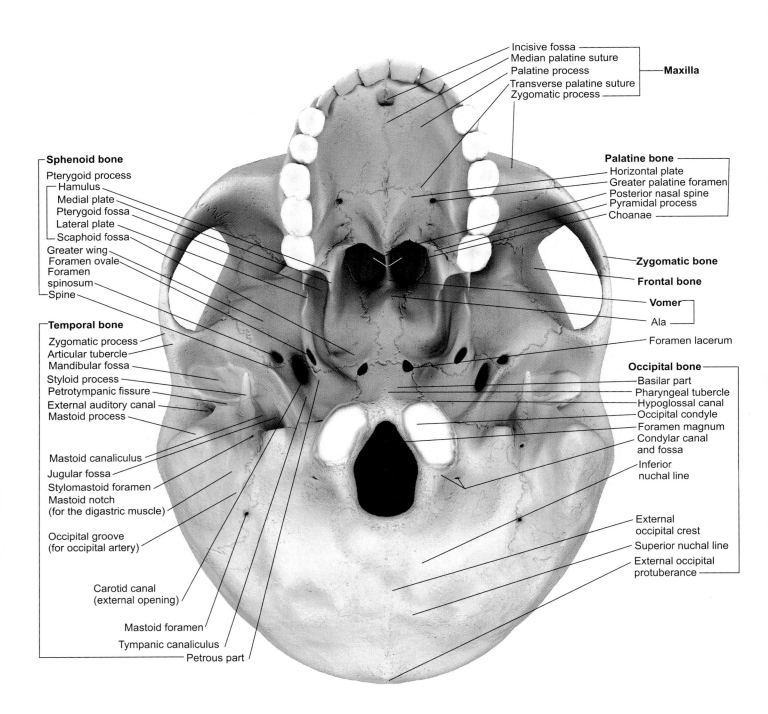

Incisive fossa
Median palatine suture
Palatine process
Transverse palatine suture
Zygomatic process

Maxilla

Sphenoid bone
Pterygoid process
Hamulus
Medial plate
Pterygoid fossa
Lateral plate
Scaphoid fossa
Greater wing
Foramen ovale
Foramen spinosum
Spine

Palatine bone
Horizontal plate
Greater palatine foramen
Posterior nasal spine
Pyramidal process
Choanae

Zygomatic bone

Frontal bone

Vomer
Ala

Foramen lacerum

Temporal bone
Zygomatic process
Articular tubercle
Mandibular fossa
Styloid process
Petrotympanic fissure
External auditory canal
Mastoid process

Occipital bone
Basilar part
Pharyngeal tubercle
Hypoglossal canal
Occipital condyle
Foramen magnum
Condylar canal and fossa
Inferior nuchal line

Mastoid canaliculus
Jugular fossa
Stylomastoid foramen
Mastoid notch (for the digastric muscle)

Occipital groove (for occipital artery)

External occipital crest
Superior nuchal line
External occipital protuberance

Carotid canal (external opening)

Mastoid foramen
Tympanic canaliculus
Petrous part

Inferior

Unit 1 Skeletal System

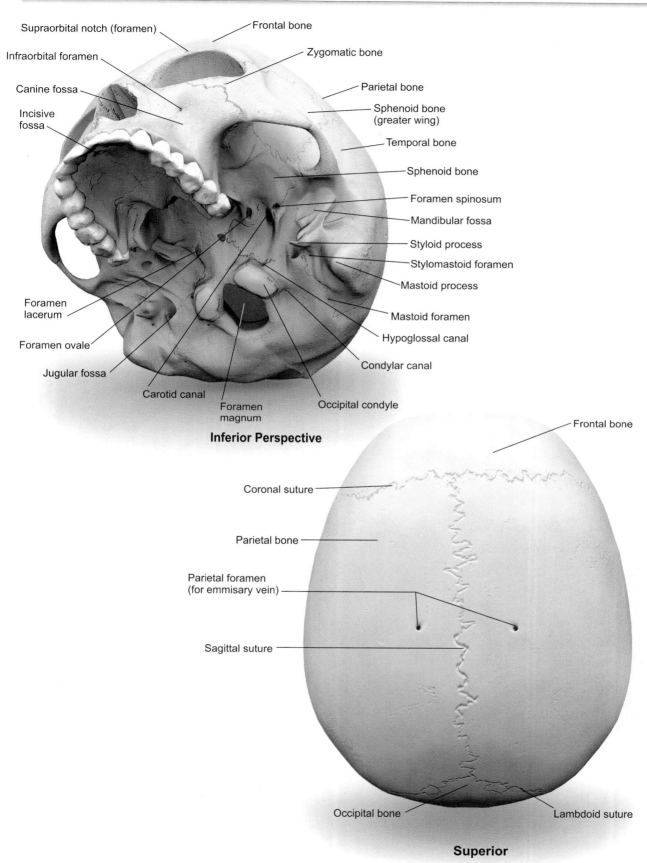

Supraorbital notch (foramen)

Frontal bone

Infraorbital foramen

Zygomatic bone

Canine fossa

Parietal bone

Incisive
fossa

Sphenoid bone
(greater wing)

Temporal bone

Sphenoid bone

Foramen spinosum

Mandibular fossa

Styloid process

Stylomastoid foramen

Mastoid process

Foramen
lacerum

Mastoid foramen

Foramen ovale

Hypoglossal canal

Jugular fossa

Condylar canal

Carotid canal

Occipital condyle

Foramen
magnum

Inferior Perspective

Frontal bone

Coronal suture

Parietal bone

Parietal foramen
(for emmisary vein)

Sagittal suture

Occipital bone

Lambdoid suture

Superior

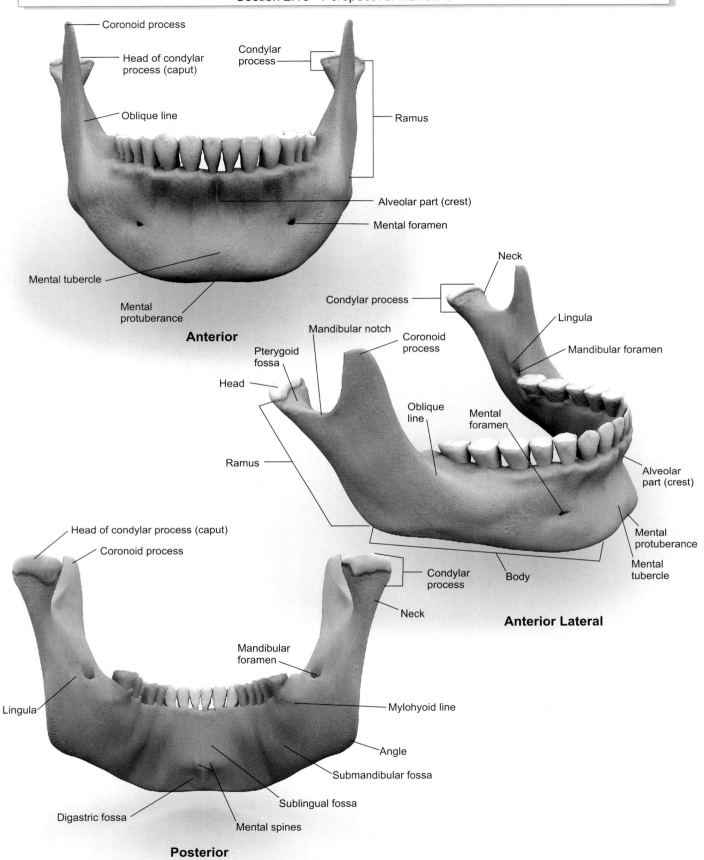

Coronoid process
Head of condylar process (caput)
Condylar process
Oblique line
Ramus
Alveolar part (crest)
Mental foramen
Mental tubercle
Mental protuberance
Anterior

Neck
Condylar process
Lingula
Mandibular foramen
Mandibular notch
Coronoid process
Pterygoid fossa
Head
Oblique line
Mental foramen
Ramus
Alveolar part (crest)
Mental protuberance
Mental tubercle
Condylar process
Body
Neck
Anterior Lateral

Head of condylar process (caput)
Coronoid process
Mandibular foramen
Lingula
Mylohyoid line
Angle
Submandibular fossa
Sublingual fossa
Digastric fossa
Mental spines
Posterior

Unit 1 Skeletal System

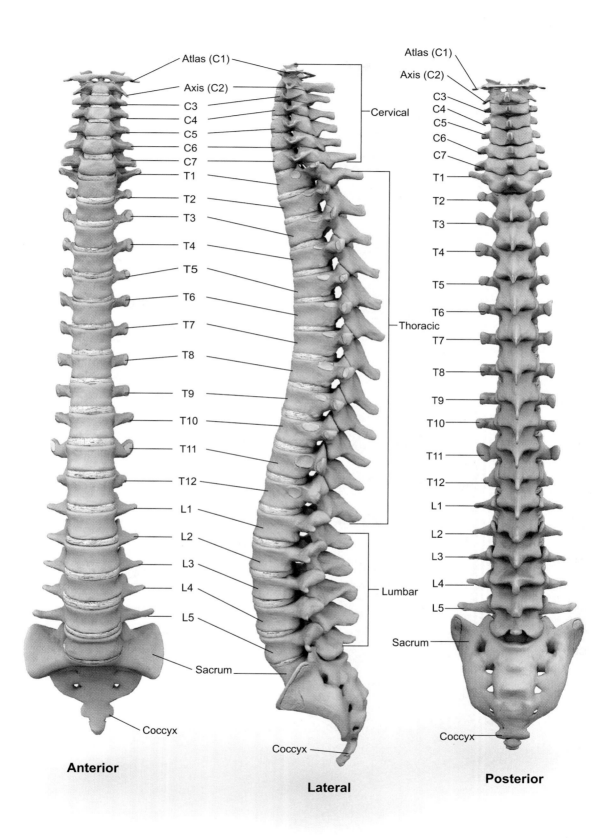

Atlas (C1)
Axis (C2)
C3
C4
C5
C6
C7
T1
T2
T3
T4
T5
T6
T7
T8
T9
T10
T11
T12
L1
L2
L3
L4
L5
Sacrum
Coccyx

Anterior

Cervical

Thoracic

Lumbar

Lateral

Coccyx

Atlas (C1)
Axis (C2)
C3
C4
C5
C6
C7
T1
T2
T3
T4
T5
T6
T7
T8
T9
T10
T11
T12
L1
L2
L3
L4
L5
Sacrum
Coccyx

Posterior

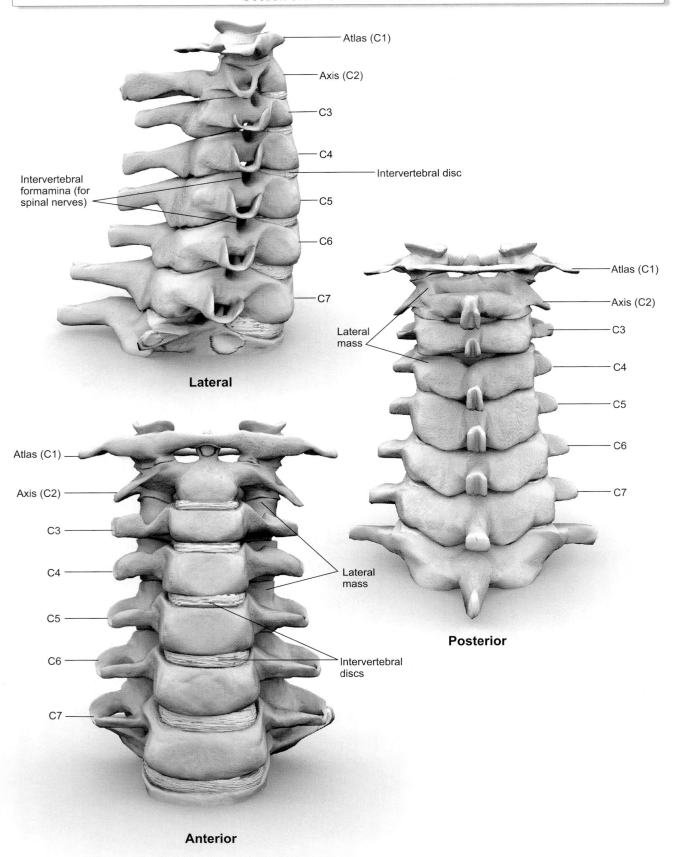

Atlas (C1)

Axis (C2)

C3

C4

Intervertebral disc

Intervertebral formamina (for spinal nerves)

C5

C6

C7

Lateral

Lateral mass

Atlas (C1)

Axis (C2)

C3

C4

C5

C6

C7

Atlas (C1)

Axis (C2)

C3

C4

C5

Lateral mass

C6

Intervertebral discs

C7

Posterior

Anterior

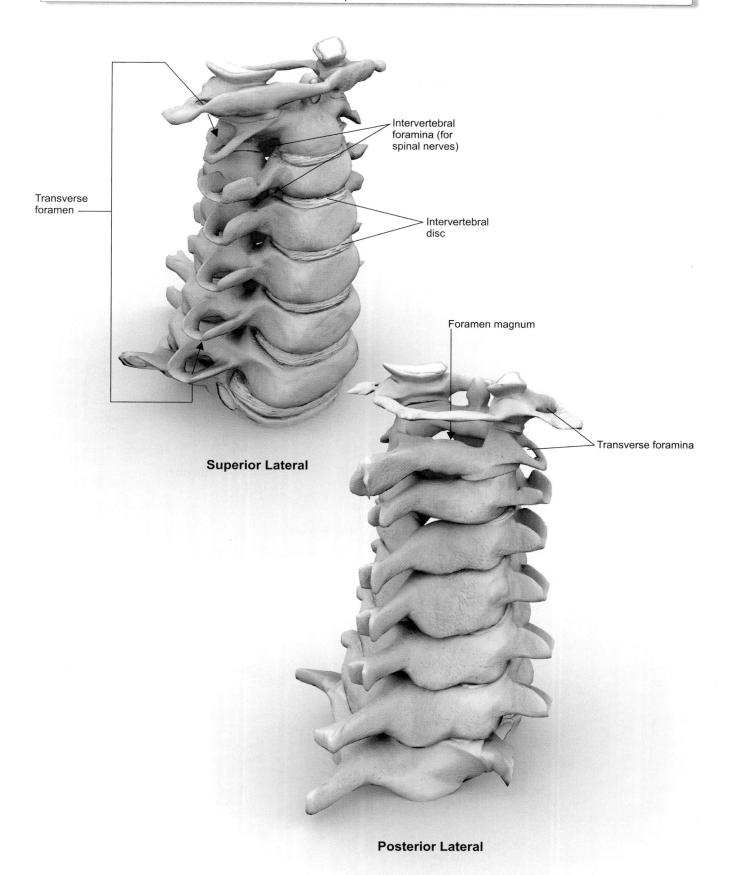

Transverse
foramen

Intervertebral
foramina (for
spinal nerves)

Intervertebral
disc

Superior Lateral

Foramen magnum

Transverse foramina

Posterior Lateral

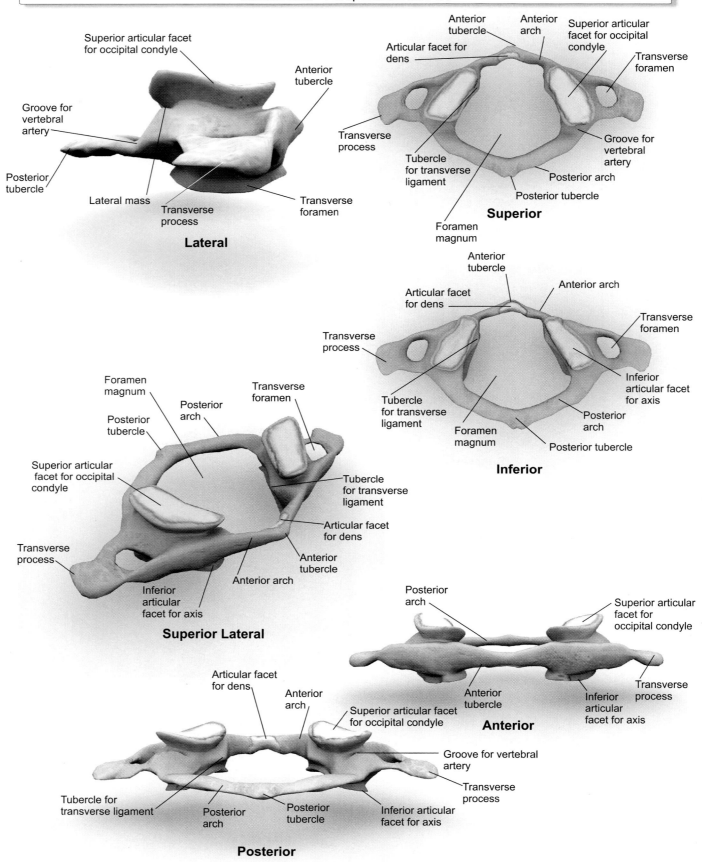

Lateral

Superior

Inferior

Superior Lateral

Anterior

Posterior

Unit 1 Skeletal System

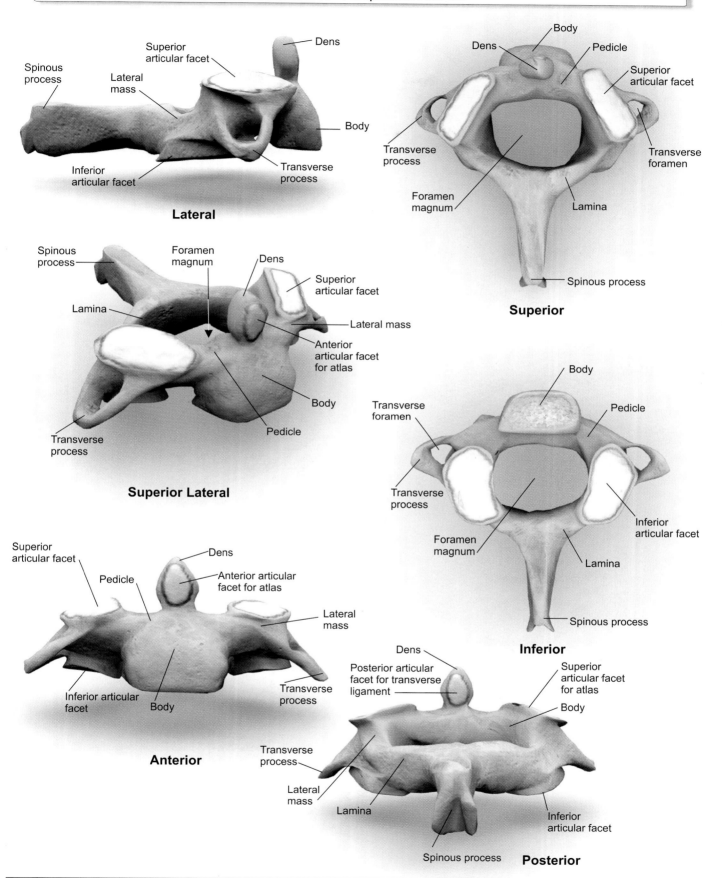

Lateral

Superior Lateral

Superior

Inferior

Anterior

Posterior

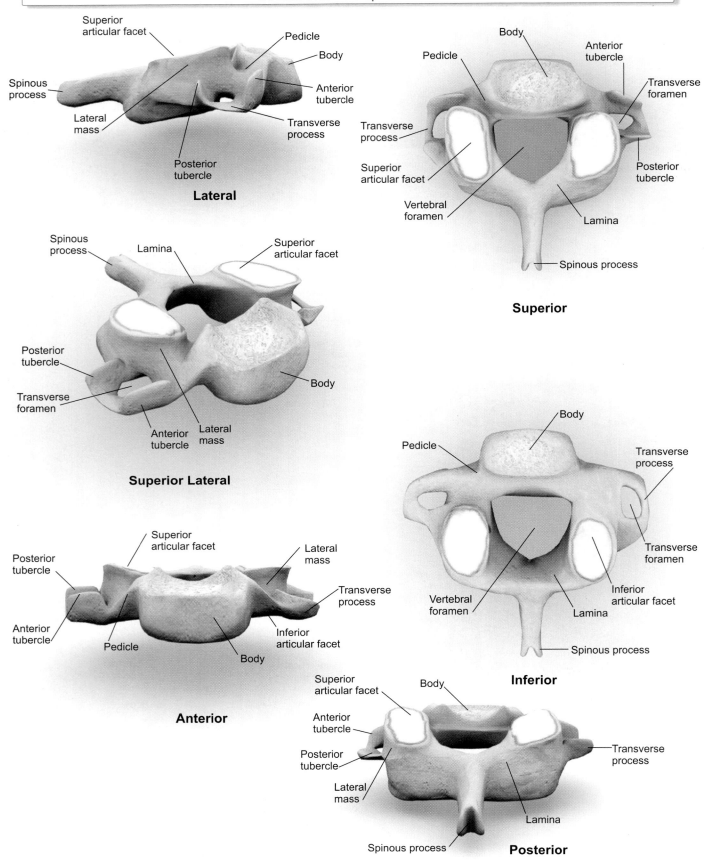

Lateral

Superior Lateral

Superior

Anterior

Inferior

Posterior

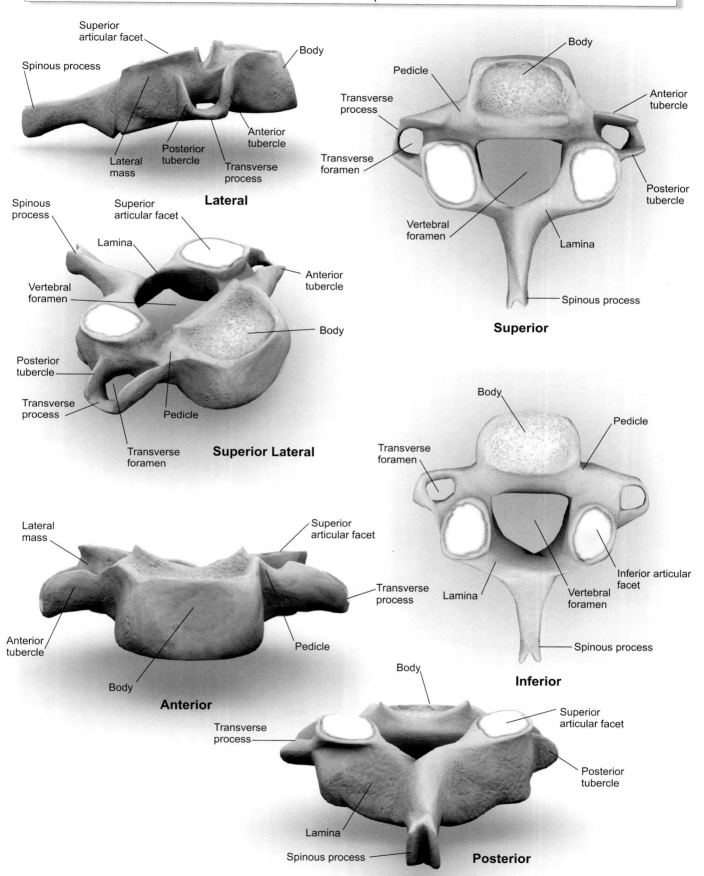

Lateral

Superior Lateral

Superior

Anterior

Inferior

Posterior

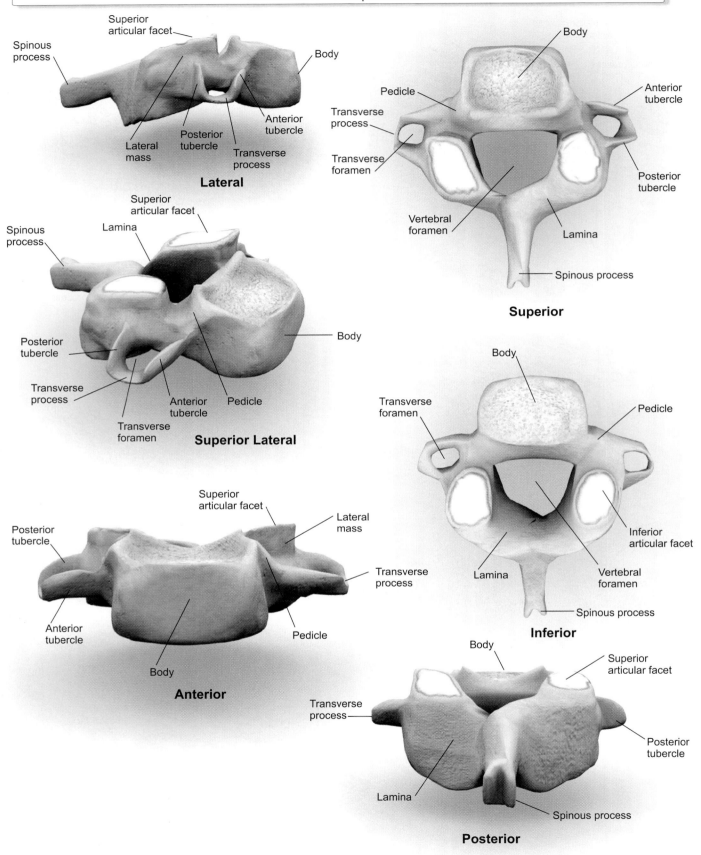

Lateral

Superior Lateral

Anterior

Superior

Inferior

Posterior

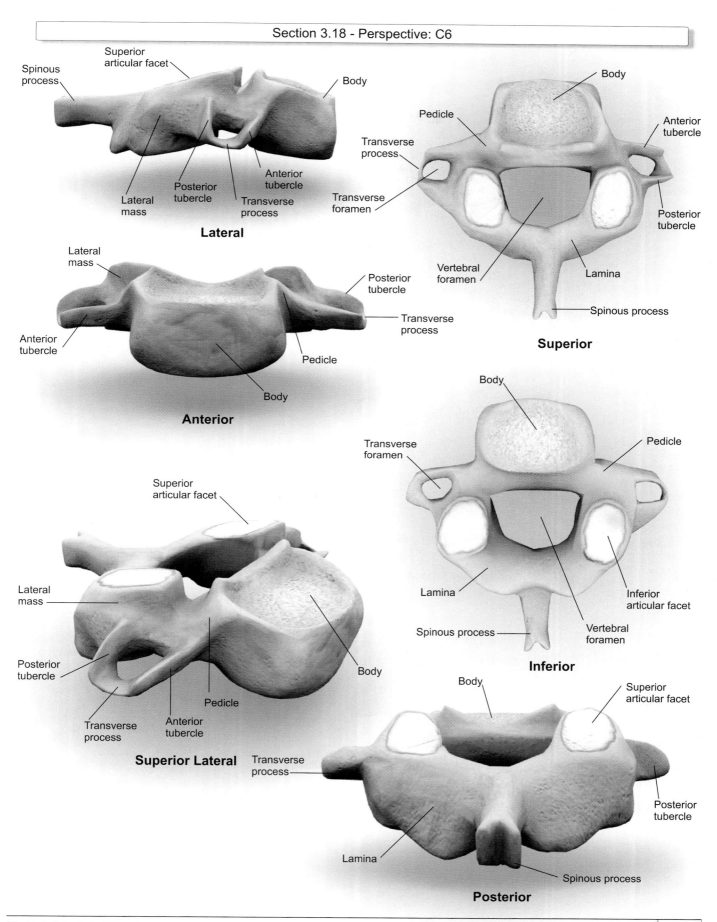

Lateral

Superior

Anterior

Superior Lateral

Inferior

Posterior

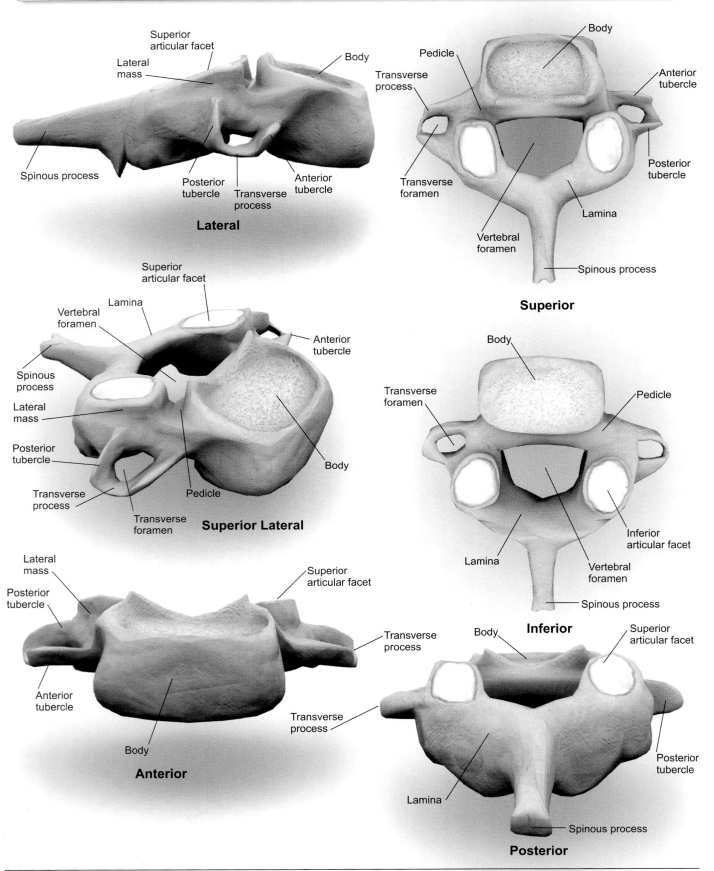

Lateral

Superior

Superior Lateral

Inferior

Anterior

Posterior

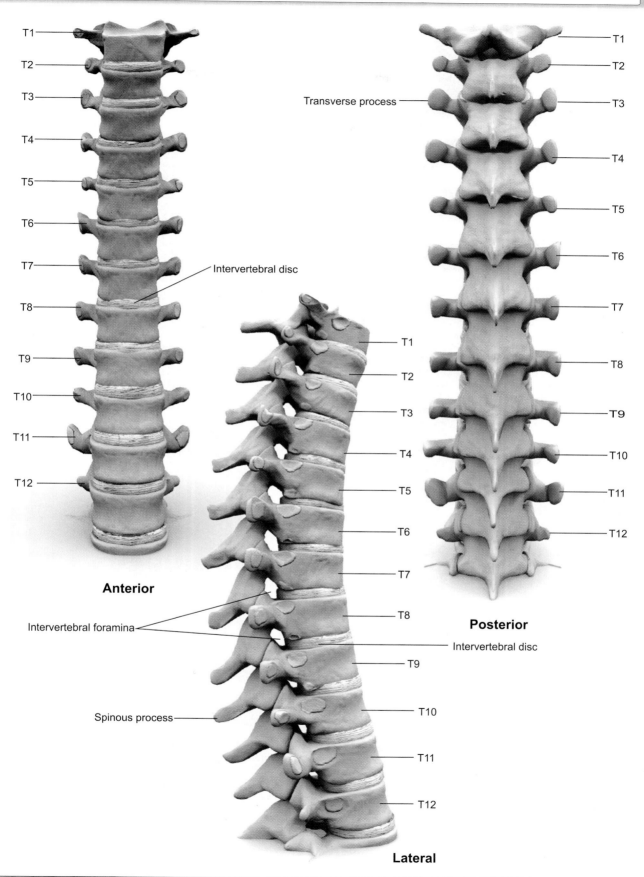

T1
T2
T3
T4
T5
T6
T7
T8
T9
T10
T11
T12

Intervertebral disc

Anterior

Intervertebral foramina

Spinous process

T1
T2
T3
T4
T5
T6
T7
T8
T9
T10
T11
T12

Lateral

Intervertebral disc

Transverse process

T1
T2
T3
T4
T5
T6
T7
T8
T9
T10
T11
T12

Posterior

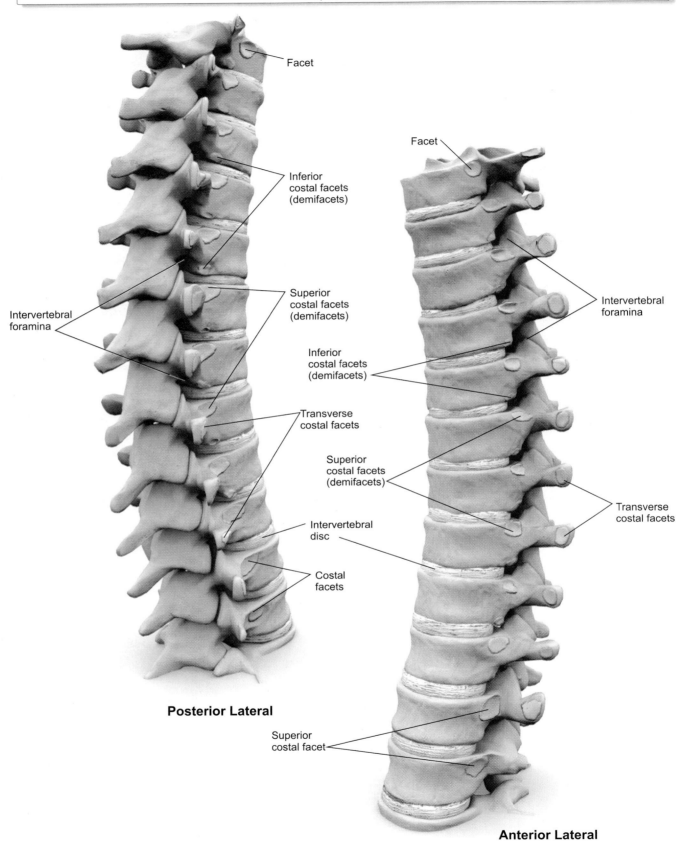

Facet

Inferior
costal facets
(demifacets)

Superior
costal facets
(demifacets)

Intervertebral
foramina

Transverse
costal facets

Intervertebral
disc

Costal
facets

Facet

Intervertebral
foramina

Inferior
costal facets
(demifacets)

Superior
costal facets
(demifacets)

Transverse
costal facets

Superior
costal facet

Posterior Lateral

Anterior Lateral

Unit 1 Skeletal System

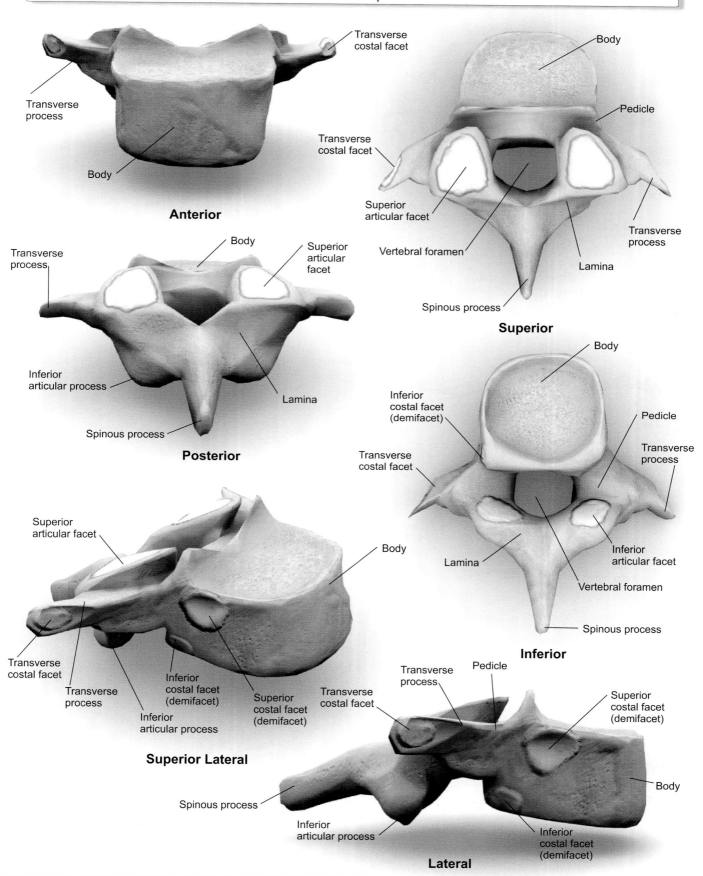

Anterior

Transverse costal facet

Transverse process

Body

Body

Pedicle

Transverse costal facet

Superior articular facet

Vertebral foramen

Transverse process

Lamina

Spinous process

Superior

Transverse process

Body

Superior articular facet

Inferior articular process

Lamina

Spinous process

Posterior

Body

Inferior costal facet (demifacet)

Pedicle

Transverse process

Transverse costal facet

Lamina

Inferior articular facet

Vertebral foramen

Spinous process

Inferior

Superior articular facet

Body

Transverse costal facet

Transverse process

Inferior costal facet (demifacet)

Superior costal facet (demifacet)

Inferior articular process

Superior Lateral

Transverse process

Pedicle

Transverse costal facet

Superior costal facet (demifacet)

Spinous process

Body

Inferior articular process

Inferior costal facet (demifacet)

Lateral

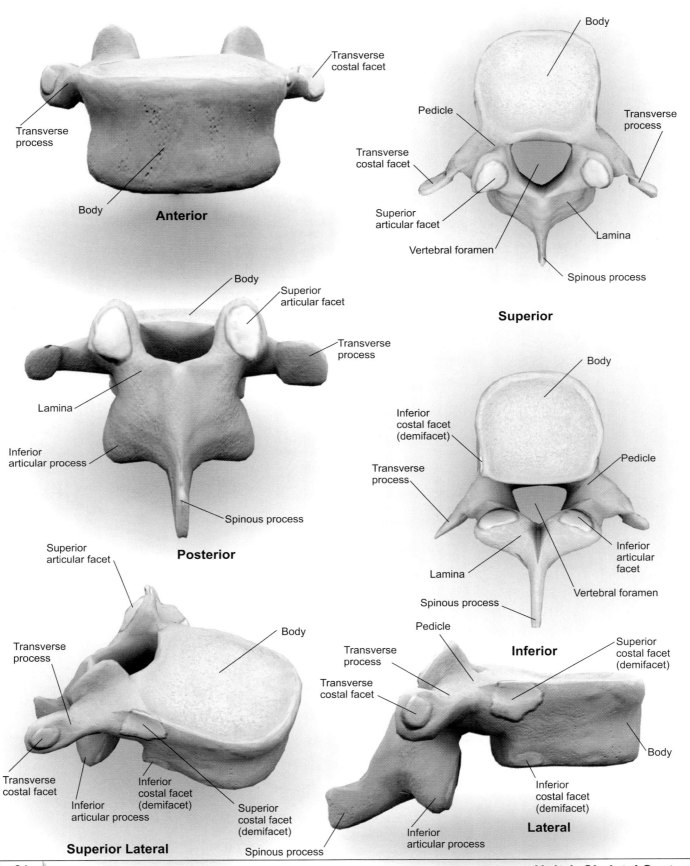

Transverse costal facet

Transverse process

Body

Anterior

Body

Pedicle

Transverse costal facet

Superior articular facet

Vertebral foramen

Transverse process

Lamina

Spinous process

Superior

Body

Superior articular facet

Transverse process

Lamina

Inferior articular process

Spinous process

Posterior

Inferior costal facet (demifacet)

Transverse process

Lamina

Spinous process

Body

Pedicle

Inferior articular facet

Vertebral foramen

Inferior

Superior articular facet

Transverse process

Transverse costal facet

Inferior articular process

Inferior costal facet (demifacet)

Superior costal facet (demifacet)

Body

Superior Lateral

Pedicle

Transverse process

Transverse costal facet

Inferior articular process

Spinous process

Superior costal facet (demifacet)

Body

Inferior costal facet (demifacet)

Lateral

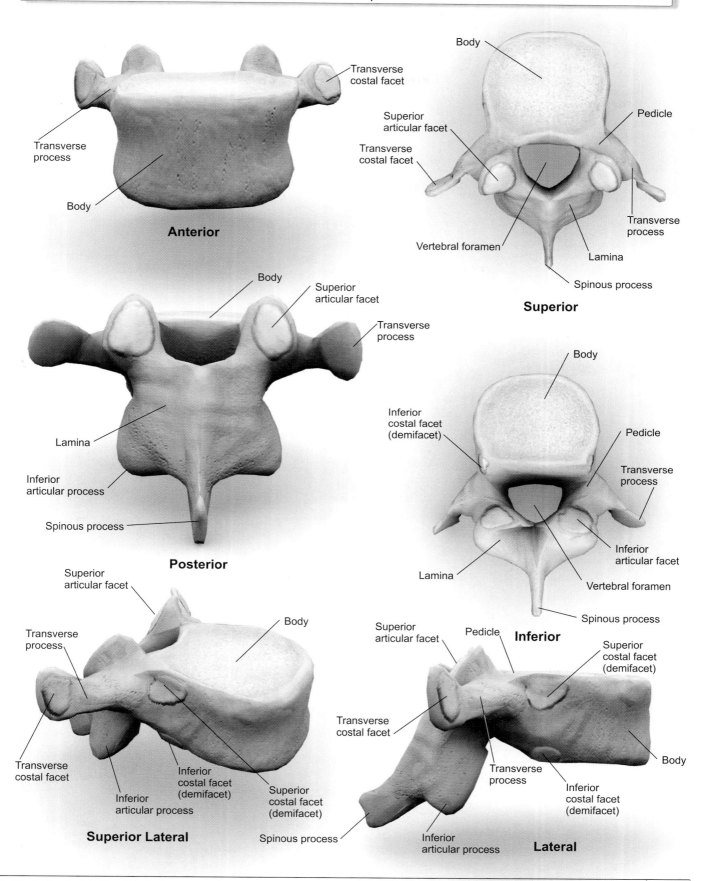

Anterior

Transverse costal facet

Transverse process

Body

Superior

Body

Pedicle

Superior articular facet

Transverse costal facet

Vertebral foramen

Lamina

Spinous process

Posterior

Body

Superior articular facet

Transverse process

Lamina

Inferior articular process

Spinous process

Inferior

Body

Inferior costal facet (demifacet)

Pedicle

Transverse process

Lamina

Inferior articular facet

Vertebral foramen

Spinous process

Superior Lateral

Superior articular facet

Transverse process

Body

Transverse costal facet

Inferior articular process

Inferior costal facet (demifacet)

Superior costal facet (demifacet)

Lateral

Superior articular facet

Pedicle

Superior costal facet (demifacet)

Transverse costal facet

Transverse process

Body

Inferior articular process

Inferior costal facet (demifacet)

Spinous process

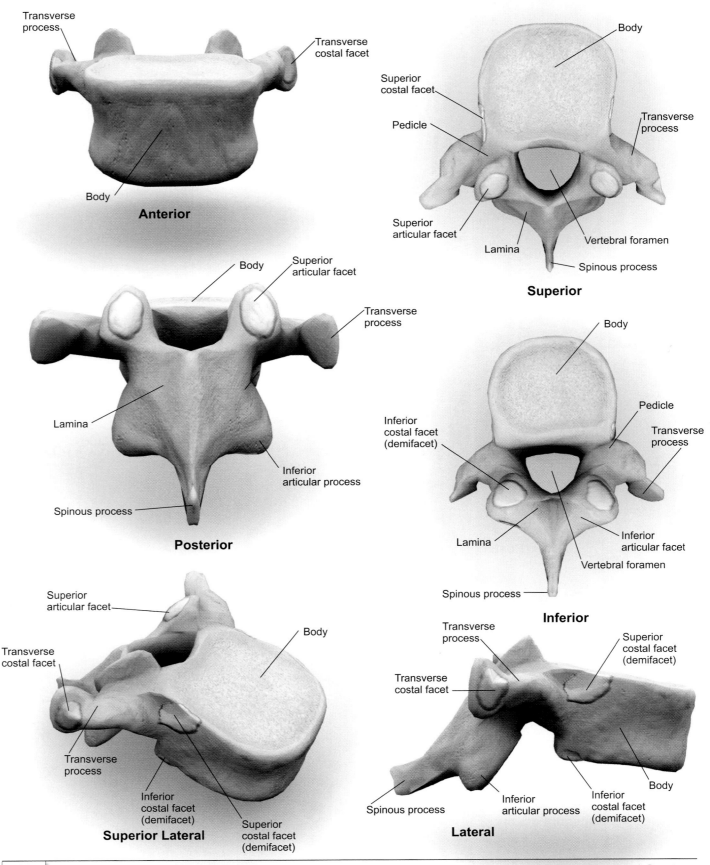

Transverse process

Transverse costal facet

Body

Anterior

Body

Superior costal facet

Pedicle

Transverse process

Superior articular facet

Lamina

Vertebral foramen

Spinous process

Superior

Body

Superior articular facet

Transverse process

Lamina

Inferior articular process

Spinous process

Posterior

Body

Inferior costal facet (demifacet)

Pedicle

Transverse process

Lamina

Inferior articular facet

Vertebral foramen

Spinous process

Inferior

Superior articular facet

Transverse costal facet

Body

Transverse process

Inferior costal facet (demifacet)

Superior costal facet (demifacet)

Superior Lateral

Transverse process

Transverse costal facet

Superior costal facet (demifacet)

Spinous process

Inferior articular process

Inferior costal facet (demifacet)

Body

Lateral

Unit 1 Skeletal System

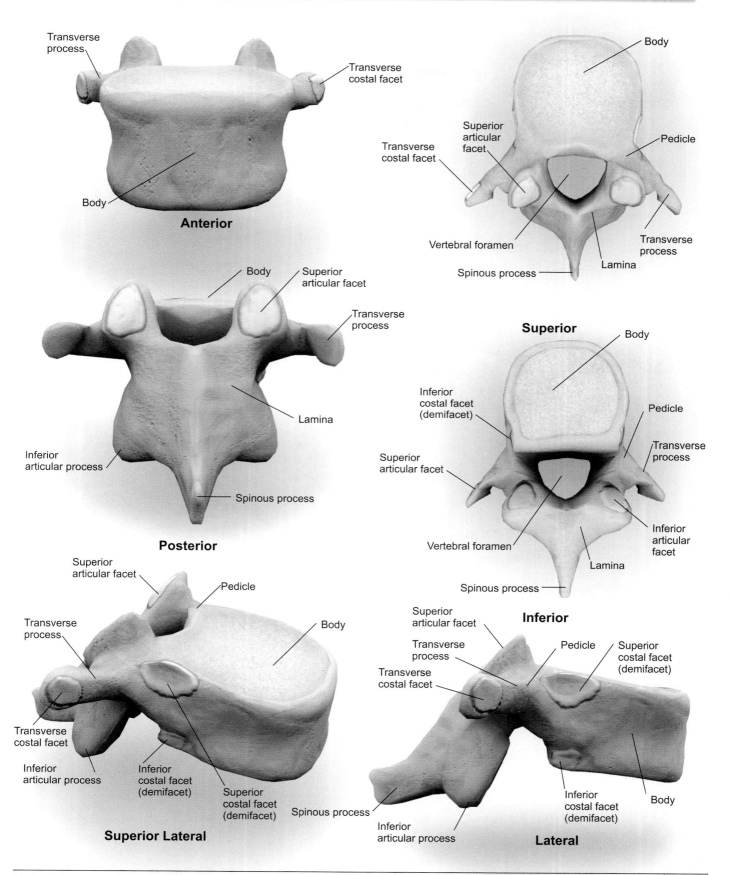

Anterior

Transverse process

Transverse costal facet

Body

Body

Superior articular facet

Transverse costal facet

Pedicle

Vertebral foramen

Transverse process

Spinous process

Lamina

Superior

Body

Superior articular facet

Transverse process

Lamina

Inferior articular process

Spinous process

Posterior

Inferior costal facet (demifacet)

Body

Pedicle

Transverse process

Superior articular facet

Vertebral foramen

Inferior articular facet

Spinous process

Lamina

Inferior

Superior articular facet

Pedicle

Transverse process

Body

Transverse costal facet

Inferior articular process

Inferior costal facet (demifacet)

Superior costal facet (demifacet)

Spinous process

Superior Lateral

Superior articular facet

Transverse process

Transverse costal facet

Pedicle

Superior costal facet (demifacet)

Inferior costal facet (demifacet)

Body

Inferior articular process

Lateral

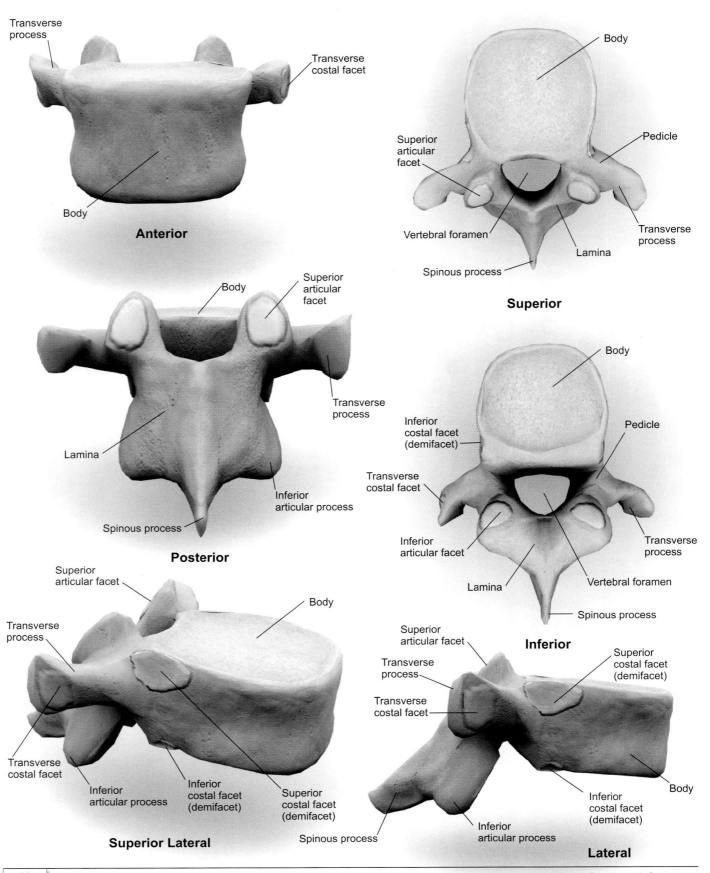

Transverse process

Transverse costal facet

Body

Anterior

Body

Superior articular facet

Pedicle

Vertebral foramen

Transverse process

Spinous process

Lamina

Superior

Body

Superior articular facet

Transverse process

Inferior articular process

Lamina

Spinous process

Posterior

Body

Inferior costal facet (demifacet)

Pedicle

Transverse costal facet

Inferior articular facet

Transverse process

Lamina

Vertebral foramen

Spinous process

Inferior

Superior articular facet

Transverse process

Body

Transverse costal facet

Inferior articular process

Inferior costal facet (demifacet)

Superior costal facet (demifacet)

Superior Lateral

Superior articular facet

Transverse process

Transverse costal facet

Superior costal facet (demifacet)

Body

Inferior costal facet (demifacet)

Inferior articular process

Spinous process

Lateral

28

Unit 1 Skeletal System

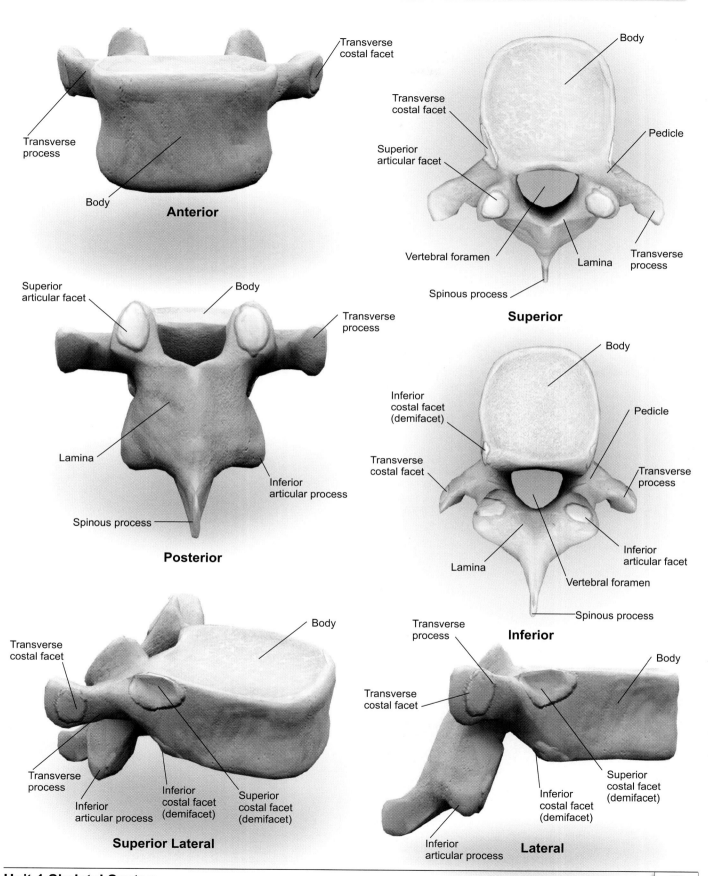

Transverse costal facet

Transverse process

Body

Anterior

Superior articular facet

Body

Transverse process

Lamina

Inferior articular process

Spinous process

Posterior

Transverse costal facet

Transverse process

Inferior articular process

Inferior costal facet (demifacet)

Superior costal facet (demifacet)

Superior Lateral

Body

Transverse costal facet

Superior articular facet

Pedicle

Vertebral foramen

Lamina

Transverse process

Spinous process

Superior

Body

Inferior costal facet (demifacet)

Transverse costal facet

Pedicle

Transverse process

Inferior articular facet

Lamina

Vertebral foramen

Spinous process

Inferior

Transverse process

Transverse costal facet

Body

Inferior costal facet (demifacet)

Superior costal facet (demifacet)

Inferior articular process

Lateral

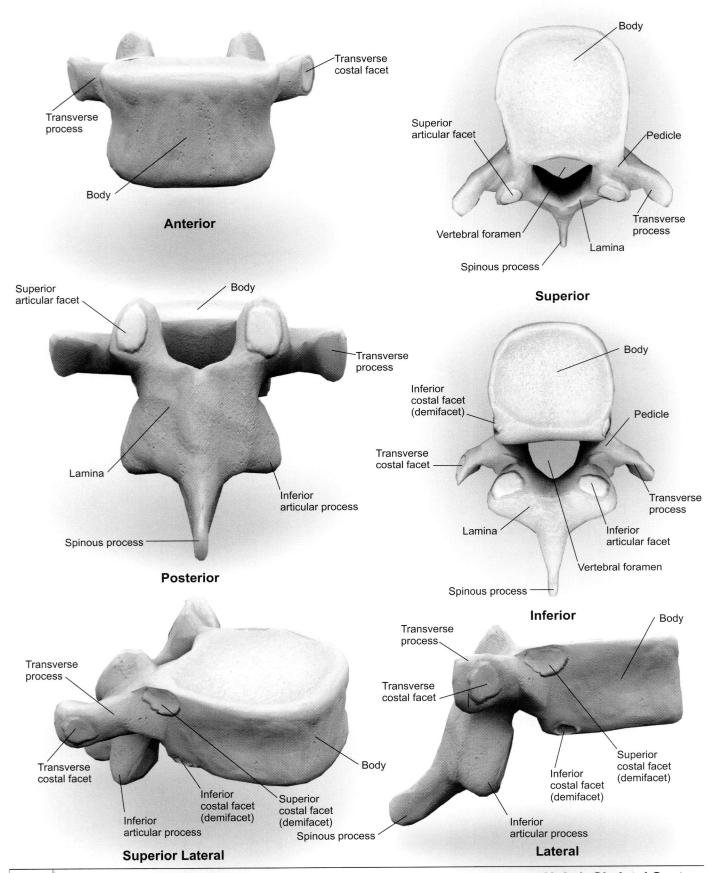

Transverse costal facet

Transverse process

Body

Anterior

Body

Superior articular facet

Pedicle

Vertebral foramen

Transverse process

Spinous process

Lamina

Superior

Superior articular facet

Body

Transverse process

Lamina

Inferior articular process

Spinous process

Posterior

Inferior costal facet (demifacet)

Body

Transverse costal facet

Pedicle

Lamina

Transverse process

Inferior articular facet

Vertebral foramen

Spinous process

Inferior

Transverse process

Transverse process

Transverse costal facet

Body

Inferior costal facet (demifacet)

Superior costal facet (demifacet)

Body

Inferior articular process

Inferior costal facet (demifacet)

Superior costal facet (demifacet)

Spinous process

Superior Lateral

Transverse process

Transverse costal facet

Body

Inferior costal facet (demifacet)

Superior costal facet (demifacet)

Inferior articular process

Lateral

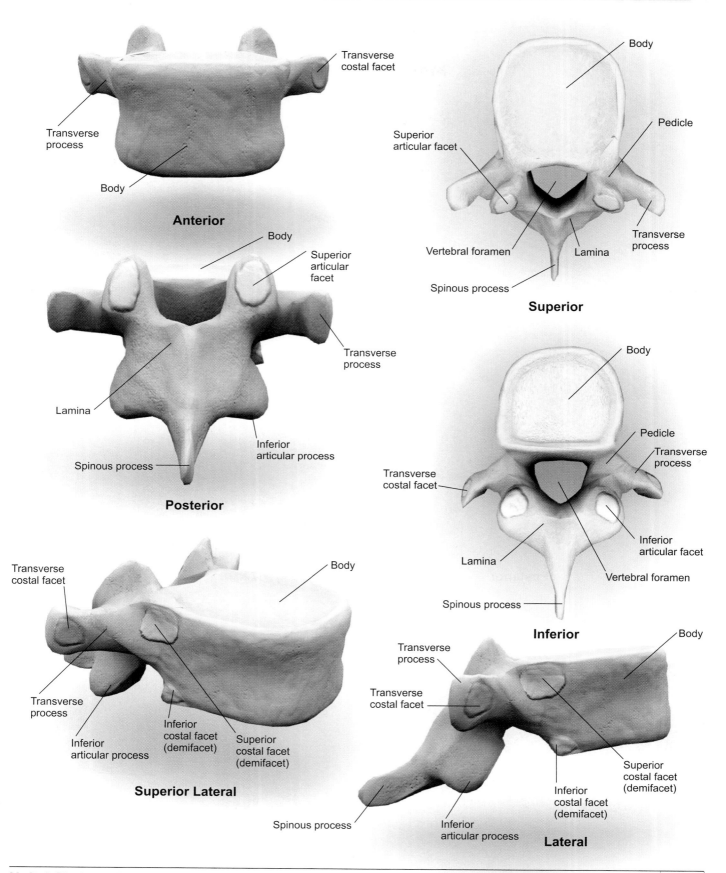

Anterior

Transverse costal facet

Transverse process

Body

Posterior

Body

Superior articular facet

Transverse process

Lamina

Spinous process

Inferior articular process

Superior

Body

Superior articular facet

Pedicle

Vertebral foramen

Lamina

Transverse process

Spinous process

Inferior

Body

Pedicle

Transverse process

Transverse costal facet

Lamina

Inferior articular facet

Vertebral foramen

Spinous process

Superior Lateral

Transverse costal facet

Body

Transverse process

Inferior articular process

Inferior costal facet (demifacet)

Superior costal facet (demifacet)

Lateral

Transverse process

Transverse costal facet

Body

Superior costal facet (demifacet)

Inferior costal facet (demifacet)

Inferior articular process

Spinous process

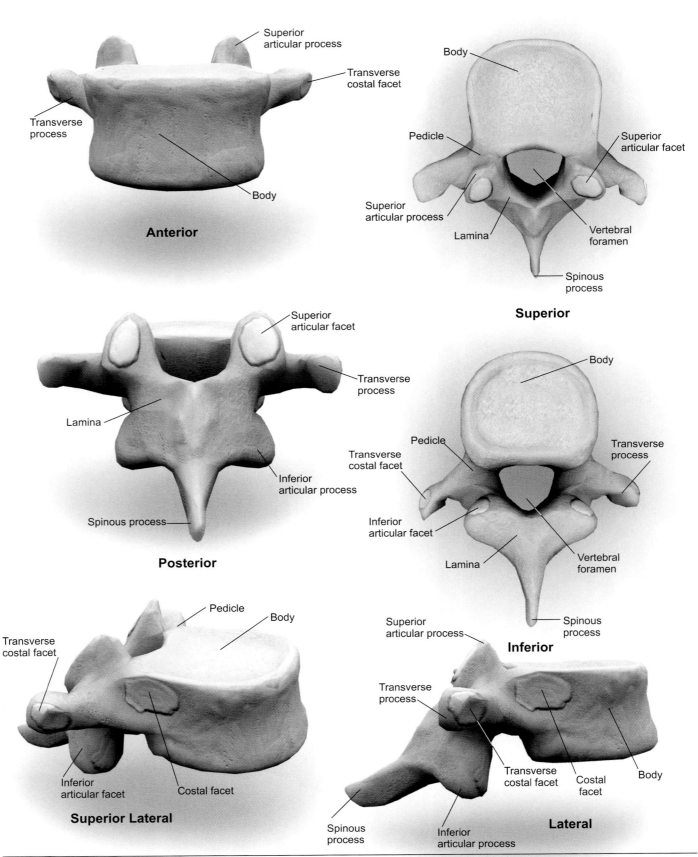

Anterior

Superior articular process

Transverse costal facet

Transverse process

Body

Body

Pedicle

Superior articular facet

Superior articular process

Lamina

Vertebral foramen

Spinous process

Superior

Superior articular facet

Transverse process

Lamina

Inferior articular process

Spinous process

Posterior

Body

Pedicle

Transverse costal facet

Transverse process

Inferior articular facet

Lamina

Vertebral foramen

Spinous process

Inferior

Pedicle

Body

Transverse costal facet

Transverse process

Inferior articular facet

Costal facet

Superior Lateral

Superior articular process

Transverse process

Transverse costal facet

Costal facet

Body

Spinous process

Inferior articular process

Lateral

Unit 1 Skeletal System

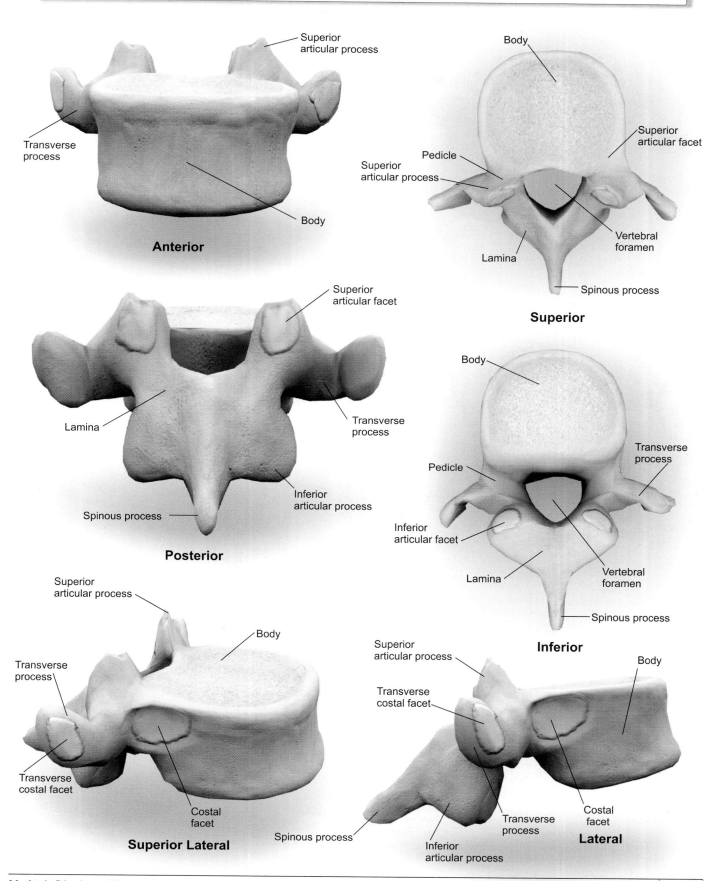

Superior
articular process

Transverse
process

Body

Anterior

Superior
articular facet

Lamina

Transverse
process

Spinous process

Inferior
articular process

Posterior

Superior
articular process

Body

Transverse
process

Transverse
costal facet

Costal
facet

Superior Lateral

Body

Superior
articular facet

Pedicle

Superior
articular process

Lamina

Vertebral
foramen

Spinous process

Superior

Body

Pedicle

Transverse
process

Inferior
articular facet

Lamina

Vertebral
foramen

Spinous process

Inferior

Superior
articular process

Body

Transverse
costal facet

Costal
facet

Spinous process

Inferior
articular process

Transverse
process

Lateral

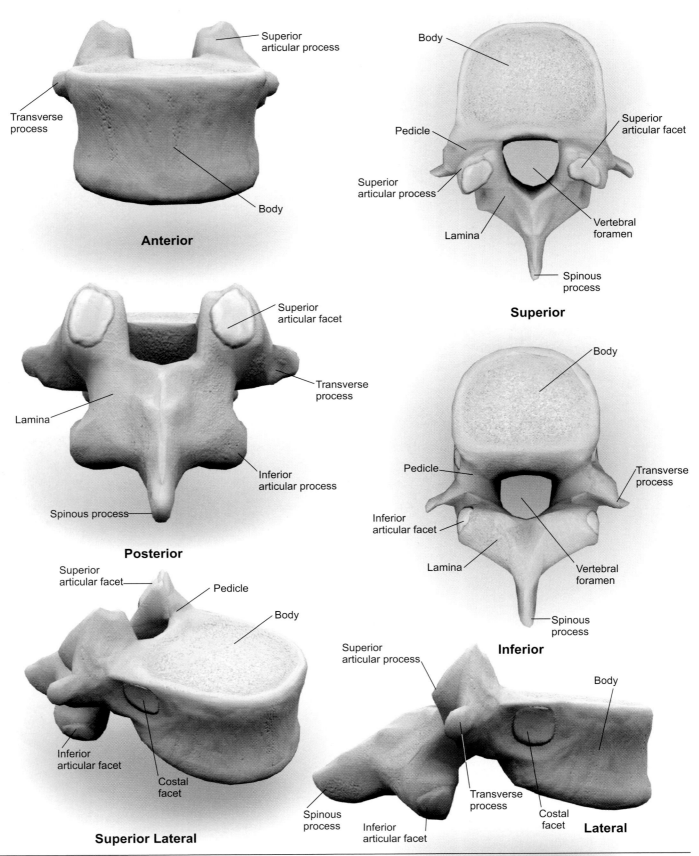

Anterior

Superior
articular process

Transverse
process

Body

Superior

Body

Pedicle

Superior
articular process

Lamina

Superior
articular facet

Vertebral
foramen

Spinous
process

Posterior

Superior
articular facet

Transverse
process

Lamina

Inferior
articular process

Spinous process

Inferior

Body

Pedicle

Inferior
articular facet

Lamina

Transverse
process

Vertebral
foramen

Spinous
process

Superior Lateral

Superior
articular facet

Pedicle

Body

Inferior
articular facet

Costal
facet

Lateral

Superior
articular process

Body

Spinous
process

Inferior
articular process

Transverse
process

Costal
facet

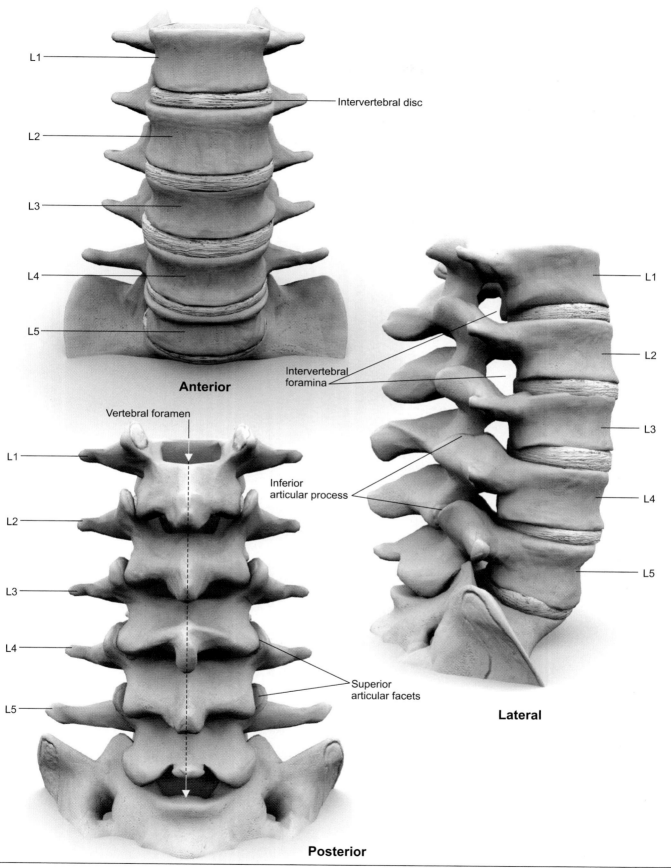

L1

L2

L3

L4

L5

Intervertebral disc

Anterior

Vertebral foramen

L1

L2

L3

L4

L5

Intervertebral foramina

Inferior articular process

Superior articular facets

Posterior

L1

L2

L3

L4

L5

Lateral

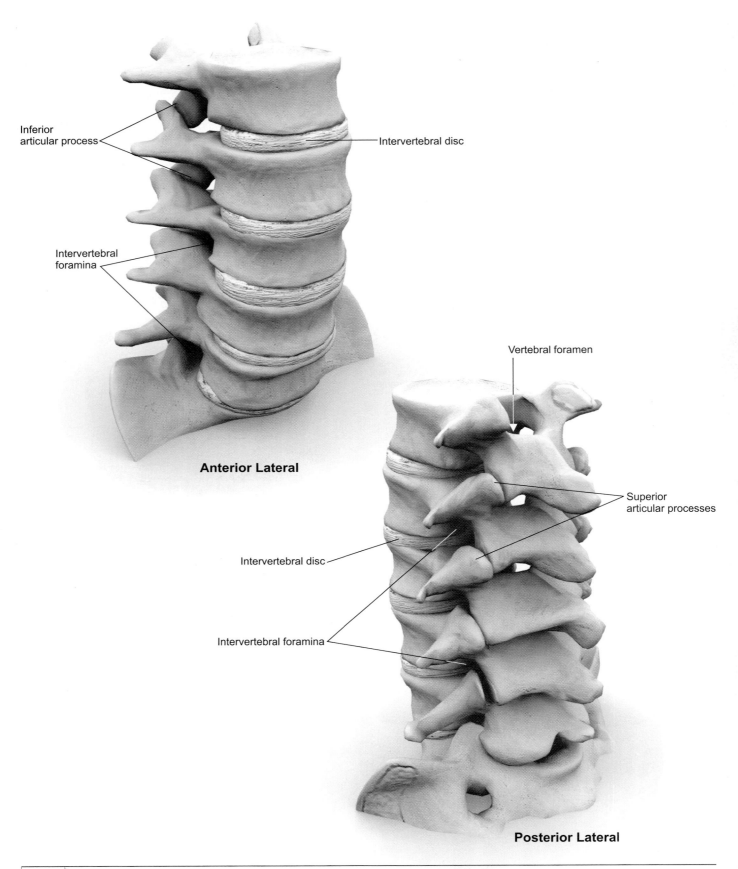

Inferior
articular process

Intervertebral disc

Intervertebral
foramina

Anterior Lateral

Vertebral foramen

Superior
articular processes

Intervertebral disc

Intervertebral foramina

Posterior Lateral

Unit 1 Skeletal System

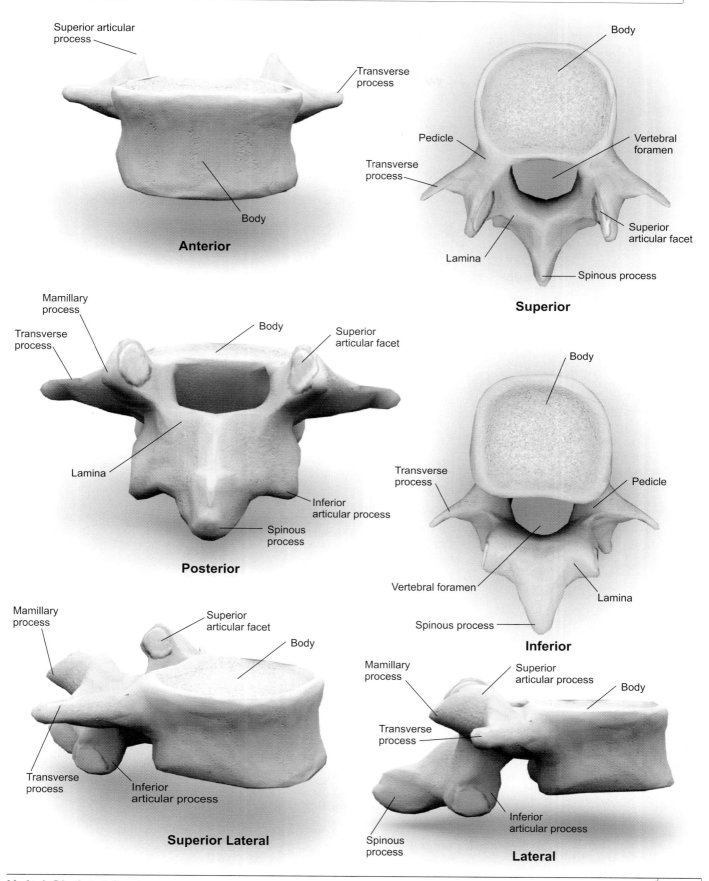

Superior articular process

Transverse process

Body

Anterior

Body

Pedicle

Vertebral foramen

Transverse process

Superior articular facet

Lamina

Spinous process

Superior

Mamillary process

Transverse process

Body

Superior articular facet

Lamina

Inferior articular process

Spinous process

Posterior

Body

Transverse process

Pedicle

Vertebral foramen

Lamina

Spinous process

Inferior

Mamillary process

Superior articular facet

Body

Transverse process

Inferior articular process

Superior Lateral

Mamillary process

Superior articular process

Body

Transverse process

Inferior articular process

Spinous process

Lateral

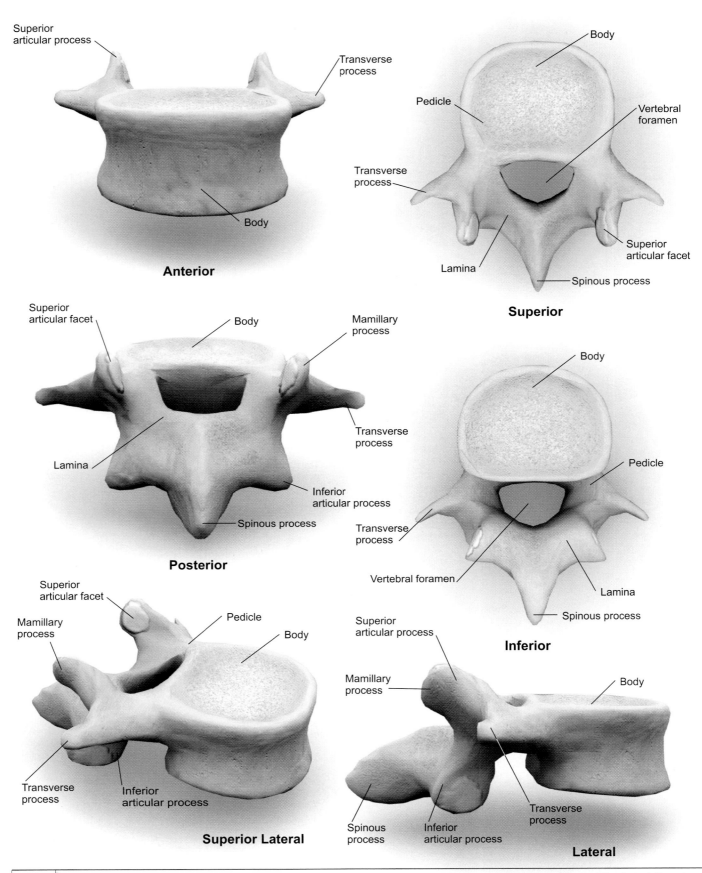

Anterior

Superior

Posterior

Inferior

Superior Lateral

Lateral

Unit 1 Skeletal System

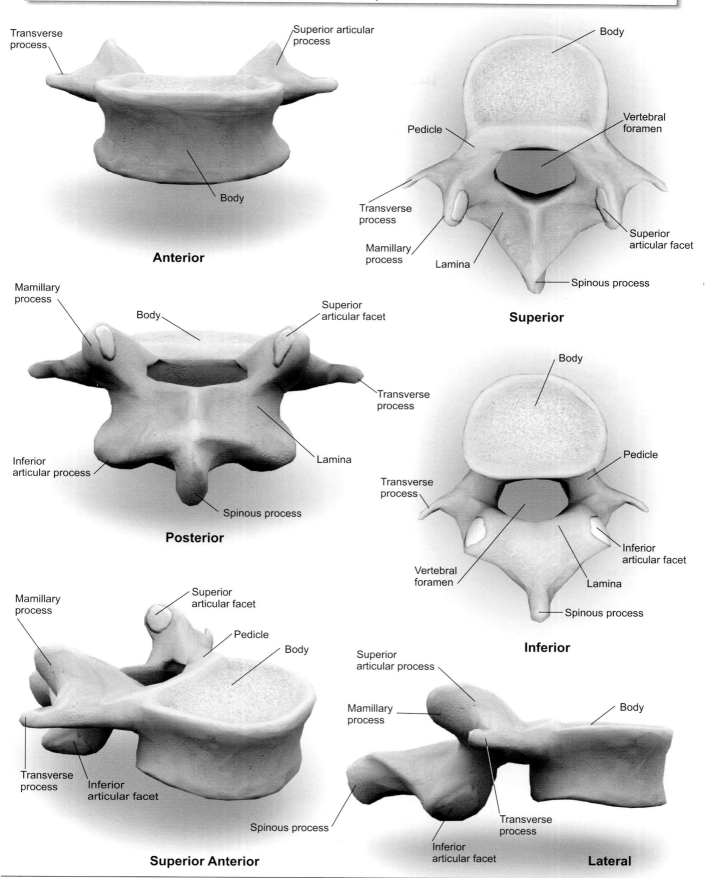

Anterior

Superior

Posterior

Inferior

Superior Anterior

Lateral

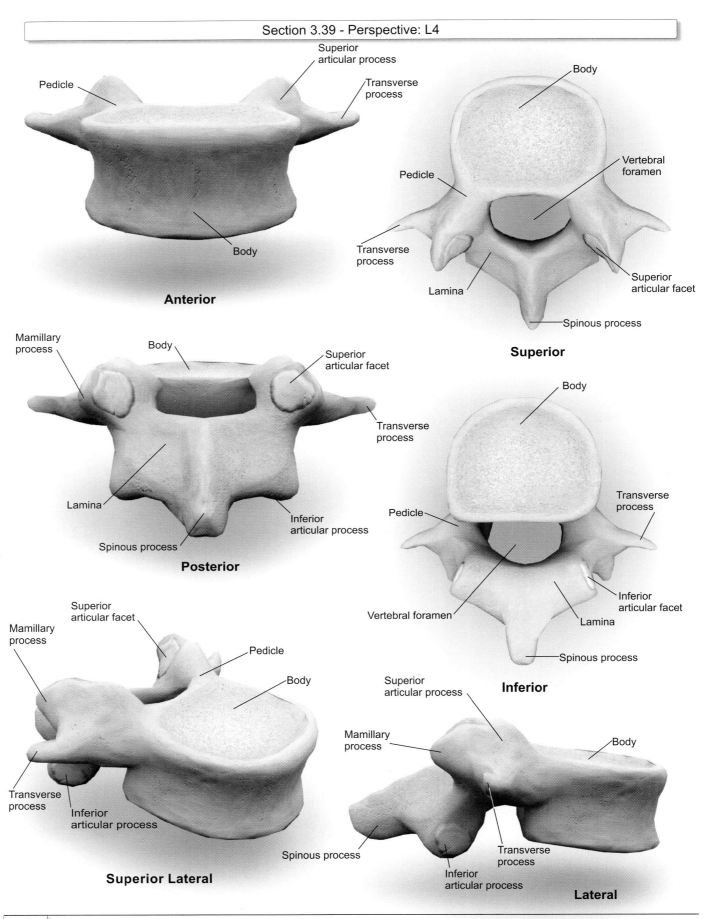

Anterior

Superior

Posterior

Inferior

Superior Lateral

Lateral

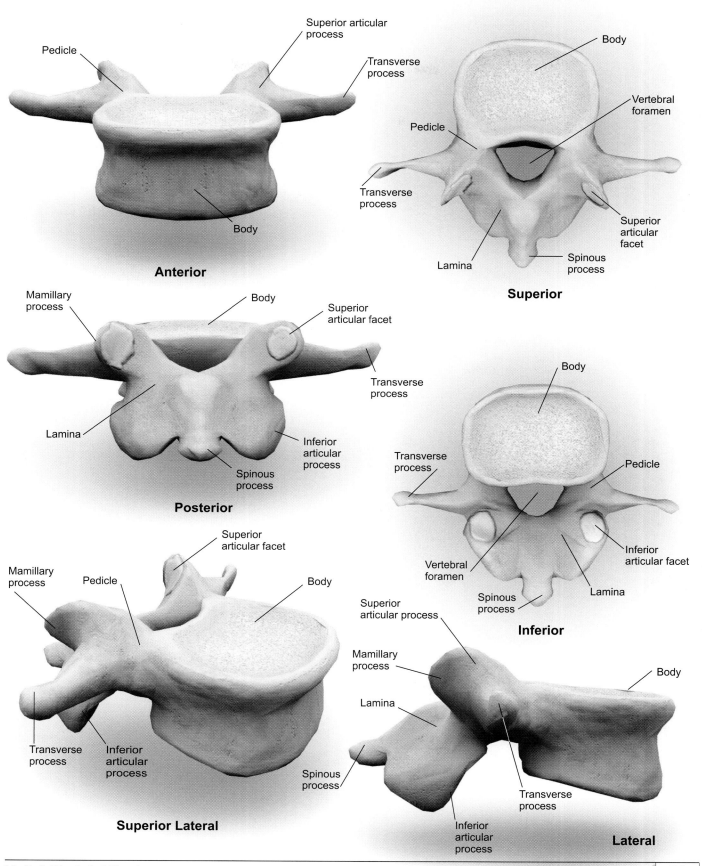

Pedicle

Superior articular process

Transverse process

Body

Body

Anterior

Pedicle

Vertebral foramen

Transverse process

Superior articular facet

Lamina

Spinous process

Superior

Mamillary process

Body

Superior articular facet

Lamina

Transverse process

Spinous process

Inferior articular process

Posterior

Body

Transverse process

Pedicle

Vertebral foramen

Spinous process

Inferior articular facet

Lamina

Inferior

Mamillary process

Pedicle

Superior articular facet

Body

Transverse process

Inferior articular process

Superior Lateral

Superior articular process

Mamillary process

Lamina

Spinous process

Body

Transverse process

Inferior articular process

Lateral

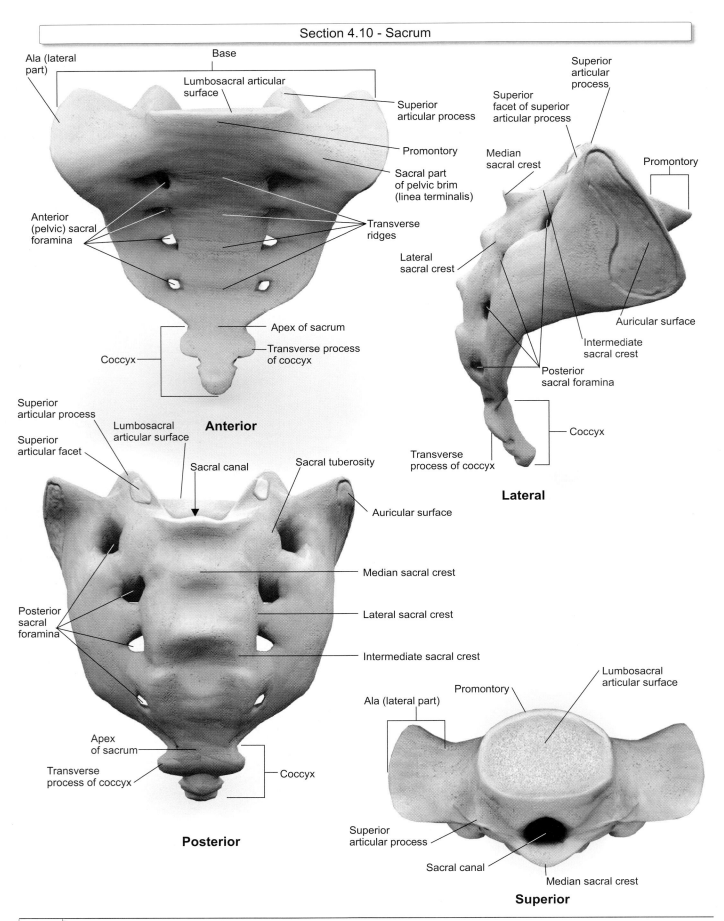

Ala (lateral part)

Base

Lumbosacral articular surface

Superior articular process

Promontory

Sacral part of pelvic brim (linea terminalis)

Anterior (pelvic) sacral foramina

Transverse ridges

Apex of sacrum

Transverse process of coccyx

Coccyx

Anterior

Superior articular process

Superior facet of superior articular process

Superior articular process

Median sacral crest

Promontory

Lateral sacral crest

Auricular surface

Intermediate sacral crest

Posterior sacral foramina

Coccyx

Transverse process of coccyx

Lateral

Superior articular process

Lumbosacral articular surface

Superior articular facet

Sacral canal

Sacral tuberosity

Auricular surface

Median sacral crest

Lateral sacral crest

Intermediate sacral crest

Posterior sacral foramina

Apex of sacrum

Transverse process of coccyx

Coccyx

Posterior

Ala (lateral part)

Promontory

Lumbosacral articular surface

Superior articular process

Sacral canal

Median sacral crest

Superior

Unit 1 Skeletal System

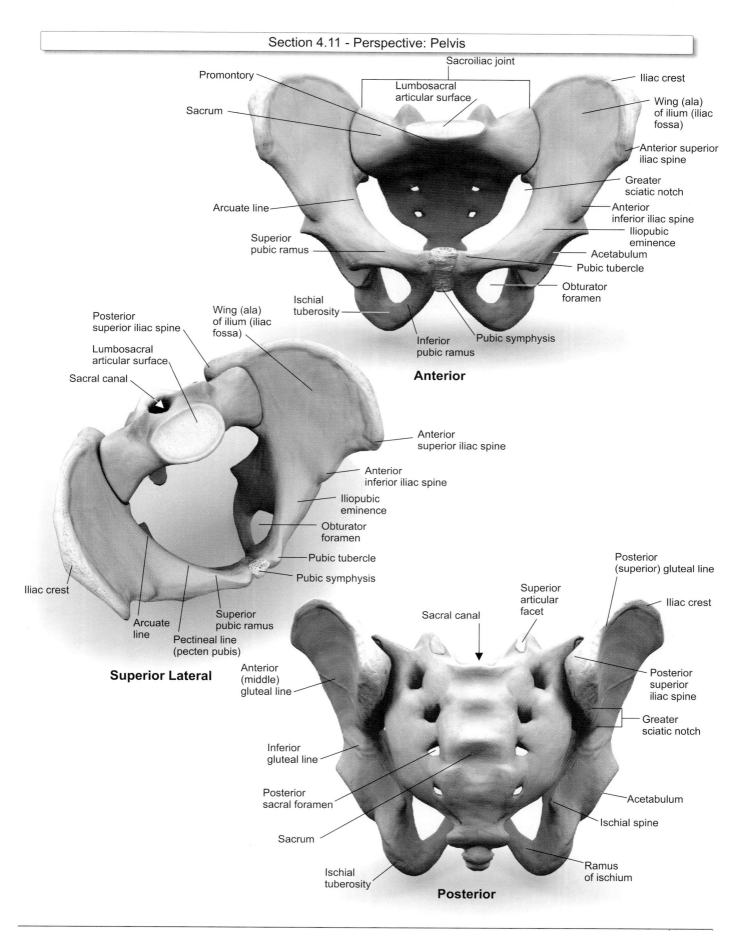

Promontory

Sacroiliac joint

Iliac crest

Lumbosacral
articular surface

Sacrum

Wing (ala)
of ilium (iliac
fossa)

Anterior superior
iliac spine

Greater
sciatic notch

Arcuate line

Anterior
inferior iliac spine

Iliopubic
eminence

Superior
pubic ramus

Acetabulum

Pubic tubercle

Obturator
foramen

Ischial
tuberosity

Inferior
pubic ramus

Pubic symphysis

Anterior

Posterior
superior iliac spine

Wing (ala)
of ilium (iliac
fossa)

Lumbosacral
articular surface

Sacral canal

Anterior
superior iliac spine

Anterior
inferior iliac spine

Iliopubic
eminence

Obturator
foramen

Pubic tubercle

Pubic symphysis

Iliac crest

Arcuate
line

Superior
pubic ramus

Pectineal line
(pecten pubis)

Superior Lateral

Posterior
(superior) gluteal line

Superior
articular
facet

Sacral canal

Iliac crest

Posterior
superior
iliac spine

Greater
sciatic notch

Anterior
(middle)
gluteal line

Inferior
gluteal line

Posterior
sacral foramen

Acetabulum

Ischial spine

Sacrum

Ramus
of ischium

Ischial
tuberosity

Posterior

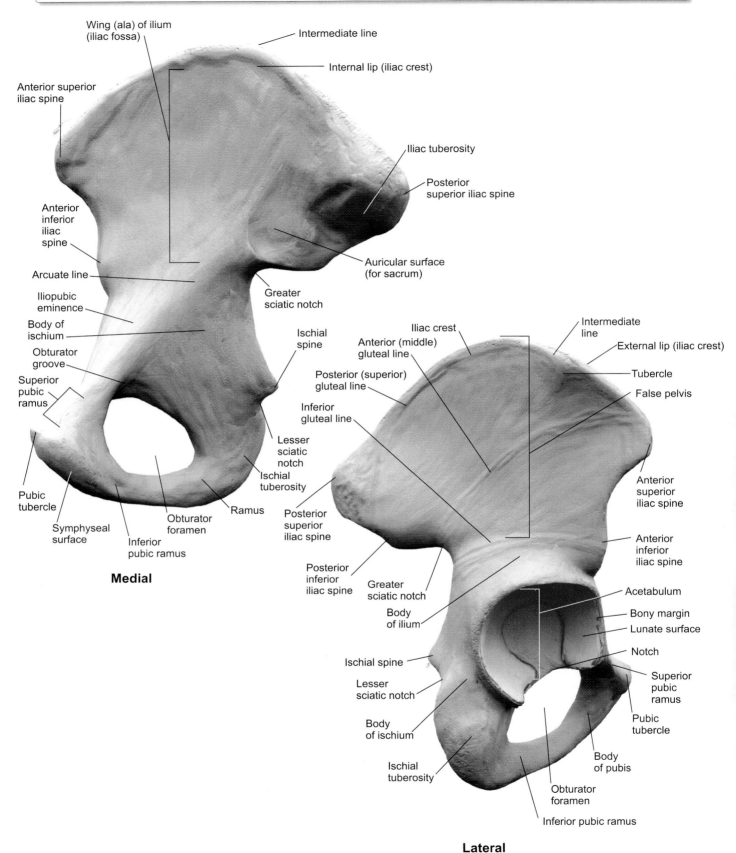

Wing (ala) of ilium
(iliac fossa)

Intermediate line

Internal lip (iliac crest)

Anterior superior
iliac spine

Iliac tuberosity

Posterior
superior iliac spine

Anterior
inferior
iliac
spine

Arcuate line

Auricular surface
(for sacrum)

Iliopubic
eminence

Greater
sciatic notch

Body of
ischium

Ischial
spine

Obturator
groove

Iliac crest

Intermediate
line

Anterior (middle)
gluteal line

External lip (iliac crest)

Superior
pubic
ramus

Posterior (superior)
gluteal line

Tubercle

False pelvis

Inferior
gluteal line

Pubic
tubercle

Lesser
sciatic
notch

Ischial
tuberosity

Anterior
superior
iliac spine

Symphyseal
surface

Ramus

Posterior
superior
iliac spine

Anterior
inferior
iliac spine

Inferior
pubic ramus

Obturator
foramen

Posterior
inferior
iliac spine

Greater
sciatic notch

Acetabulum

Bony margin

Medial

Body
of ilium

Lunate surface

Notch

Ischial spine

Superior
pubic
ramus

Lesser
sciatic notch

Pubic
tubercle

Body
of ischium

Body
of pubis

Ischial
tuberosity

Obturator
foramen

Inferior pubic ramus

Lateral

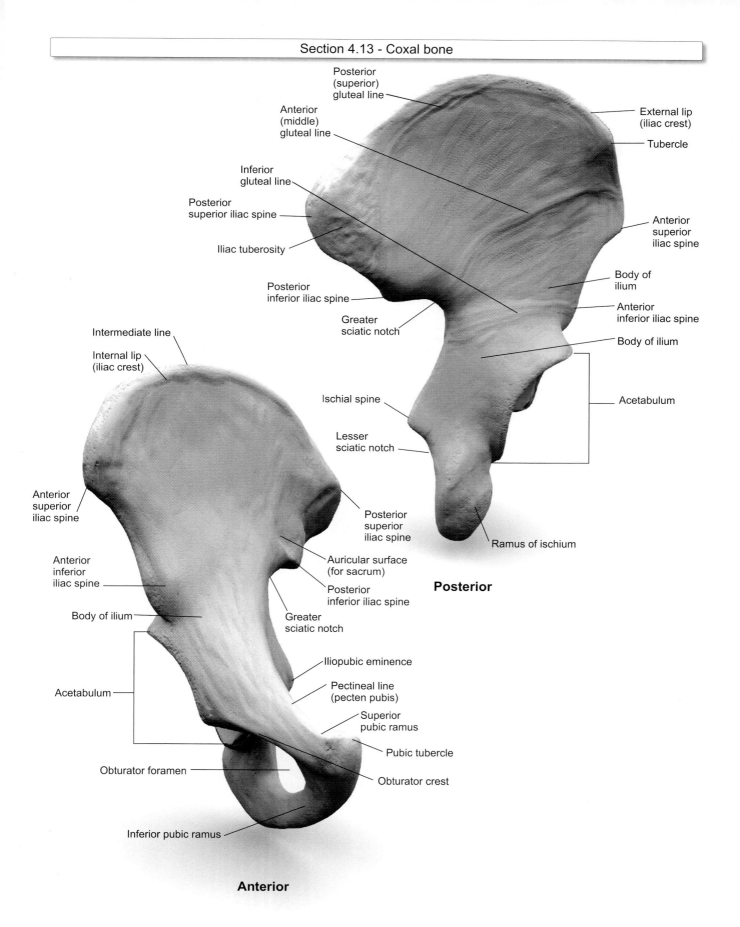

Posterior (superior) gluteal line

Anterior (middle) gluteal line

Inferior gluteal line

Posterior superior iliac spine

Iliac tuberosity

Posterior inferior iliac spine

Greater sciatic notch

External lip (iliac crest)

Tubercle

Anterior superior iliac spine

Body of ilium

Anterior inferior iliac spine

Body of ilium

Acetabulum

Ischial spine

Lesser sciatic notch

Ramus of ischium

Posterior

Intermediate line

Internal lip (iliac crest)

Anterior superior iliac spine

Anterior inferior iliac spine

Body of ilium

Acetabulum

Obturator foramen

Inferior pubic ramus

Posterior superior iliac spine

Auricular surface (for sacrum)

Posterior inferior iliac spine

Greater sciatic notch

Iliopubic eminence

Pectineal line (pecten pubis)

Superior pubic ramus

Pubic tubercle

Obturator crest

Anterior

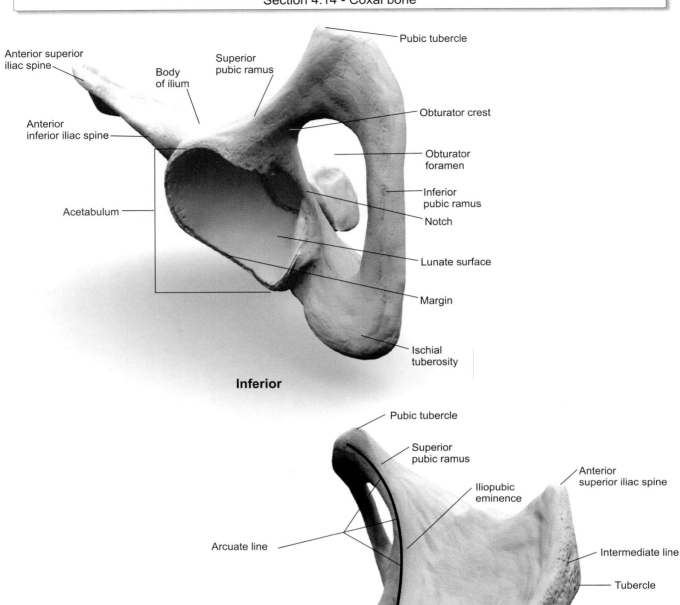

Pubic tubercle

Anterior superior
iliac spine

Body
of ilium

Superior
pubic ramus

Obturator crest

Anterior
inferior iliac spine

Obturator
foramen

Inferior
pubic ramus

Acetabulum

Notch

Lunate surface

Margin

Ischial
tuberosity

Inferior

Pubic tubercle

Superior
pubic ramus

Iliopubic
eminence

Anterior
superior iliac spine

Arcuate line

Intermediate line

Tubercle

Ischial spine

External lip (iliac crest)

Auricular
surface (for sacrum)

Internal lip
(iliac crest)

Posterior
superior iliac spine

Superior

Unit 1 Skeletal System

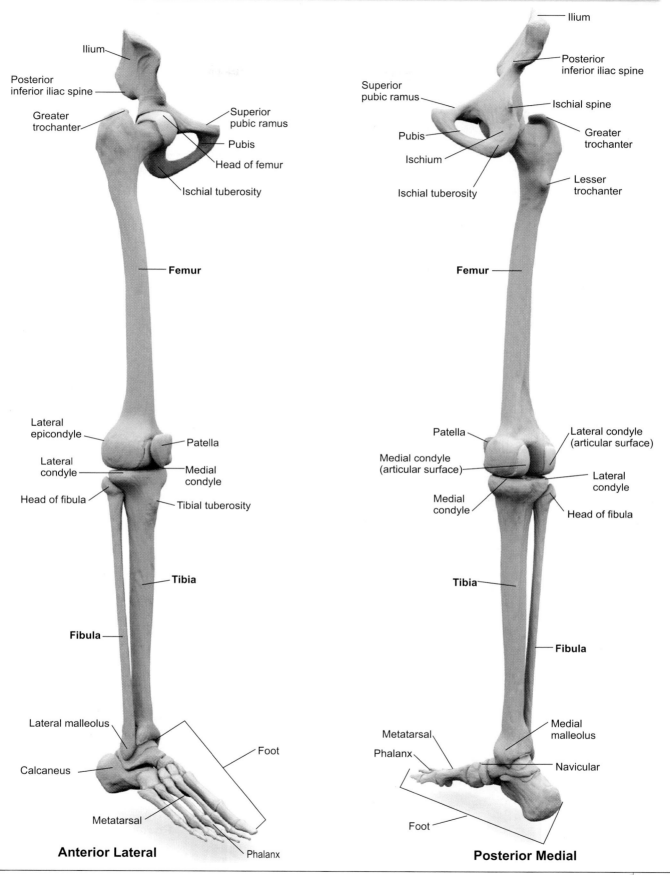

Ilium

Posterior
inferior iliac spine

Greater
trochanter

Superior
pubic ramus

Pubis

Head of femur

Ischial tuberosity

Femur

Lateral
epicondyle

Patella

Lateral
condyle

Medial
condyle

Head of fibula

Tibial tuberosity

Tibia

Fibula

Lateral malleolus

Foot

Calcaneus

Metatarsal

Phalanx

Anterior Lateral

Ilium

Posterior
inferior iliac spine

Superior
pubic ramus

Ischial spine

Pubis

Greater
trochanter

Ischium

Ischial tuberosity

Lesser
trochanter

Femur

Patella

Lateral condyle
(articular surface)

Medial condyle
(articular surface)

Lateral
condyle

Medial
condyle

Head of fibula

Tibia

Fibula

Metatarsal

Medial
malleolus

Phalanx

Navicular

Foot

Posterior Medial

Unit 1 Skeletal System

47

Femur

Greater trochanter

Intertrochanteric line

Neck

Head

Lesser trochanter

Femur

Shaft

Patellar surface

Lateral epicondyle

Lateral condyle

Adductor tubercle

Medial epicondyle

Medial condyle

Anterior

Trochanteric fossa

Fovea of head

Head

Greater trochanter

Intertrochanteric crest

Neck

Calcar

Lesser trochanter

Pectineal line

Gluteal tuberosity

Linea aspera (medial lip)

Linea aspera (lateral lip)

Linea aspera

Shaft

Femur

Adductor tubercle

Medial epicondyle

Medial condyle

Lateral epicondyle

Intercondylar fossa

Posterior

Patella

Anterior surface

Anterior

Articular surface of patella

Posterior

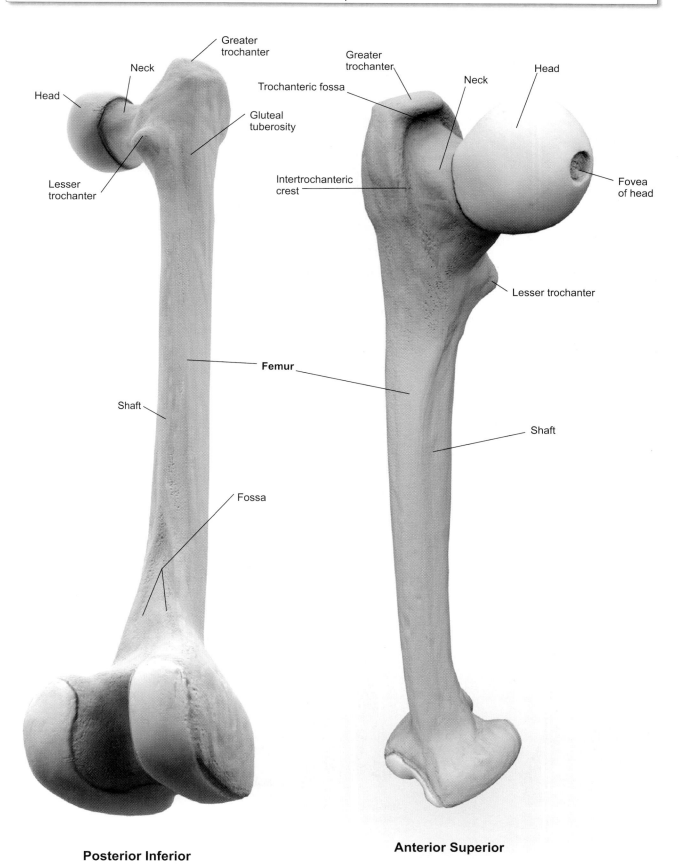

Head

Neck

Greater
trochanter

Greater
trochanter

Neck

Head

Trochanteric fossa

Gluteal
tuberosity

Fovea
of head

Lesser
trochanter

Intertrochanteric
crest

Lesser trochanter

Femur

Shaft

Shaft

Fossa

Posterior Inferior

Anterior Superior

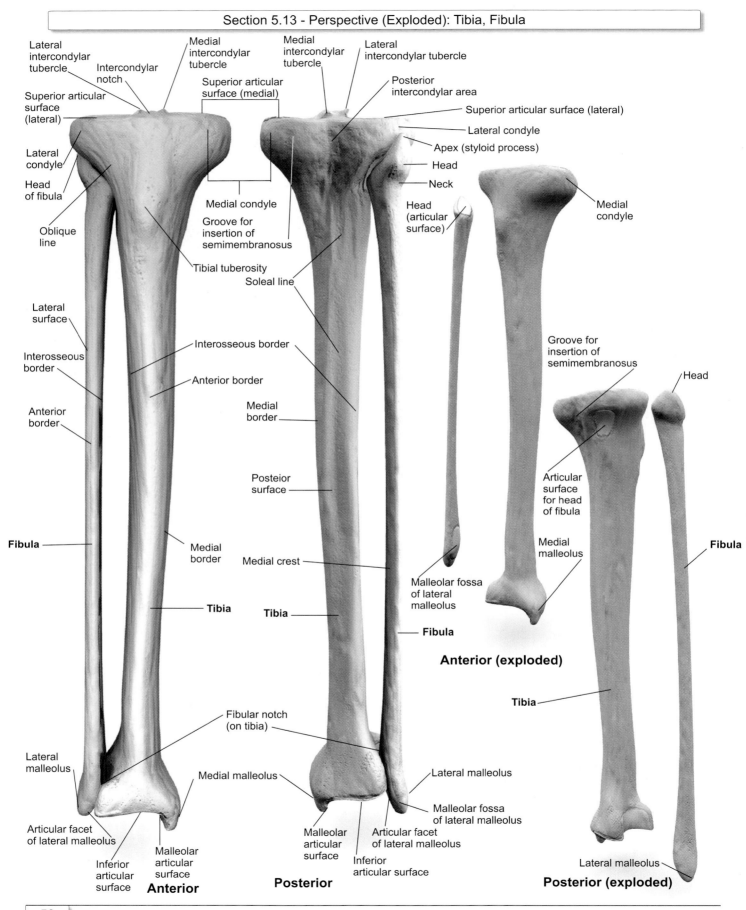

Lateral intercondylar tubercle
Intercondylar notch
Medial intercondylar tubercle
Medial intercondylar tubercle
Lateral intercondylar tubercle
Superior articular surface (medial)
Posterior intercondylar area
Superior articular surface (lateral)
Lateral condyle
Apex (styloid process)
Superior articular surface (lateral)
Lateral condyle
Head of fibula
Head
Neck
Medial condyle
Oblique line
Head (articular surface)
Lateral surface
Medial condyle
Groove for insertion of semimembranosus
Tibial tuberosity
Soleal line
Interosseous border
Anterior border
Medial border
Groove for insertion of semimembranosus
Head
Interosseous border
Anterior border
Articular surface for head of fibula
Anterior border
Posterior surface
Fibula
Medial malleolus
Fibula
Medial border
Medial crest
Tibia
Tibia
Fibula
Malleolar fossa of lateral malleolus
Fibular notch (on tibia)
Tibia
Lateral malleolus
Medial malleolus
Lateral malleolus
Articular facet of lateral malleolus
Malleolar articular surface
Malleolar fossa of lateral malleolus
Inferior articular surface
Malleolar articular surface
Malleolar articular surface
Articular facet of lateral malleolus
Lateral malleolus
Anterior
Inferior articular surface
Posterior
Inferior articular surface
Anterior (exploded)
Posterior (exploded)

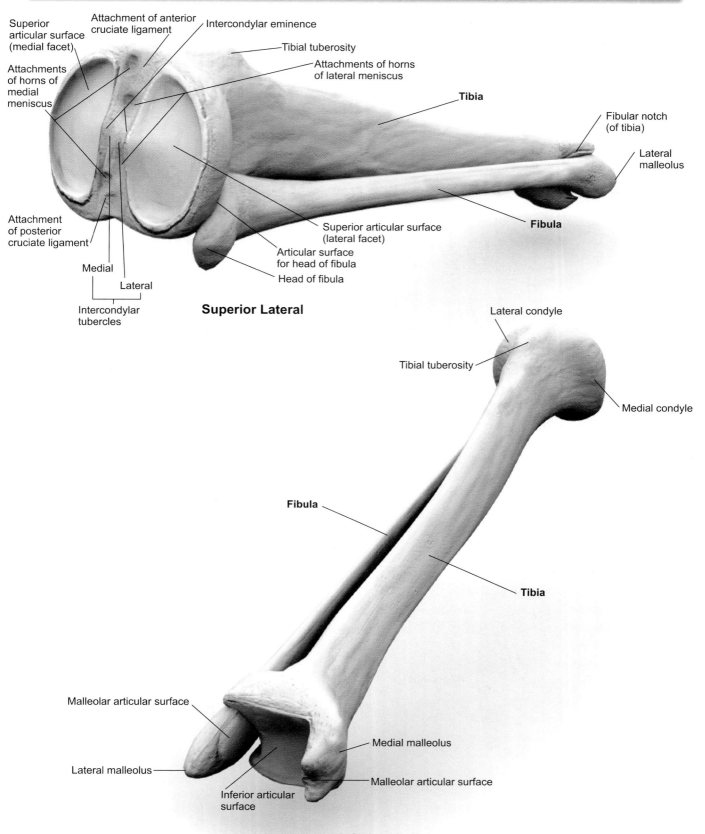

Superior articular surface (medial facet)

Attachment of anterior cruciate ligament

Intercondylar eminence

Tibial tuberosity

Attachments of horns of lateral meniscus

Attachments of horns of medial meniscus

Tibia

Fibular notch (of tibia)

Lateral malleolus

Attachment of posterior cruciate ligament

Superior articular surface (lateral facet)

Fibula

Medial

Lateral

Articular surface for head of fibula

Head of fibula

Intercondylar tubercles

Superior Lateral

Lateral condyle

Tibial tuberosity

Medial condyle

Fibula

Tibia

Malleolar articular surface

Medial malleolus

Lateral malleolus

Malleolar articular surface

Inferior articular surface

Inferior Medial

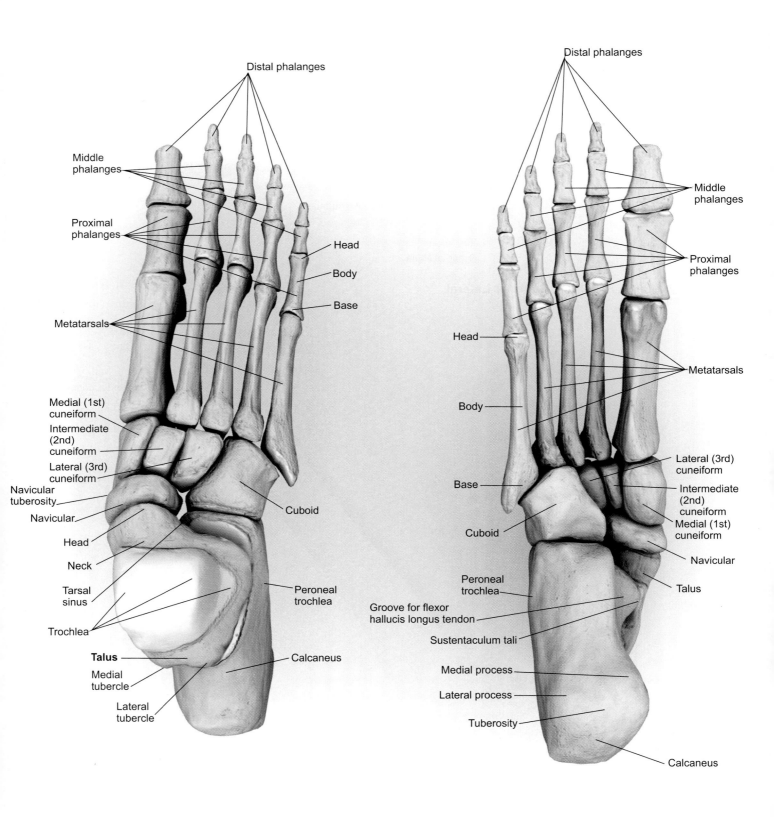

Distal phalanges

Middle phalanges

Proximal phalanges

Head

Body

Base

Metatarsals

Medial (1st) cuneiform

Intermediate (2nd) cuneiform

Lateral (3rd) cuneiform

Navicular tuberosity

Navicular

Head

Neck

Tarsal sinus

Trochlea

Cuboid

Peroneal trochlea

Talus

Medial tubercle

Lateral tubercle

Calcaneus

Superior

Distal phalanges

Middle phalanges

Proximal phalanges

Head

Body

Base

Metatarsals

Lateral (3rd) cuneiform

Intermediate (2nd) cuneiform

Medial (1st) cuneiform

Navicular

Talus

Cuboid

Peroneal trochlea

Groove for flexor hallucis longus tendon

Sustentaculum tali

Medial process

Lateral process

Tuberosity

Calcaneus

Inferior

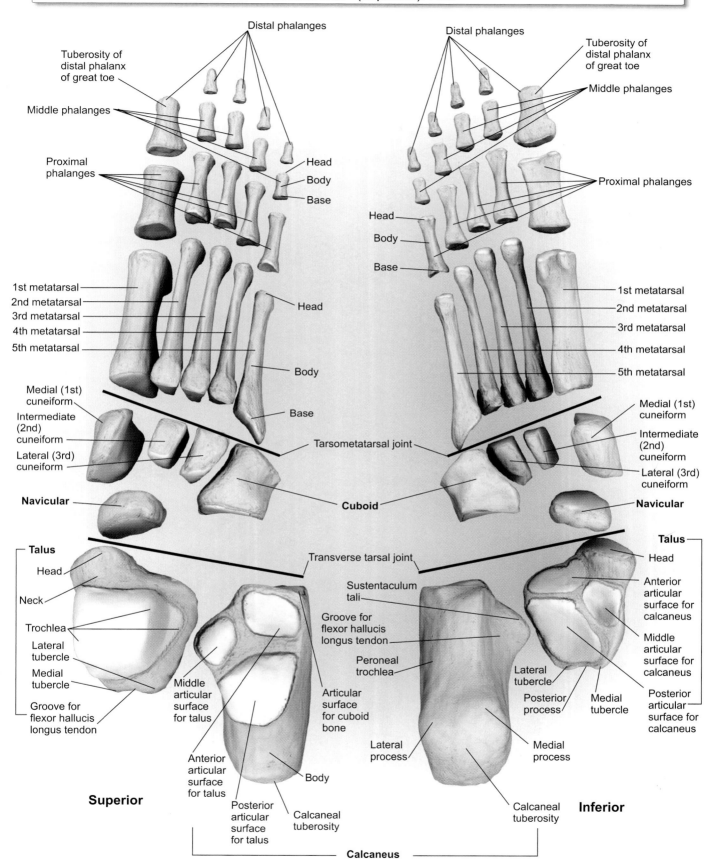

Distal phalanges

Tuberosity of
distal phalanx
of great toe

Middle phalanges

Proximal
phalanges

Head
Body
Base

1st metatarsal
2nd metatarsal
3rd metatarsal
4th metatarsal
5th metatarsal

Head

Body

Base

Medial (1st)
cuneiform

Intermediate
(2nd)
cuneiform

Lateral (3rd)
cuneiform

Navicular

Tarsometatarsal joint

Cuboid

Talus

Head

Neck

Trochlea

Lateral
tubercle

Medial
tubercle

Groove for
flexor hallucis
longus tendon

Middle
articular
surface
for talus

Anterior
articular
surface
for talus

Posterior
articular
surface
for talus

Body

Calcaneal
tuberosity

Transverse tarsal joint

Sustentaculum
tali

Groove for
flexor hallucis
longus tendon

Peroneal
trochlea

Articular
surface
for cuboid
bone

Lateral
process

Medial
process

Calcaneal
tuberosity

Superior

Calcaneus

Distal phalanges

Tuberosity of
distal phalanx
of great toe

Middle phalanges

Proximal phalanges

Head
Body
Base

1st metatarsal
2nd metatarsal
3rd metatarsal
4th metatarsal
5th metatarsal

Medial (1st)
cuneiform

Intermediate
(2nd)
cuneiform

Lateral (3rd)
cuneiform

Navicular

Talus

Head

Anterior
articular
surface for
calcaneus

Middle
articular
surface for
calcaneus

Posterior
articular
surface for
calcaneus

Lateral
tubercle

Posterior
process

Medial
tubercle

Inferior

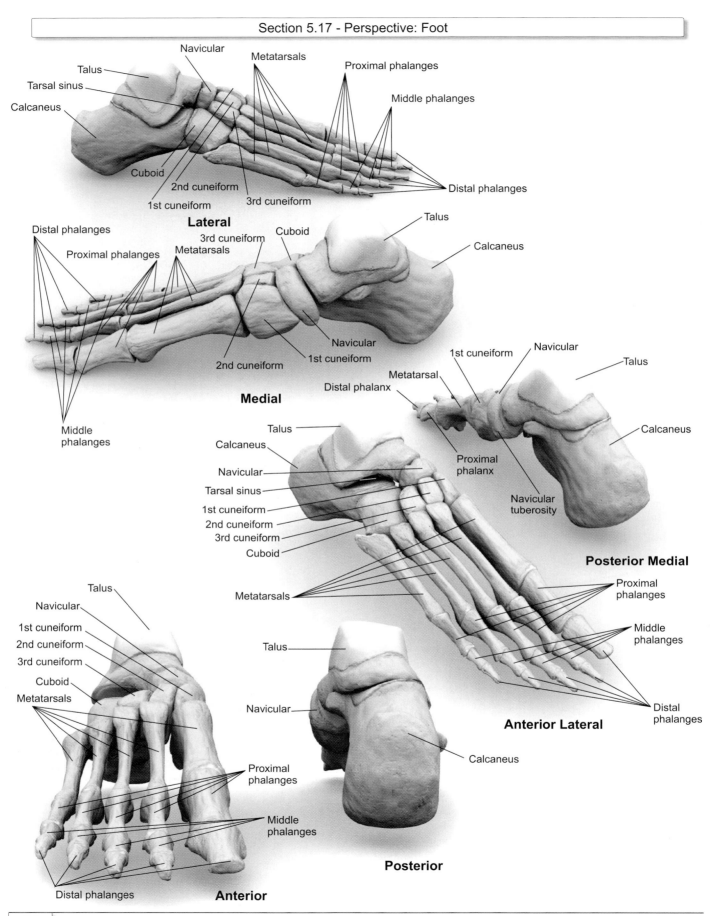

Lateral

Talus
Tarsal sinus
Calcaneus
Navicular
Metatarsals
Proximal phalanges
Middle phalanges
Distal phalanges
Cuboid
2nd cuneiform
1st cuneiform
3rd cuneiform

Medial

Distal phalanges
Proximal phalanges
3rd cuneiform
Cuboid
Metatarsals
Talus
Calcaneus
Middle phalanges
2nd cuneiform
1st cuneiform
Navicular

Posterior Medial

1st cuneiform
Navicular
Metatarsal
Distal phalanx
Proximal phalanx
Navicular tuberosity
Talus
Calcaneus

Anterior Lateral

Talus
Calcaneus
Navicular
Tarsal sinus
1st cuneiform
2nd cuneiform
3rd cuneiform
Cuboid
Metatarsals
Proximal phalanges
Middle phalanges
Distal phalanges

Anterior

Talus
Navicular
1st cuneiform
2nd cuneiform
3rd cuneiform
Cuboid
Metatarsals
Proximal phalanges
Middle phalanges
Distal phalanges

Posterior

Talus
Navicular
Calcaneus

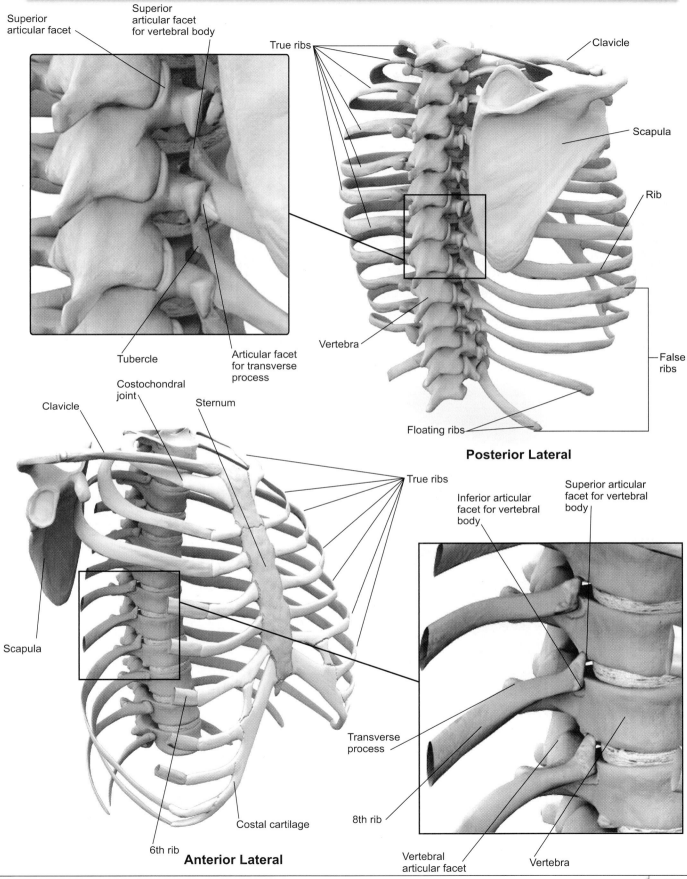

Superior articular facet

Superior articular facet for vertebral body

True ribs

Clavicle

Scapula

Rib

Tubercle

Articular facet for transverse process

Vertebra

False ribs

Floating ribs

Posterior Lateral

Costochondral joint

Sternum

Clavicle

True ribs

Inferior articular facet for vertebral body

Superior articular facet for vertebral body

Scapula

Transverse process

8th rib

Costal cartilage

6th rib

Anterior Lateral

Vertebral articular facet

Vertebra

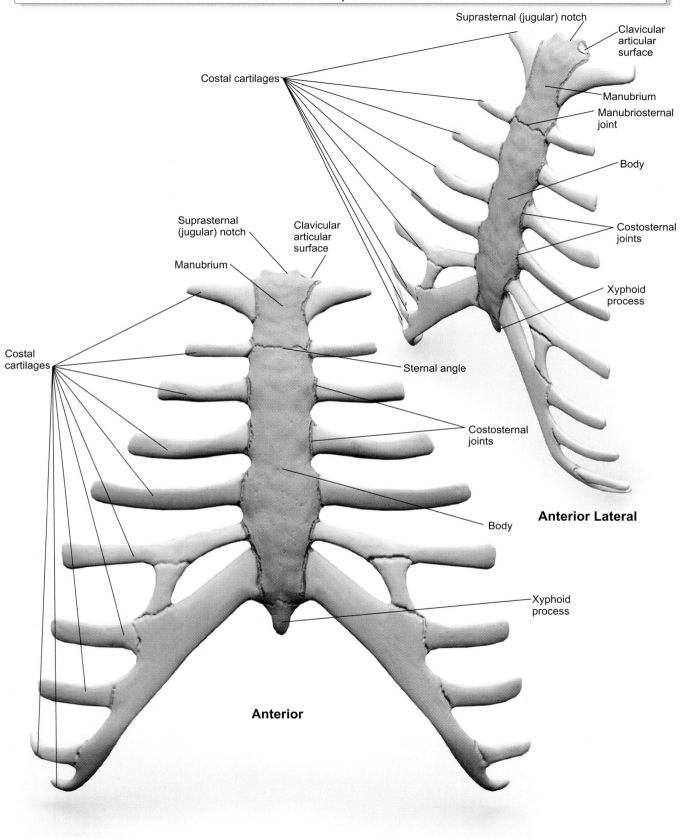

Suprasternal (jugular) notch

Clavicular articular surface

Manubrium

Manubriosternal joint

Body

Costosternal joints

Xyphoid process

Costal cartilages

Suprasternal (jugular) notch

Clavicular articular surface

Manubrium

Sternal angle

Costosternal joints

Costal cartilages

Body

Anterior Lateral

Xyphoid process

Anterior

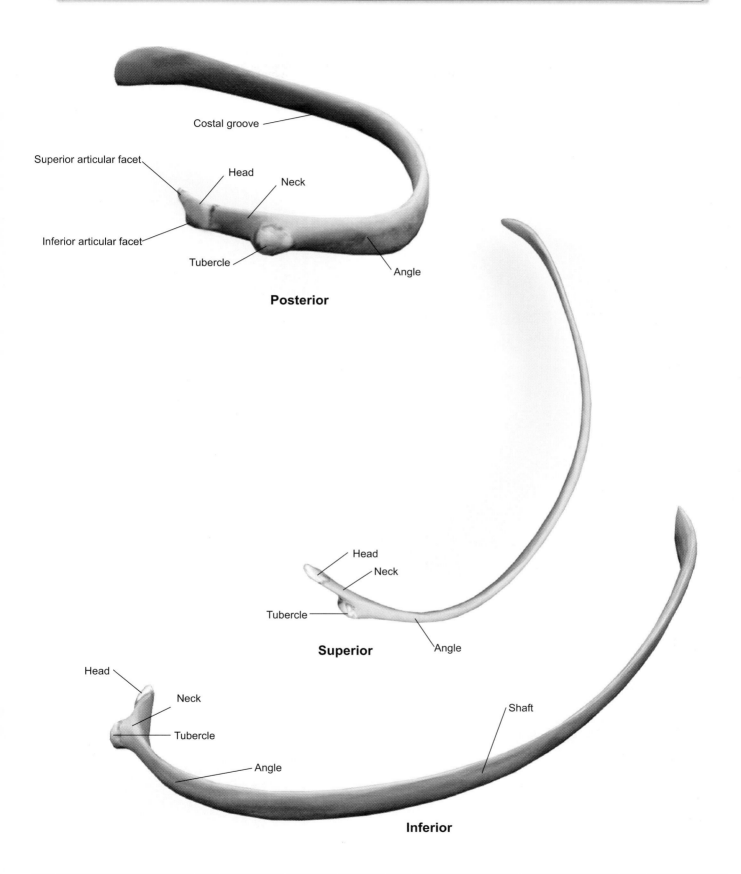

Costal groove

Superior articular facet

Head

Neck

Inferior articular facet

Tubercle

Angle

Posterior

Head

Neck

Tubercle

Angle

Superior

Head

Neck

Tubercle

Shaft

Angle

Inferior

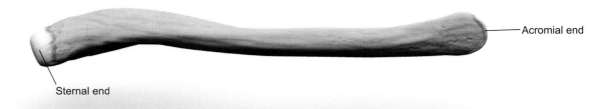

Anterior

Acromial end

Sternal end

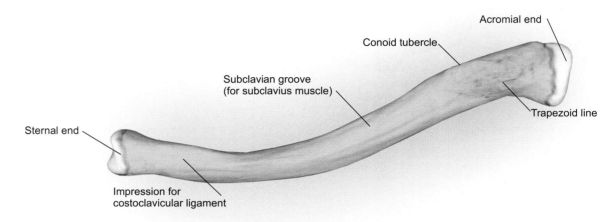

Acromial end

Conoid tubercle

Subclavian groove
(for subclavius muscle)

Trapezoid line

Sternal end

Impression for
costoclavicular ligament

Inferior

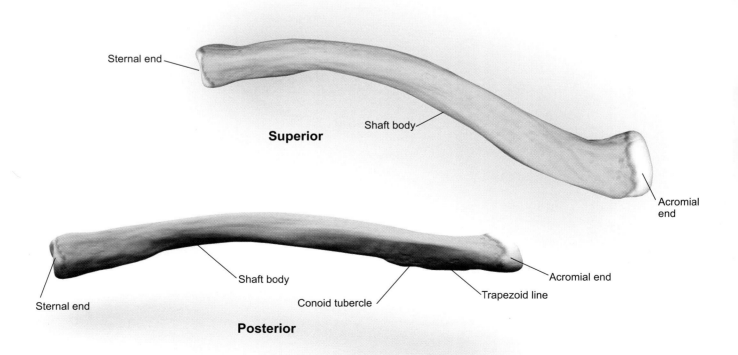

Sternal end

Shaft body

Superior

Acromial
end

Shaft body

Conoid tubercle

Trapezoid line

Acromial end

Sternal end

Posterior

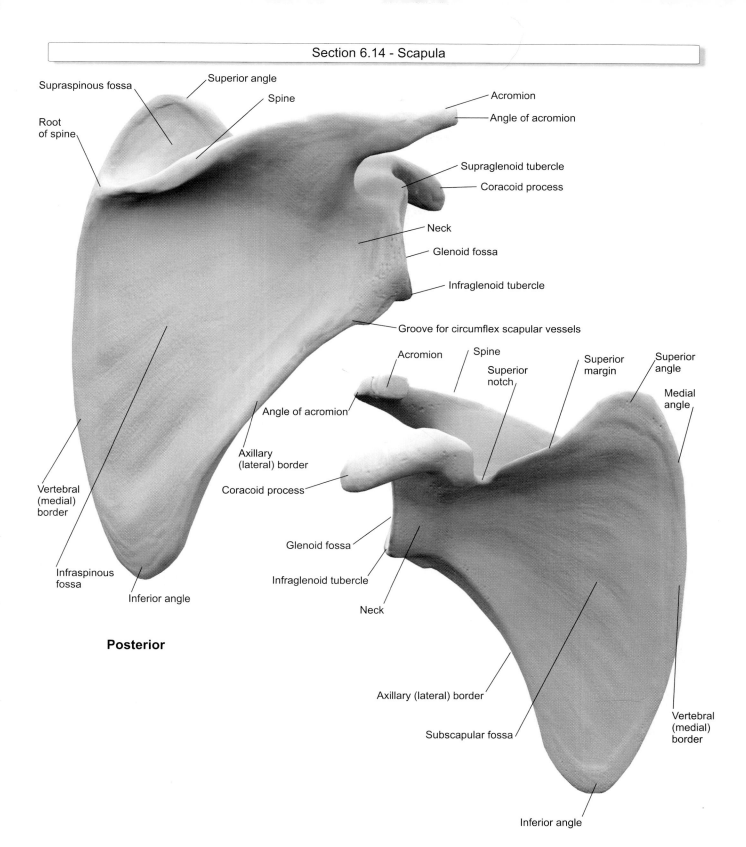

Supraspinous fossa

Superior angle

Spine

Acromion

Angle of acromion

Root
of spine

Supraglenoid tubercle

Coracoid process

Neck

Glenoid fossa

Infraglenoid tubercle

Groove for circumflex scapular vessels

Acromion

Spine

Superior
notch

Superior
margin

Superior
angle

Medial
angle

Angle of acromion

Vertebral
(medial)
border

Axillary
(lateral) border

Coracoid process

Glenoid fossa

Infraspinous
fossa

Infraglenoid tubercle

Inferior angle

Neck

Posterior

Axillary (lateral) border

Subscapular fossa

Vertebral
(medial)
border

Inferior angle

Anterior

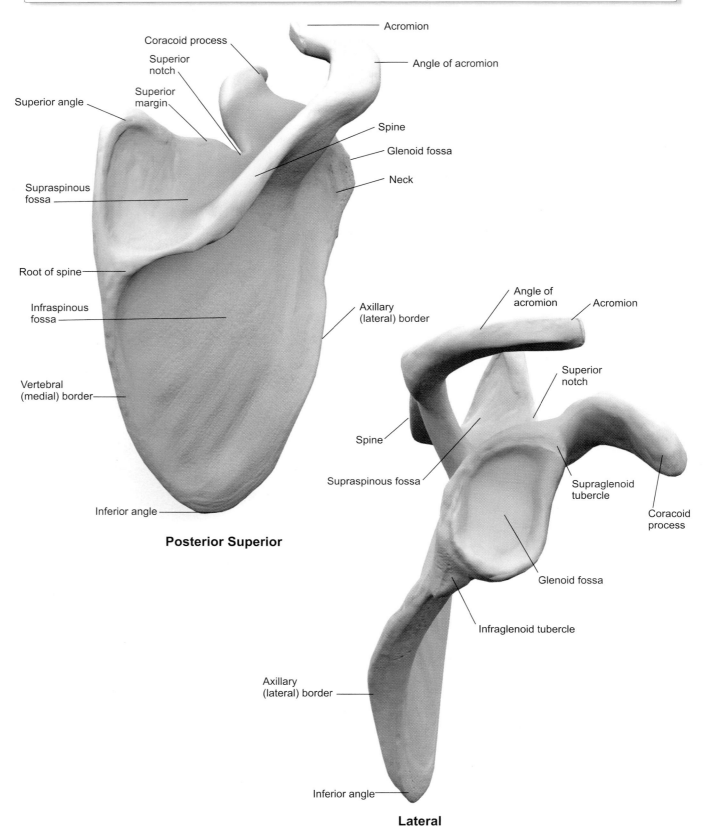

Acromion

Coracoid process

Superior notch

Angle of acromion

Superior margin

Superior angle

Spine

Glenoid fossa

Neck

Supraspinous fossa

Root of spine

Infraspinous fossa

Axillary (lateral) border

Vertebral (medial) border

Inferior angle

Posterior Superior

Angle of acromion

Acromion

Superior notch

Spine

Supraspinous fossa

Supraglenoid tubercle

Coracoid process

Glenoid fossa

Infraglenoid tubercle

Axillary (lateral) border

Inferior angle

Lateral

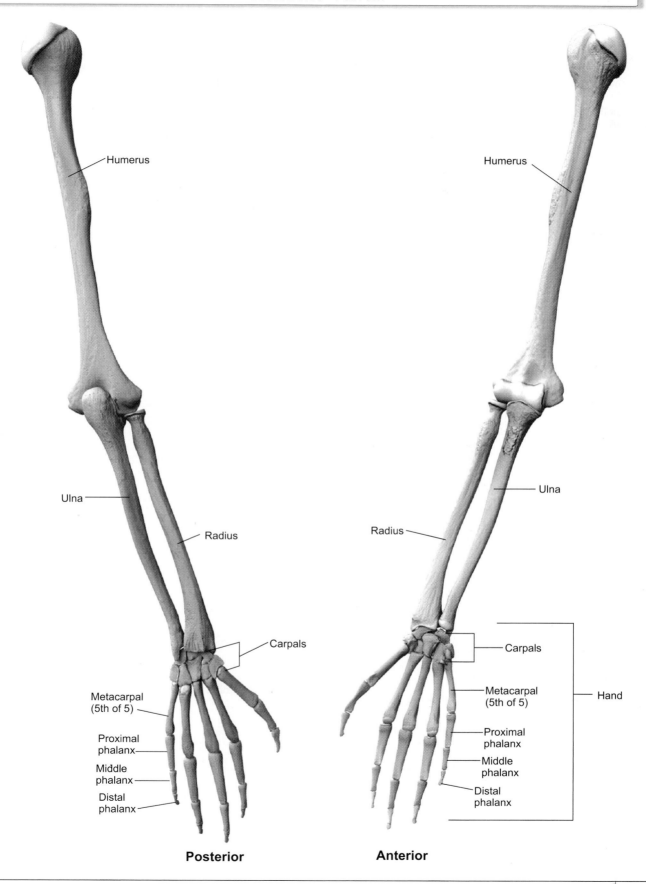

Humerus

Humerus

Ulna

Ulna

Radius

Radius

Carpals

Carpals

Metacarpal
(5th of 5)

Metacarpal
(5th of 5)

Hand

Proximal
phalanx

Proximal
phalanx

Middle
phalanx

Middle
phalanx

Distal
phalanx

Distal
phalanx

Posterior

Anterior

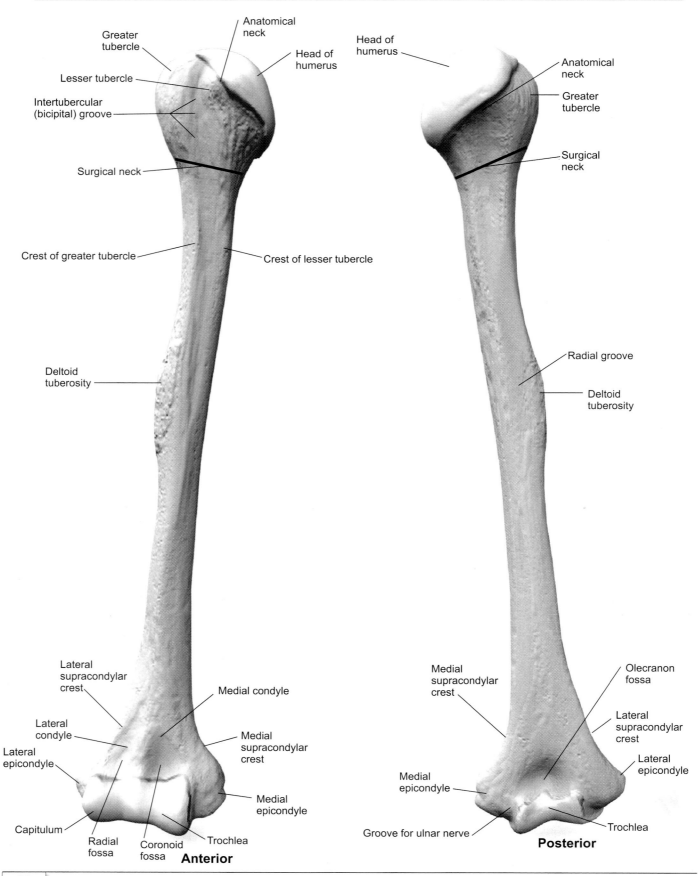

Greater tubercle

Anatomical neck

Head of humerus

Lesser tubercle

Intertubercular (bicipital) groove

Surgical neck

Crest of greater tubercle

Crest of lesser tubercle

Deltoid tuberosity

Lateral supracondylar crest

Medial condyle

Lateral condyle

Medial supracondylar crest

Lateral epicondyle

Capitulum

Radial fossa

Coronoid fossa

Trochlea

Medial epicondyle

Anterior

Head of humerus

Anatomical neck

Greater tubercle

Surgical neck

Radial groove

Deltoid tuberosity

Medial supracondylar crest

Olecranon fossa

Lateral supracondylar crest

Lateral epicondyle

Medial epicondyle

Groove for ulnar nerve

Trochlea

Posterior

Unit 1 Skeletal System

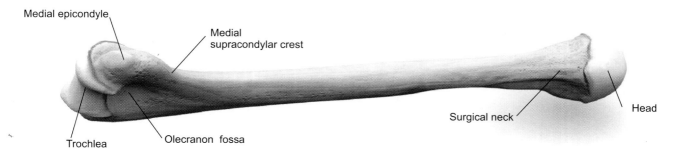

Medial epicondyle

Medial
supracondylar crest

Trochlea

Olecranon fossa

Surgical neck

Head

Superior Medial

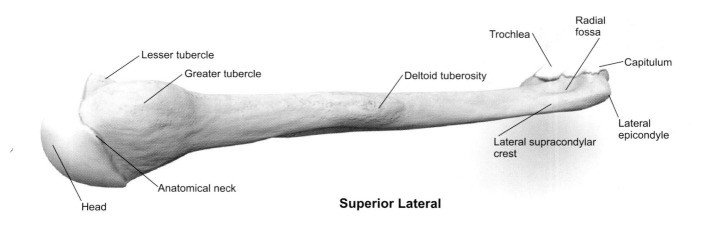

Lesser tubercle

Greater tubercle

Deltoid tuberosity

Trochlea

Radial
fossa

Capitulum

Lateral
epicondyle

Lateral supracondylar
crest

Anatomical neck

Head

Superior Lateral

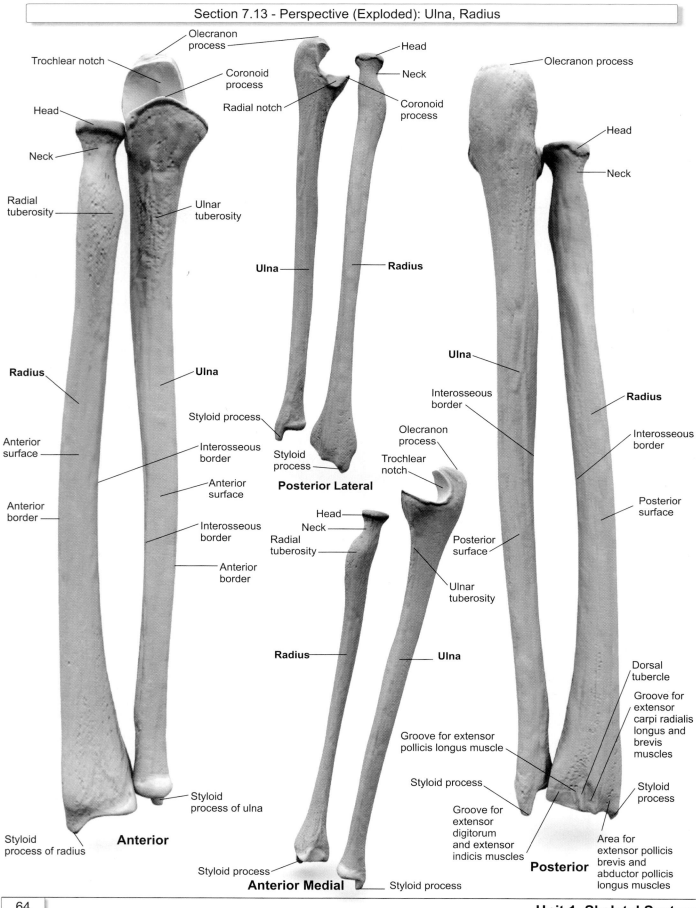

Olecranon process

Trochlear notch

Coronoid process

Radial notch

Head

Neck

Coronoid process

Head

Neck

Radial tuberosity

Ulnar tuberosity

Ulna

Radius

Radius

Ulna

Anterior surface

Interosseous border

Anterior surface

Anterior border

Interosseous border

Anterior border

Styloid process of ulna

Styloid process of radius

Anterior

Styloid process

Styloid process

Posterior Lateral

Head
Neck
Radial tuberosity

Olecranon process

Trochlear notch

Posterior surface

Ulnar tuberosity

Radius

Ulna

Groove for extensor pollicis longus muscle

Styloid process

Groove for extensor digitorum and extensor indicis muscles

Styloid process

Anterior Medial

Olecranon process

Head

Neck

Ulna

Interosseous border

Radius

Interosseous border

Posterior surface

Dorsal tubercle

Groove for extensor carpi radialis longus and brevis muscles

Styloid process

Area for extensor pollicis brevis and abductor pollicis longus muscles

Posterior

Unit 1 Skeletal System

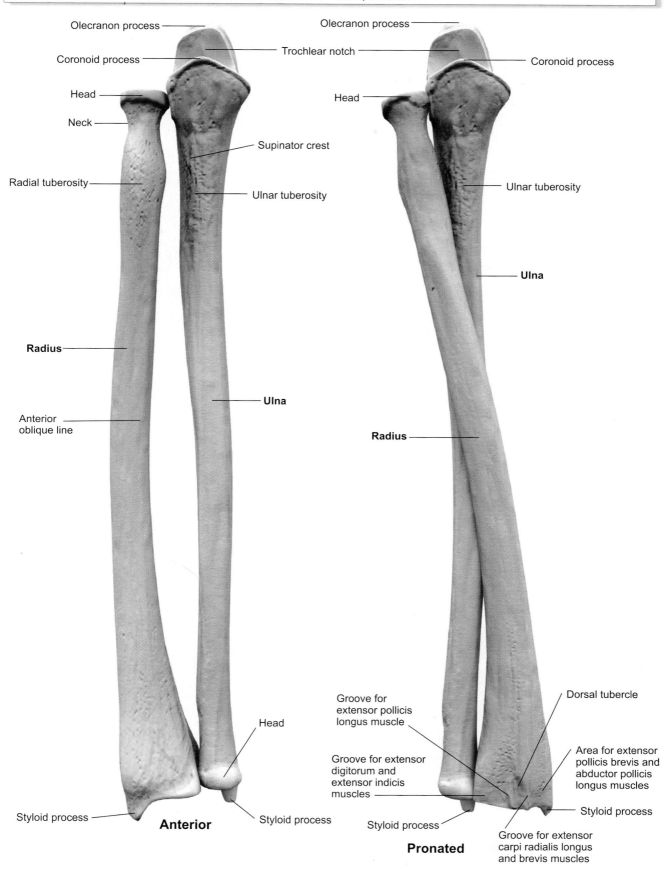

Olecranon process

Olecranon process

Coronoid process

Trochlear notch

Coronoid process

Head

Head

Neck

Supinator crest

Radial tuberosity

Ulnar tuberosity

Ulnar tuberosity

Ulna

Radius

Radius

Anterior oblique line

Ulna

Head

Groove for extensor pollicis longus muscle

Dorsal tubercle

Groove for extensor digitorum and extensor indicis muscles

Area for extensor pollicis brevis and abductor pollicis longus muscles

Styloid process

Anterior

Styloid process

Styloid process

Styloid process

Pronated

Groove for extensor carpi radialis longus and brevis muscles

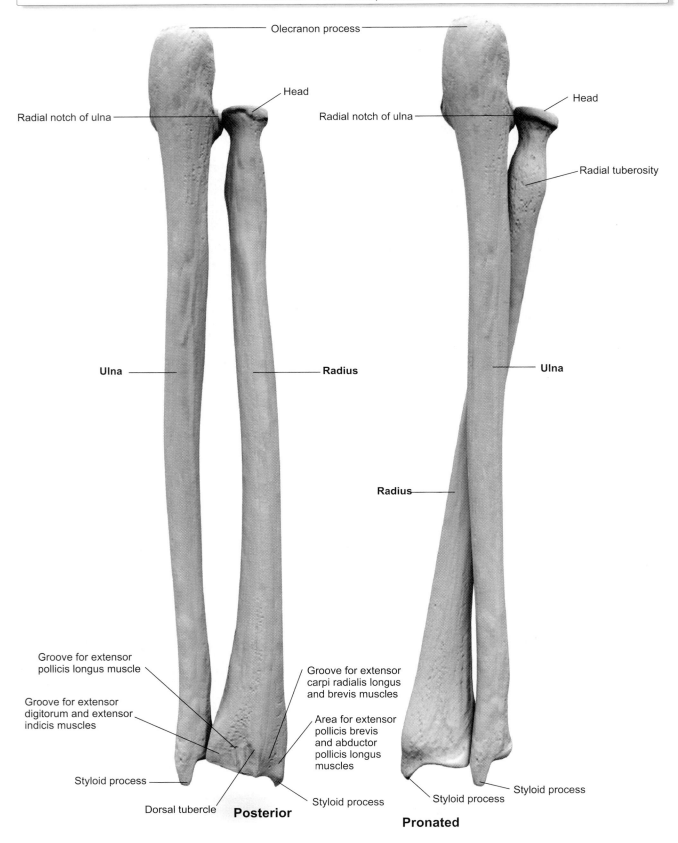

Olecranon process

Head

Radial notch of ulna

Radial notch of ulna

Head

Radial tuberosity

Ulna

Radius

Ulna

Radius

Groove for extensor pollicis longus muscle

Groove for extensor carpi radialis longus and brevis muscles

Groove for extensor digitorum and extensor indicis muscles

Area for extensor pollicis brevis and abductor pollicis longus muscles

Styloid process

Dorsal tubercle

Posterior

Styloid process

Styloid process

Styloid process

Pronated

Unit 1 Skeletal System

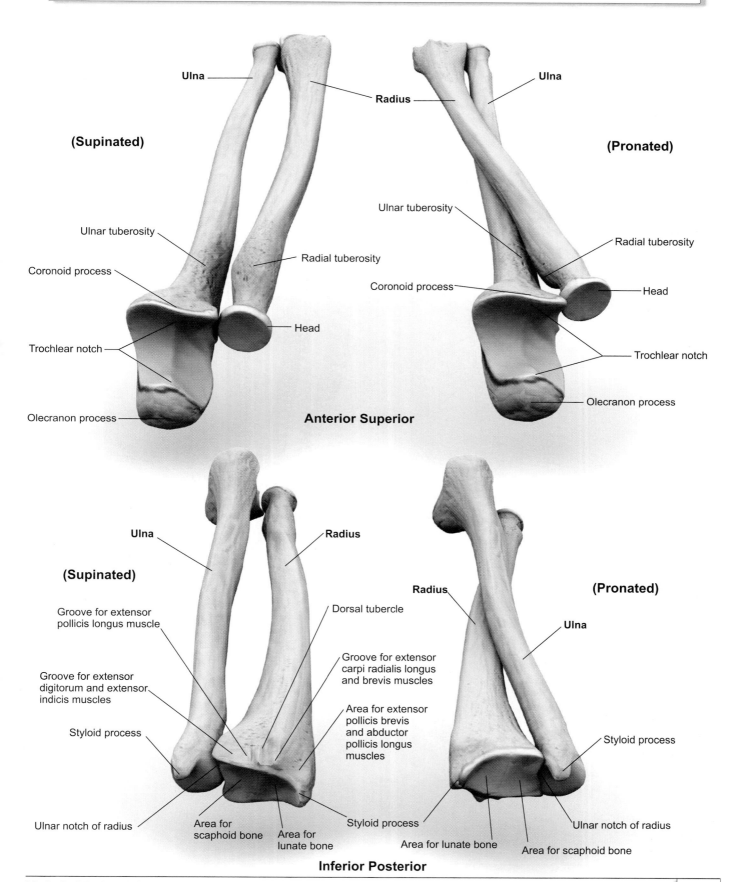

Ulna

Radius

(Supinated)

(Pronated)

Ulnar tuberosity

Coronoid process

Ulnar tuberosity

Radial tuberosity

Radial tuberosity

Coronoid process

Head

Trochlear notch

Head

Trochlear notch

Olecranon process

Olecranon process

Anterior Superior

Ulna

Radius

(Supinated)

(Pronated)

Groove for extensor pollicis longus muscle

Dorsal tubercle

Radius

Ulna

Groove for extensor carpi radialis longus and brevis muscles

Groove for extensor digitorum and extensor indicis muscles

Area for extensor pollicis brevis and abductor pollicis longus muscles

Styloid process

Styloid process

Ulnar notch of radius

Area for scaphoid bone

Area for lunate bone

Styloid process

Area for lunate bone

Area for scaphoid bone

Ulnar notch of radius

Inferior Posterior

Unit 1 Skeletal System

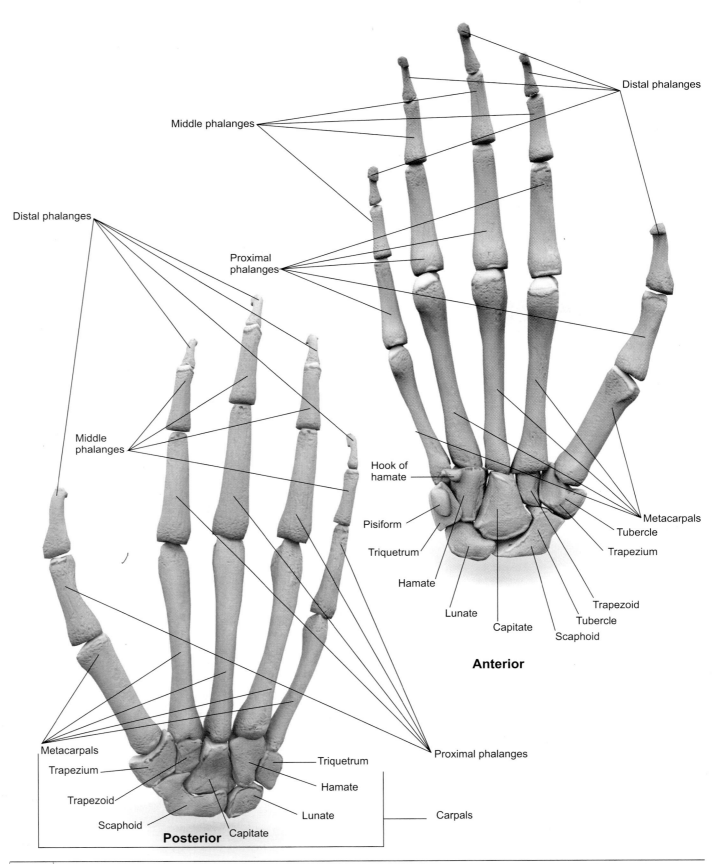

Distal phalanges

Middle phalanges

Proximal phalanges

Distal phalanges

Middle phalanges

Proximal phalanges

Hook of hamate

Pisiform

Triquetrum

Hamate

Lunate

Capitate

Metacarpals

Tubercle

Trapezium

Trapezoid

Tubercle

Scaphoid

Anterior

Metacarpals

Trapezium

Trapezoid

Scaphoid

Capitate

Lunate

Hamate

Triquetrum

Carpals

Posterior

Unit 1 Skeletal System

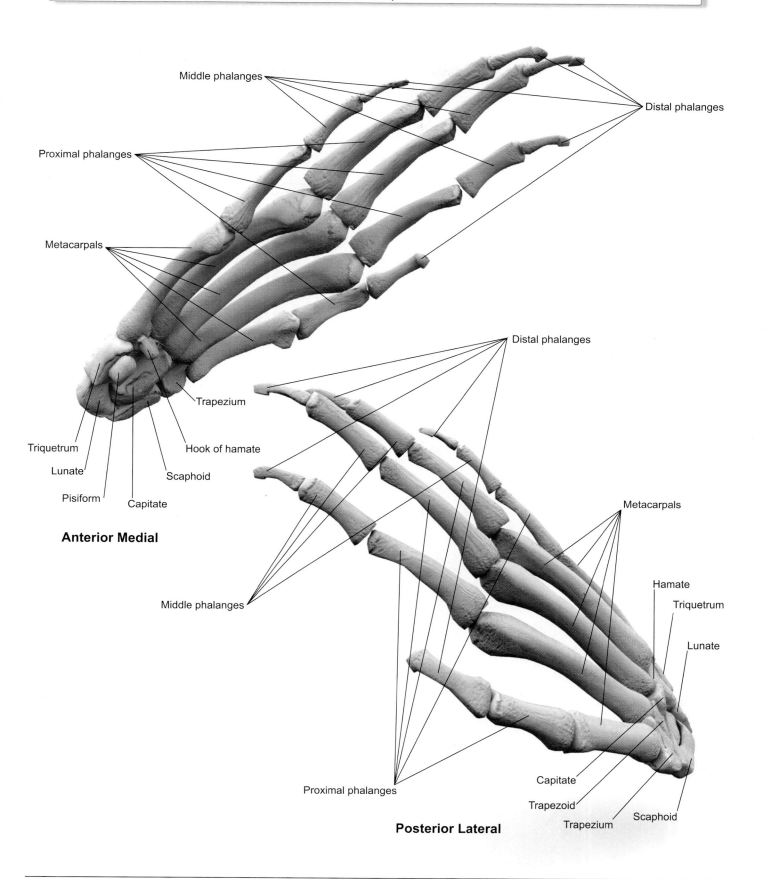

Middle phalanges

Distal phalanges

Proximal phalanges

Metacarpals

Trapezium

Triquetrum

Hook of hamate

Lunate

Scaphoid

Pisiform

Capitate

Anterior Medial

Distal phalanges

Metacarpals

Hamate

Triquetrum

Lunate

Middle phalanges

Proximal phalanges

Capitate

Trapezoid

Scaphoid

Trapezium

Posterior Lateral

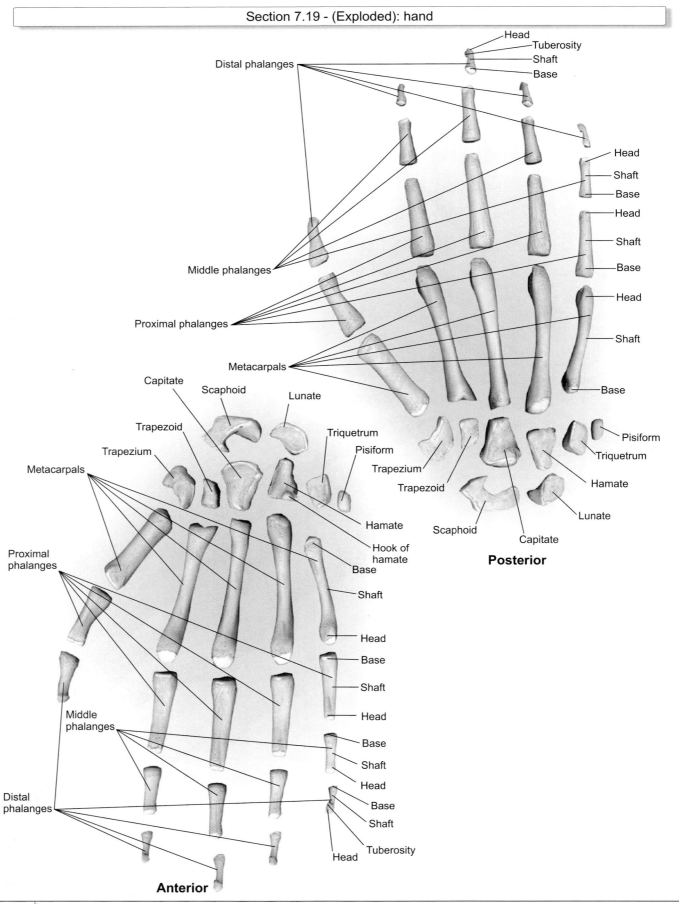

Head
Tuberosity
Shaft
Base

Distal phalanges

Head
Shaft
Base
Head
Shaft
Base
Head
Shaft

Middle phalanges

Proximal phalanges

Metacarpals

Base

Capitate   Scaphoid   Lunate

Trapezoid   Triquetrum
                        Pisiform
Trapezium

Metacarpals   Pisiform
                       Triquetrum
Trapezium
Trapezoid   Hamate

Scaphoid   Capitate   Lunate

Hamate

Posterior

Proximal
phalanges

Hook of
hamate
Base

Shaft

Head

Base

Shaft

Head

Middle
phalanges

Base

Shaft

Head

Distal
phalanges

Base
Shaft

Head   Tuberosity

Anterior

Unit 1 Skeletal System

Ligaments

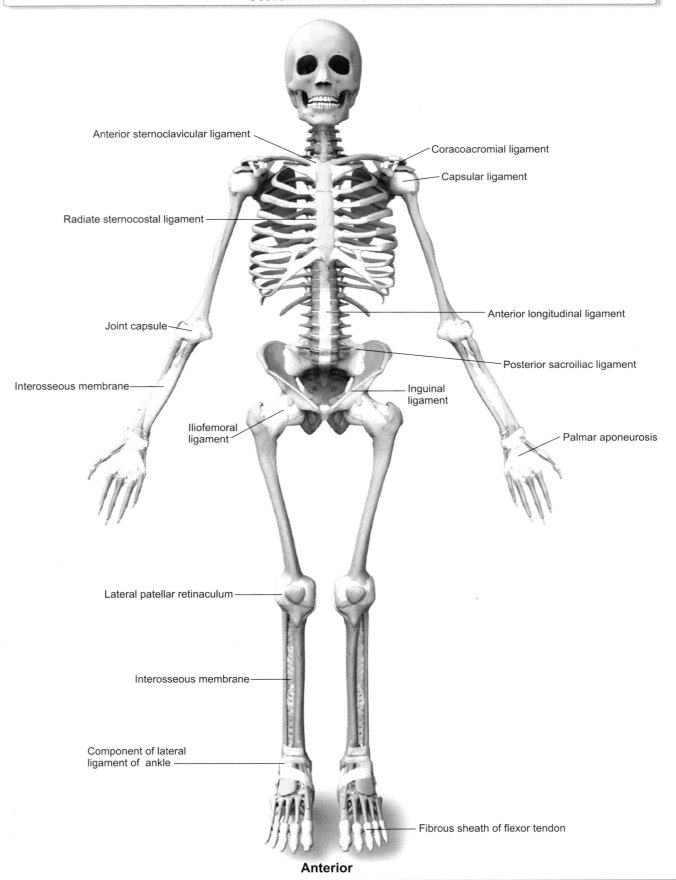

Anterior sternoclavicular ligament

Coracoacromial ligament

Capsular ligament

Radiate sternocostal ligament

Anterior longitudinal ligament

Joint capsule

Posterior sacroiliac ligament

Interosseous membrane

Inguinal ligament

Iliofemoral ligament

Palmar aponeurosis

Lateral patellar retinaculum

Interosseous membrane

Component of lateral ligament of ankle

Fibrous sheath of flexor tendon

Anterior

Unit 2   Ligaments

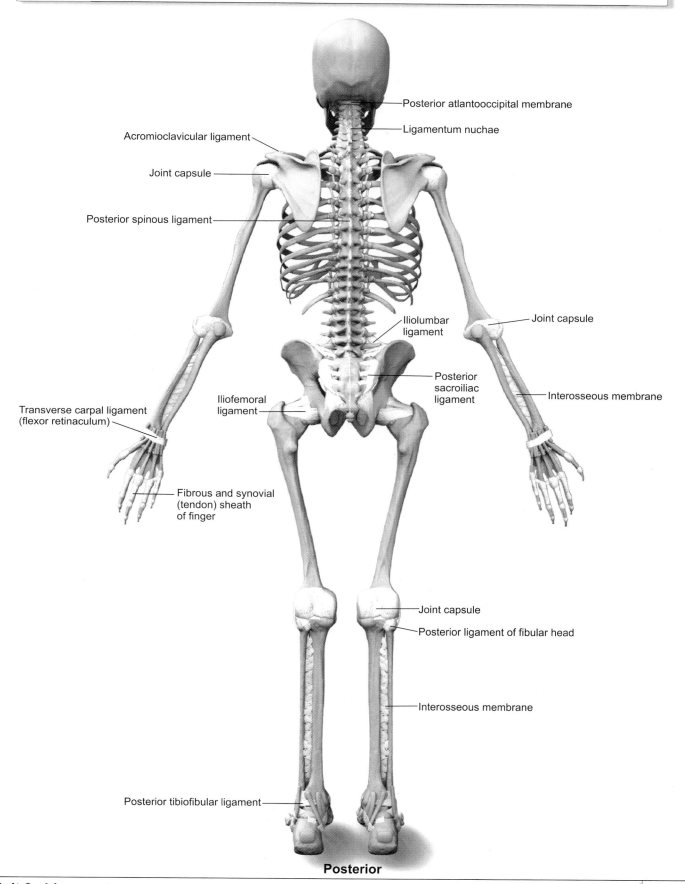

Posterior atlantooccipital membrane

Ligamentum nuchae

Acromioclavicular ligament

Joint capsule

Posterior spinous ligament

Iliolumbar ligament

Joint capsule

Posterior sacroiliac ligament

Interosseous membrane

Transverse carpal ligament (flexor retinaculum)

Iliofemoral ligament

Fibrous and synovial (tendon) sheath of finger

Joint capsule

Posterior ligament of fibular head

Interosseous membrane

Posterior tibiofibular ligament

Posterior

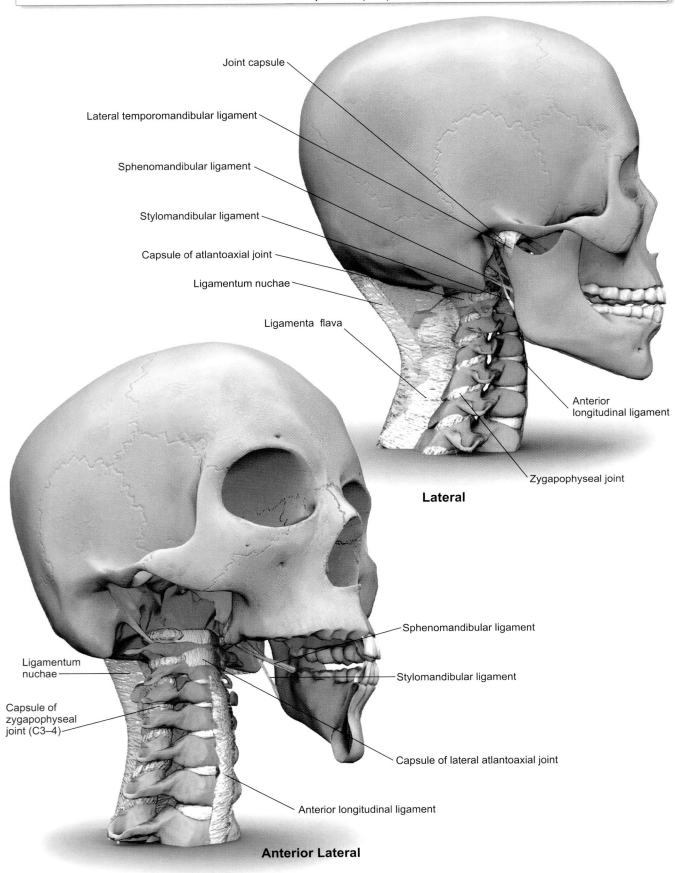

Joint capsule

Lateral temporomandibular ligament

Sphenomandibular ligament

Stylomandibular ligament

Capsule of atlantoaxial joint

Ligamentum nuchae

Ligamenta flava

Anterior longitudinal ligament

Zygapophyseal joint

Lateral

Ligamentum nuchae

Capsule of zygapophyseal joint (C3–4)

Sphenomandibular ligament

Stylomandibular ligament

Capsule of lateral atlantoaxial joint

Anterior longitudinal ligament

Anterior Lateral

Unit 2   Ligaments

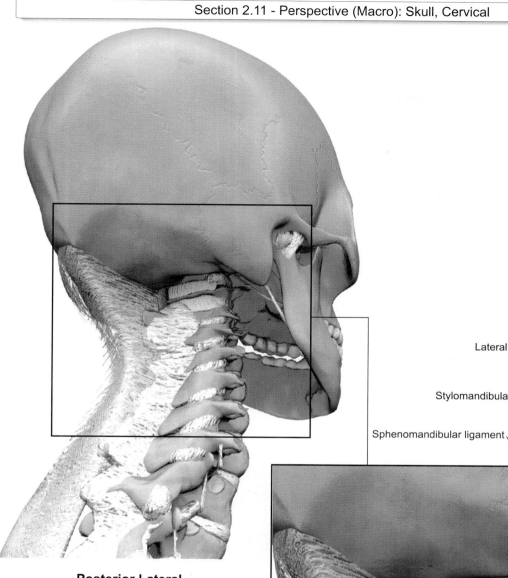

Posterior Lateral

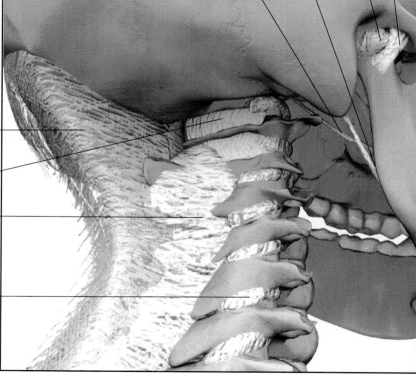

Lateral temporomandibular ligament

Joint capsule

Stylomandibular ligament

Sphenomandibular ligament

Ligamentum nuchae

Capsule of atlantooccipital joint

Ligamenta flava

Capsule of zygapophyseal joint (C5–6)

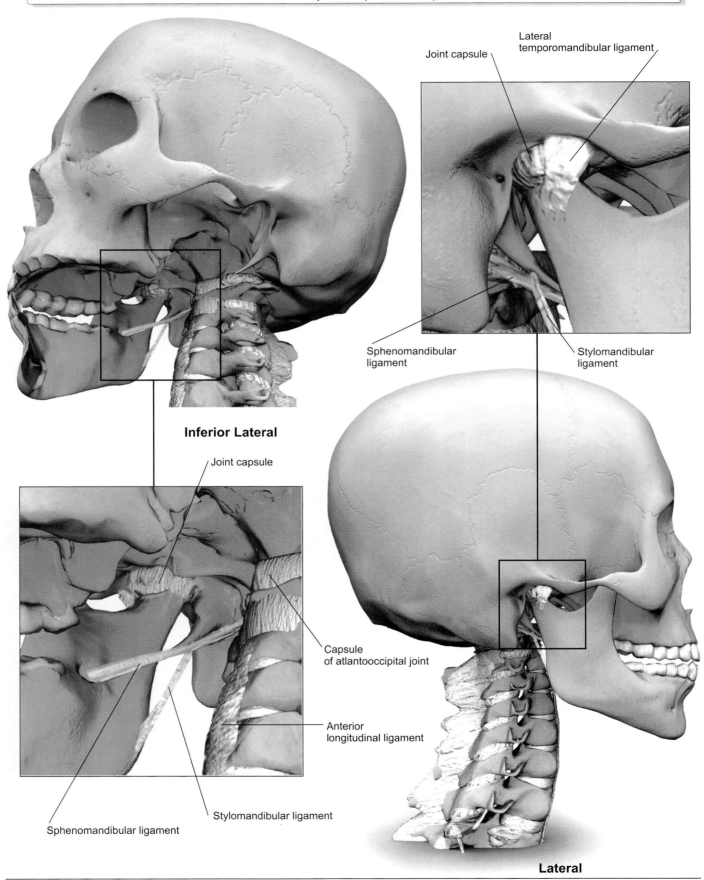

Joint capsule

Lateral
temporomandibular ligament

Sphenomandibular
ligament

Stylomandibular
ligament

Inferior Lateral

Joint capsule

Capsule
of atlantooccipital joint

Anterior
longitudinal ligament

Stylomandibular ligament

Sphenomandibular ligament

Lateral

Unit 2 Ligaments

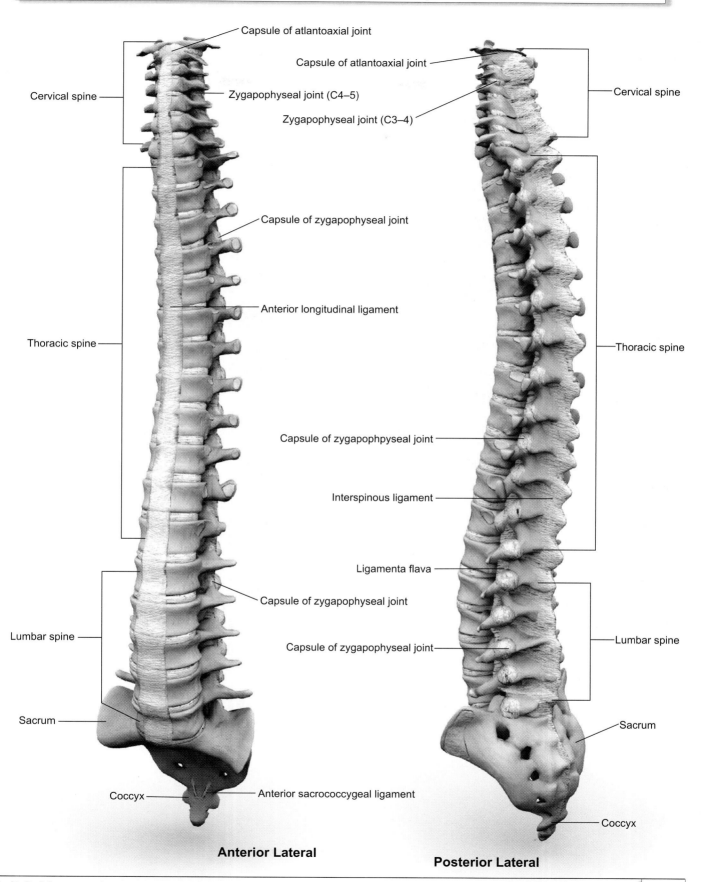

Capsule of atlantoaxial joint

Capsule of atlantoaxial joint

Cervical spine

Zygapophyseal joint (C4–5)

Cervical spine

Zygapophyseal joint (C3–4)

Capsule of zygapophyseal joint

Anterior longitudinal ligament

Thoracic spine

Thoracic spine

Capsule of zygapophpyseal joint

Interspinous ligament

Ligamenta flava

Capsule of zygapophyseal joint

Capsule of zygapophyseal joint

Lumbar spine

Lumbar spine

Sacrum

Sacrum

Coccyx

Anterior sacrococcygeal ligament

Coccyx

Anterior Lateral

Posterior Lateral

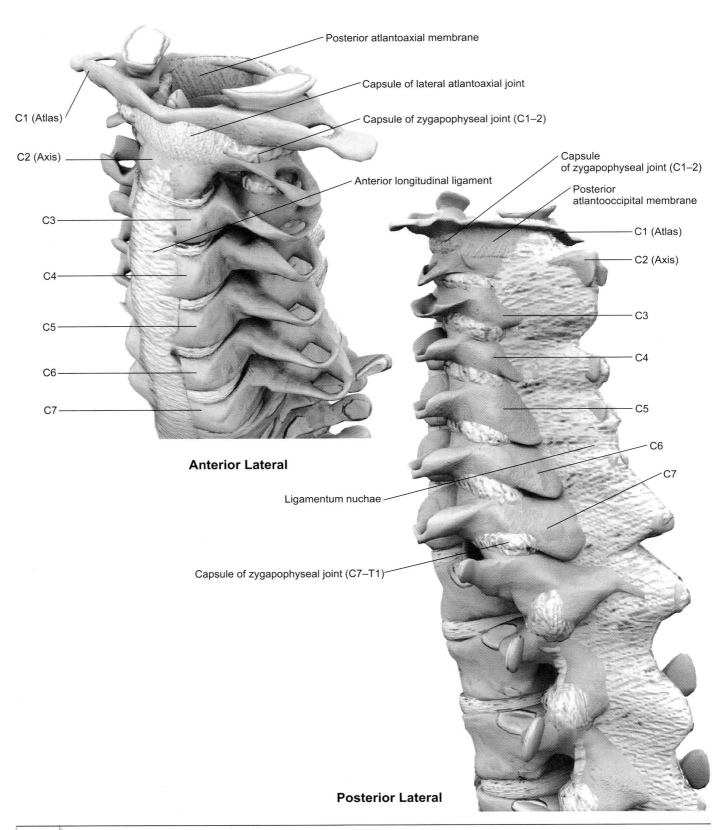

Posterior atlantoaxial membrane

Capsule of lateral atlantoaxial joint

Capsule of zygapophyseal joint (C1–2)

Anterior longitudinal ligament

C1 (Atlas)

C2 (Axis)

C3

C4

C5

C6

C7

Capsule
of zygapophyseal joint (C1–2)

Posterior
atlantooccipital membrane

C1 (Atlas)

C2 (Axis)

C3

C4

C5

C6

C7

Anterior Lateral

Ligamentum nuchae

Capsule of zygapophyseal joint (C7–T1)

Posterior Lateral

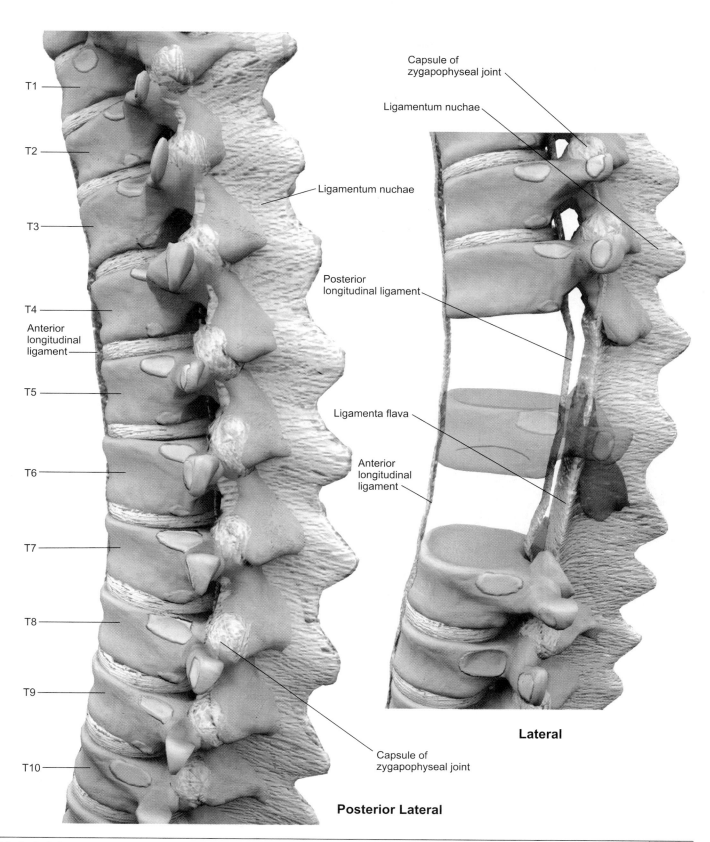

T1

T2

T3

T4

Anterior
longitudinal
ligament

T5

T6

T7

T8

T9

T10

Ligamentum nuchae

Posterior
longitudinal ligament

Capsule of
zygapophyseal joint

Posterior Lateral

Capsule of
zygapophyseal joint

Ligamentum nuchae

Ligamenta flava

Anterior
longitudinal
ligament

Lateral

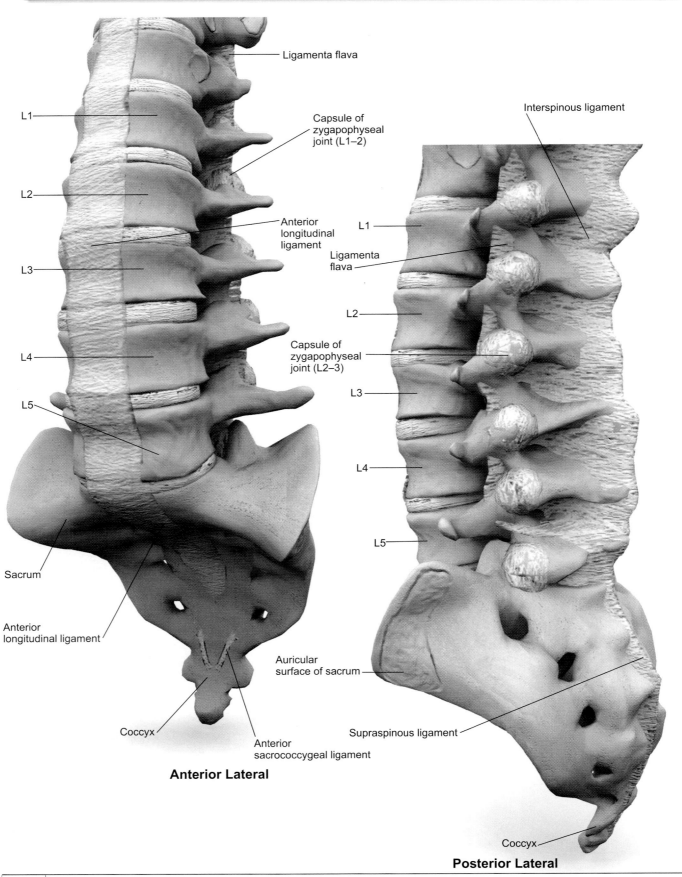

Ligamenta flava

L1

Capsule of
zygapophyseal
joint (L1–2)

L2

Anterior
longitudinal
ligament

L3

L4

L5

Sacrum

Anterior
longitudinal ligament

Coccyx

Anterior
sacrococcygeal ligament

Anterior Lateral

Interspinous ligament

L1

Ligamenta
flava

L2

Capsule of
zygapophyseal
joint (L2–3)

L3

L4

L5

Auricular
surface of sacrum

Supraspinous ligament

Coccyx

Posterior Lateral

Unit 2 Ligaments

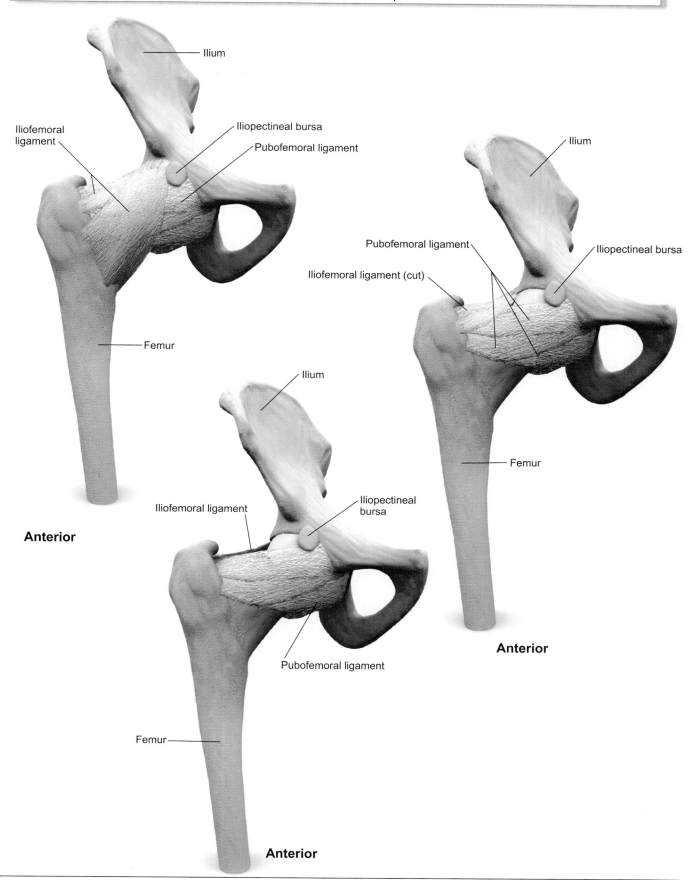

Ilium

Iliofemoral ligament

Iliopectineal bursa

Pubofemoral ligament

Femur

Anterior

Ilium

Pubofemoral ligament

Iliofemoral ligament (cut)

Iliopectineal bursa

Femur

Anterior

Ilium

Iliofemoral ligament

Iliopectineal bursa

Femur

Pubofemoral ligament

Anterior

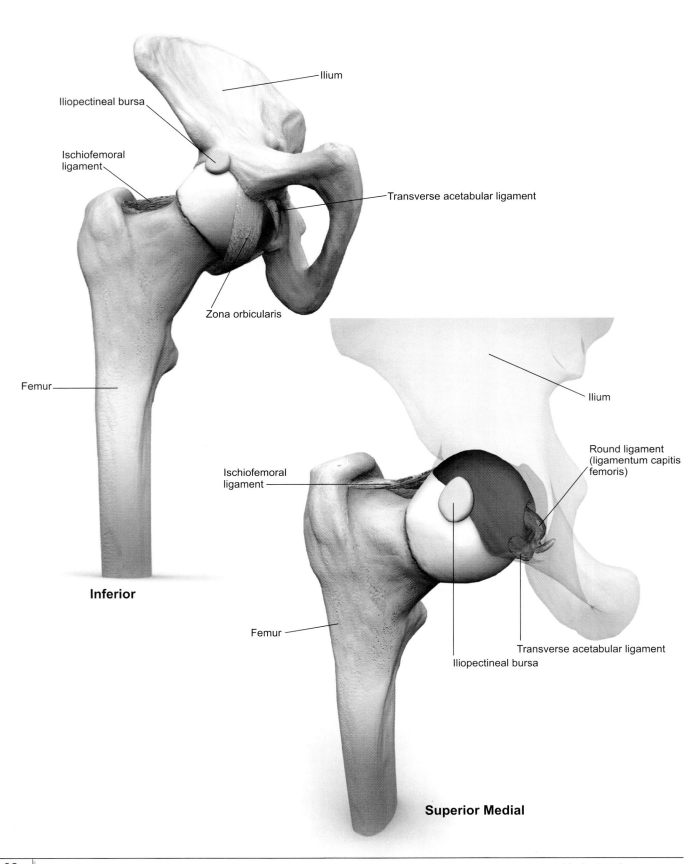

Ilium

Iliopectineal bursa

Ischiofemoral ligament

Transverse acetabular ligament

Zona orbicularis

Femur

Inferior

Ilium

Ischiofemoral ligament

Round ligament (ligamentum capitis femoris)

Femur

Transverse acetabular ligament

Iliopectineal bursa

Superior Medial

Unit 2 Ligaments

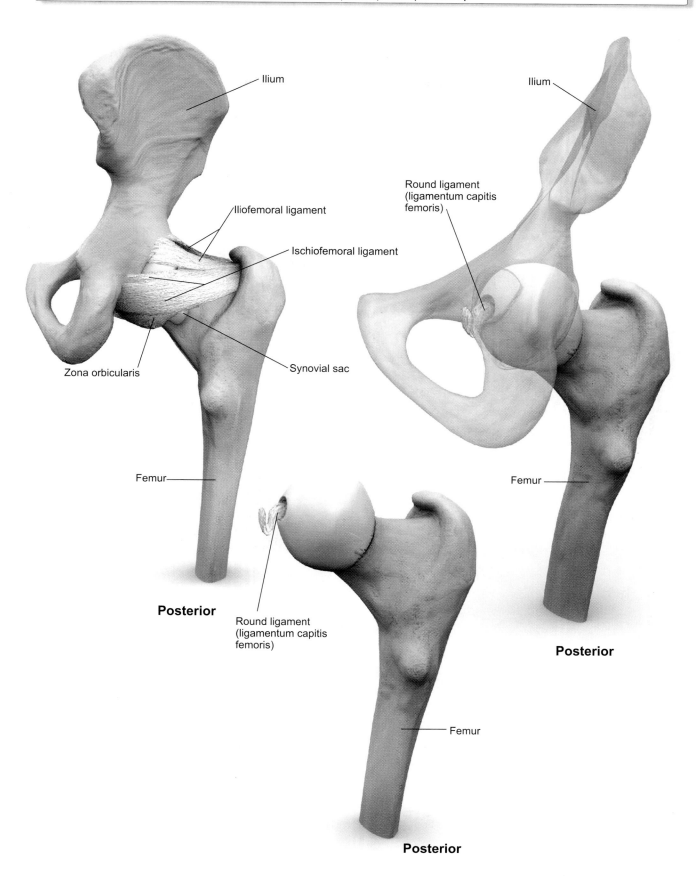

Ilium

Iliofemoral ligament

Ischiofemoral ligament

Zona orbicularis

Synovial sac

Femur

Posterior

Ilium

Round ligament
(ligamentum capitis
femoris)

Femur

Posterior

Round ligament
(ligamentum capitis
femoris)

Femur

Posterior

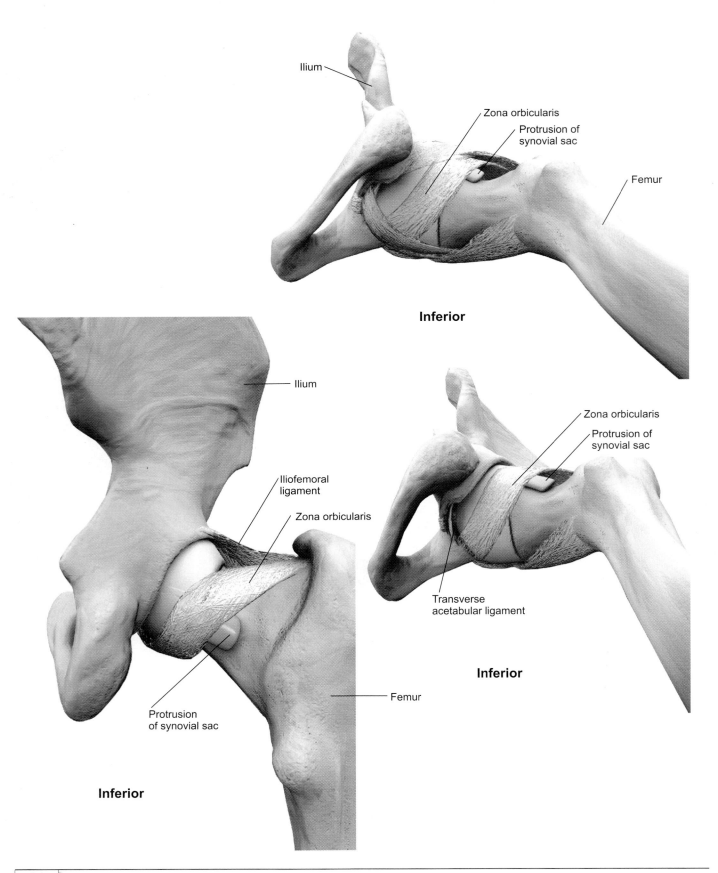

Ilium

Zona orbicularis

Protrusion of
synovial sac

Femur

Inferior

Ilium

Iliofemoral
ligament

Zona orbicularis

Zona orbicularis

Protrusion of
synovial sac

Protrusion
of synovial sac

Femur

Transverse
acetabular ligament

Inferior

Inferior

Femur

Patella

Joint capsule

Medial
collateral ligament

Coronary
ligament

Tibia

Anterior Medial

Femur

Medial
collateral ligament

Transverse ligament of knee

Coronary ligament

Tibia

Medial
meniscus

Anterior Medial

Femur

Posterior
cruciate
ligament

Lateral collateral ligament

Anterior cruciate ligament

Transverse ligament of knee

Coronary ligament

Medial
collateral ligament

Medial
meniscus

Tibia

Anterior Medial

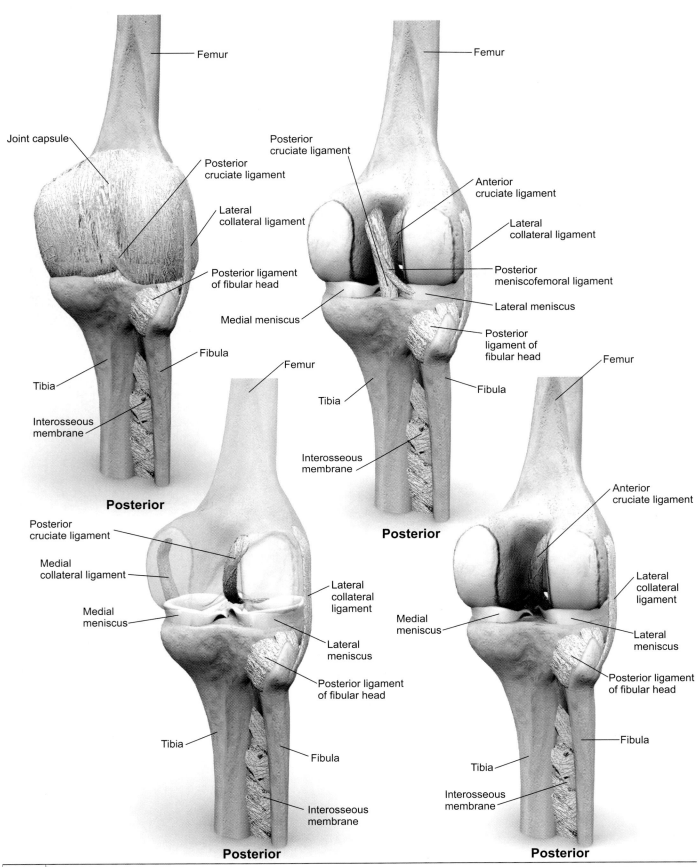

Femur

Joint capsule

Posterior
cruciate ligament

Posterior
cruciate ligament

Lateral
collateral ligament

Posterior ligament
of fibular head

Medial meniscus

Fibula

Tibia

Interosseous
membrane

Posterior

Femur

Anterior
cruciate ligament

Lateral
collateral ligament

Posterior
meniscofemoral ligament

Lateral meniscus

Posterior
ligament of
fibular head

Femur

Fibula

Tibia

Interosseous
membrane

Posterior

Posterior
cruciate ligament

Medial
collateral ligament

Medial
meniscus

Lateral
collateral
ligament

Lateral
meniscus

Posterior ligament
of fibular head

Tibia

Fibula

Interosseous
membrane

Posterior

Anterior
cruciate ligament

Lateral
collateral
ligament

Medial
meniscus

Lateral
meniscus

Posterior ligament
of fibular head

Fibula

Tibia

Interosseous
membrane

Posterior

Unit 2 Ligaments

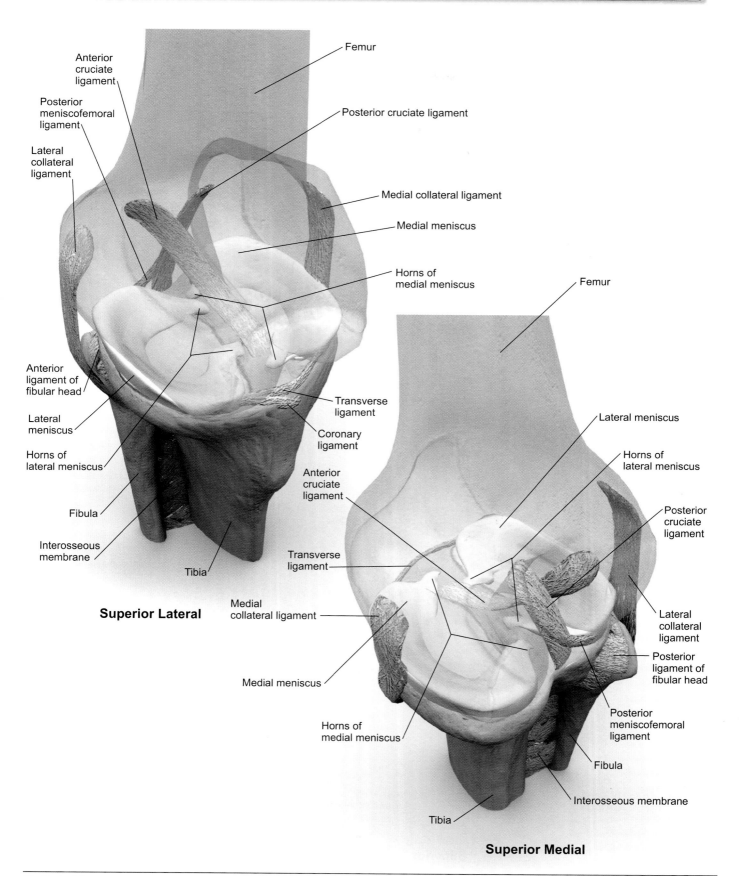

Anterior cruciate ligament

Posterior meniscofemoral ligament

Lateral collateral ligament

Femur

Posterior cruciate ligament

Medial collateral ligament

Medial meniscus

Horns of medial meniscus

Anterior ligament of fibular head

Lateral meniscus

Horns of lateral meniscus

Fibula

Interosseous membrane

Transverse ligament

Coronary ligament

Anterior cruciate ligament

Tibia

Superior Lateral

Medial collateral ligament

Medial meniscus

Transverse ligament

Horns of medial meniscus

Femur

Lateral meniscus

Horns of lateral meniscus

Posterior cruciate ligament

Lateral collateral ligament

Posterior ligament of fibular head

Posterior meniscofemoral ligament

Fibula

Interosseous membrane

Tibia

Superior Medial

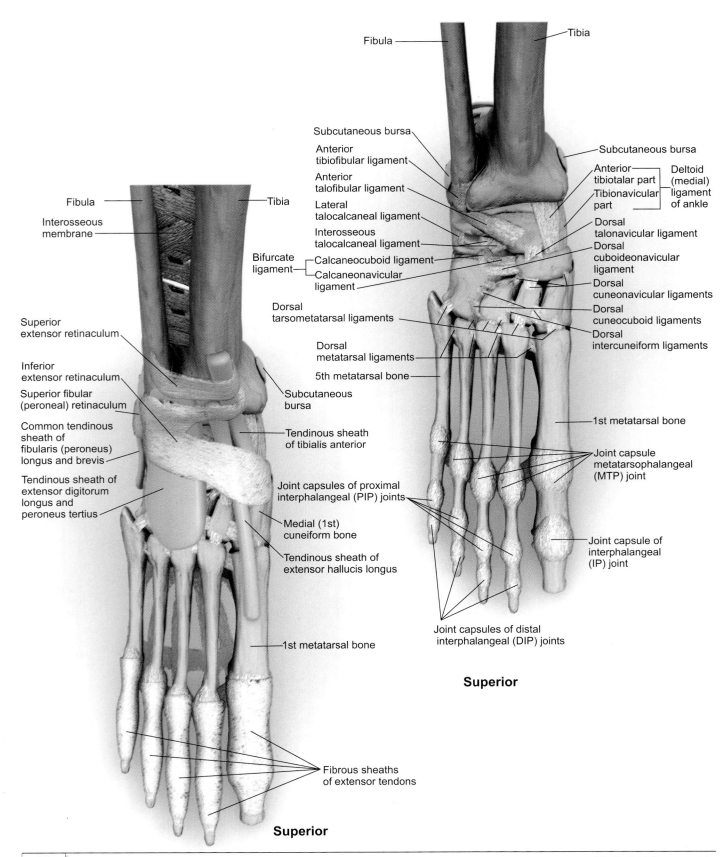

Fibula

Tibia

Subcutaneous bursa

Anterior tibiofibular ligament

Anterior talofibular ligament

Lateral talocalcaneal ligament

Interosseous talocalcaneal ligament

Bifurcate ligament
Calcaneocuboid ligament
Calcaneonavicular ligament

Dorsal tarsometatarsal ligaments

Dorsal metatarsal ligaments

5th metatarsal bone

Subcutaneous bursa

Anterior tibiotalar part
Tibionavicular part
Deltoid (medial) ligament of ankle

Dorsal talonavicular ligament

Dorsal cuboideonavicular ligament

Dorsal cuneonavicular ligaments

Dorsal cuneocuboid ligaments

Dorsal intercuneiform ligaments

1st metatarsal bone

Joint capsule metatarsophalangeal (MTP) joint

Joint capsule of interphalangeal (IP) joint

Joint capsules of distal interphalangeal (DIP) joints

Superior

Fibula

Tibia

Interosseous membrane

Superior extensor retinaculum

Inferior extensor retinaculum

Superior fibular (peroneal) retinaculum

Common tendinous sheath of fibularis (peroneus) longus and brevis

Tendinous sheath of extensor digitorum longus and peroneus tertius

Subcutaneous bursa

Tendinous sheath of tibialis anterior

Joint capsules of proximal interphalangeal (PIP) joints

Medial (1st) cuneiform bone

Tendinous sheath of extensor hallucis longus

1st metatarsal bone

Fibrous sheaths of extensor tendons

Superior

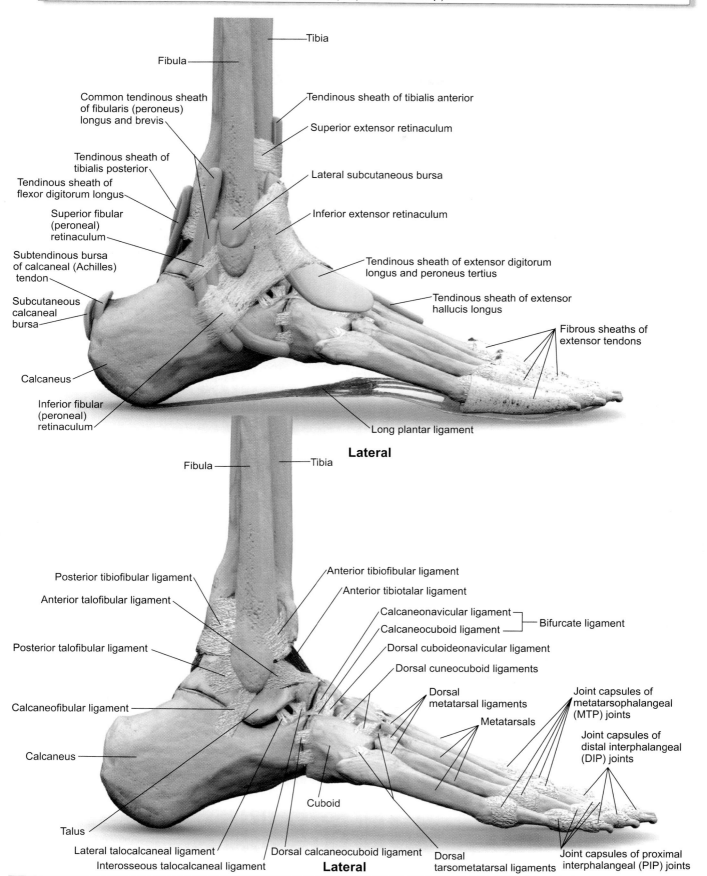

Tibia

Fibula

Common tendinous sheath of fibularis (peroneus) longus and brevis

Tendinous sheath of tibialis posterior

Tendinous sheath of flexor digitorum longus

Superior fibular (peroneal) retinaculum

Subtendinous bursa of calcaneal (Achilles) tendon

Subcutaneous calcaneal bursa

Calcaneus

Inferior fibular (peroneal) retinaculum

Tendinous sheath of tibialis anterior

Superior extensor retinaculum

Lateral subcutaneous bursa

Inferior extensor retinaculum

Tendinous sheath of extensor digitorum longus and peroneus tertius

Tendinous sheath of extensor hallucis longus

Fibrous sheaths of extensor tendons

Long plantar ligament

Lateral

Fibula

Tibia

Posterior tibiofibular ligament

Anterior talofibular ligament

Posterior talofibular ligament

Calcaneofibular ligament

Calcaneus

Talus

Lateral talocalcaneal ligament

Interosseous talocalcaneal ligament

Anterior tibiofibular ligament

Anterior tibiotalar ligament

Calcaneonavicular ligament

Calcaneocuboid ligament

Bifurcate ligament

Dorsal cuboideonavicular ligament

Dorsal cuneocuboid ligaments

Dorsal metatarsal ligaments

Metatarsals

Joint capsules of metatarsophalangeal (MTP) joints

Joint capsules of distal interphalangeal (DIP) joints

Cuboid

Dorsal calcaneocuboid ligament

Dorsal tarsometatarsal ligaments

Joint capsules of proximal interphalangeal (PIP) joints

Lateral

Unit 2 Ligaments

89

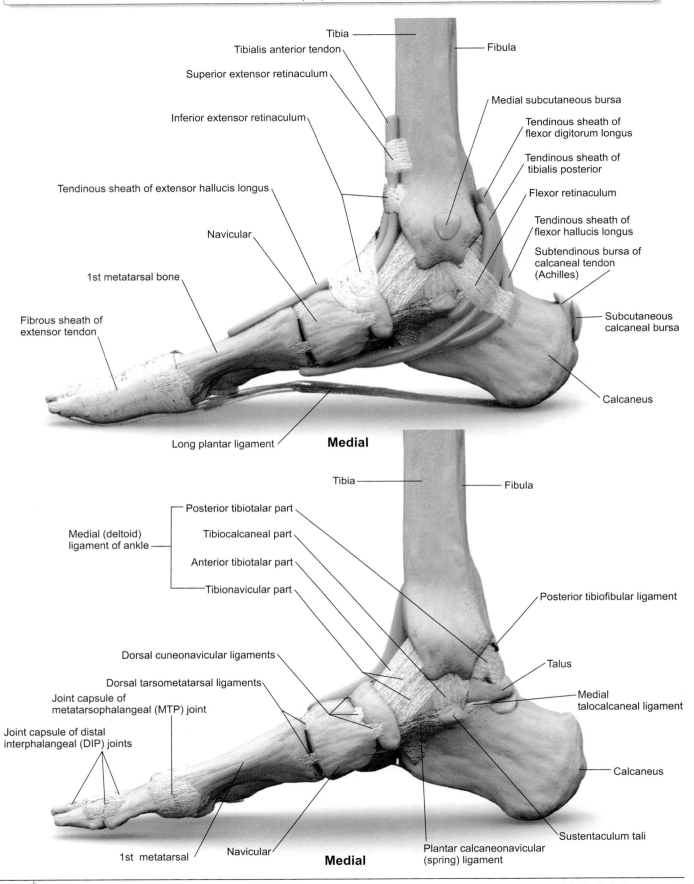

Tibia

Tibialis anterior tendon

Superior extensor retinaculum

Inferior extensor retinaculum

Tendinous sheath of extensor hallucis longus

Navicular

1st metatarsal bone

Fibrous sheath of extensor tendon

Long plantar ligament

Medial

Fibula

Medial subcutaneous bursa

Tendinous sheath of flexor digitorum longus

Tendinous sheath of tibialis posterior

Flexor retinaculum

Tendinous sheath of flexor hallucis longus

Subtendinous bursa of calcaneal tendon (Achilles)

Subcutaneous calcaneal bursa

Calcaneus

Tibia

Fibula

Posterior tibiotalar part

Tibiocalcaneal part

Medial (deltoid) ligament of ankle

Anterior tibiotalar part

Tibionavicular part

Dorsal cuneonavicular ligaments

Dorsal tarsometatarsal ligaments

Joint capsule of metatarsophalangeal (MTP) joint

Joint capsule of distal interphalangeal (DIP) joints

Posterior tibiofibular ligament

Talus

Medial talocalcaneal ligament

Calcaneus

Sustentaculum tali

1st metatarsal

Navicular

Medial

Plantar calcaneonavicular (spring) ligament

Unit 2 Ligaments

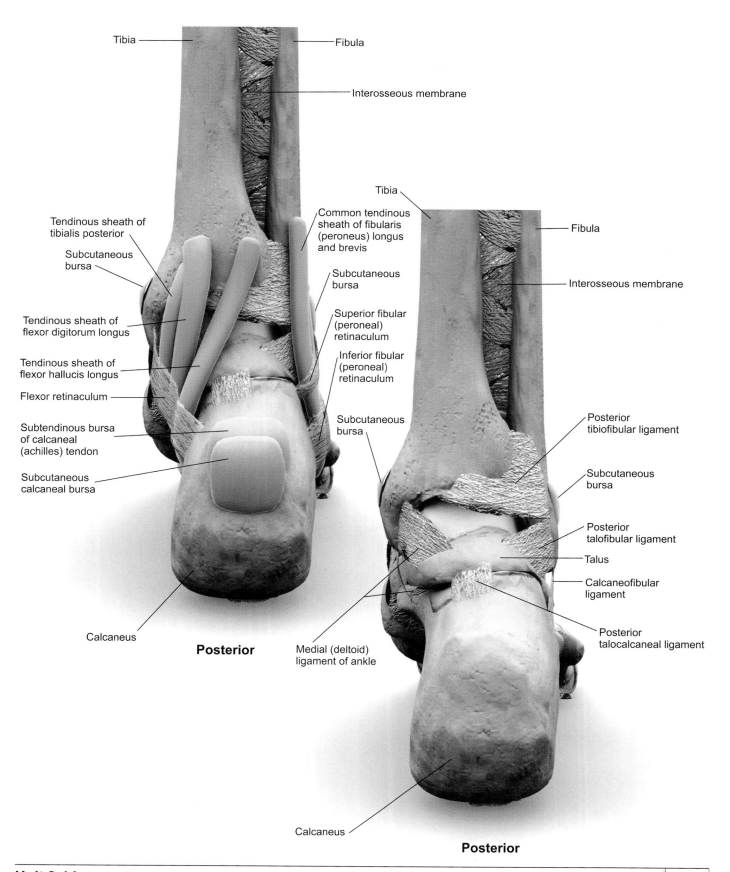

Tibia

Fibula

Interosseous membrane

Tibia

Common tendinous sheath of fibularis (peroneus) longus and brevis

Fibula

Tendinous sheath of tibialis posterior

Interosseous membrane

Subcutaneous bursa

Subcutaneous bursa

Tendinous sheath of flexor digitorum longus

Superior fibular (peroneal) retinaculum

Tendinous sheath of flexor hallucis longus

Inferior fibular (peroneal) retinaculum

Flexor retinaculum

Posterior tibiofibular ligament

Subcutaneous bursa

Subtendinous bursa of calcaneal (achilles) tendon

Subcutaneous bursa

Subcutaneous calcaneal bursa

Posterior talofibular ligament

Talus

Calcaneofibular ligament

Posterior talocalcaneal ligament

Calcaneus

Posterior

Medial (deltoid) ligament of ankle

Calcaneus

Posterior

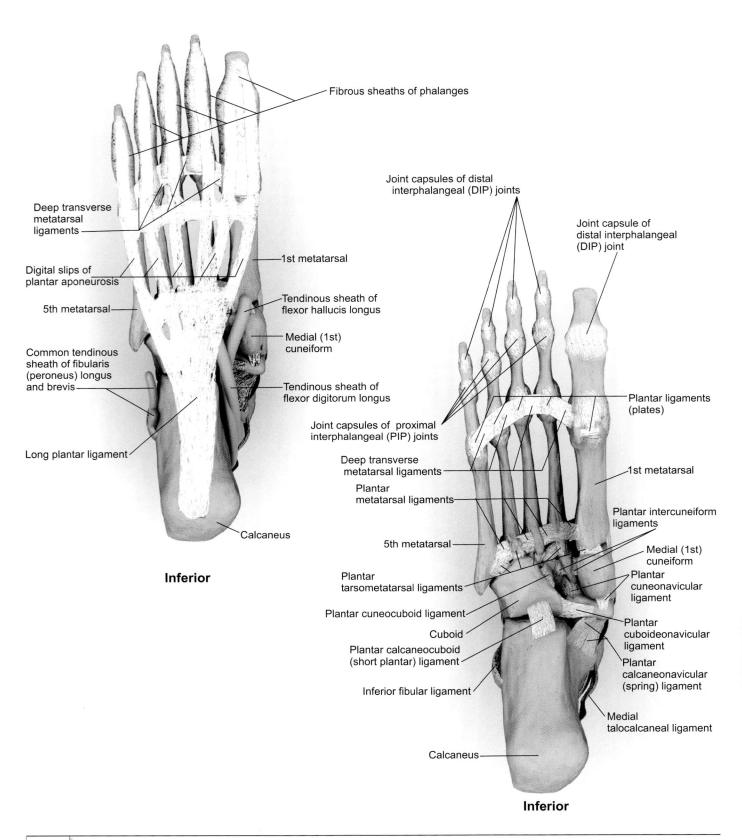

Fibrous sheaths of phalanges

Deep transverse metatarsal ligaments

Digital slips of plantar aponeurosis

5th metatarsal

Common tendinous sheath of fibularis (peroneus) longus and brevis

Long plantar ligament

1st metatarsal

Tendinous sheath of flexor hallucis longus

Medial (1st) cuneiform

Tendinous sheath of flexor digitorum longus

Calcaneus

Inferior

Joint capsules of distal interphalangeal (DIP) joints

Joint capsule of distal interphalangeal (DIP) joint

Plantar ligaments (plates)

1st metatarsal

Plantar intercuneiform ligaments

Medial (1st) cuneiform

Plantar cuneonavicular ligament

Plantar cuboideonavicular ligament

Plantar calcaneonavicular (spring) ligament

Medial talocalcaneal ligament

Joint capsules of proximal interphalangeal (PIP) joints

Deep transverse metatarsal ligaments

Plantar metatarsal ligaments

5th metatarsal

Plantar tarsometatarsal ligaments

Plantar cuneocuboid ligament

Cuboid

Plantar calcaneocuboid (short plantar) ligament

Inferior fibular ligament

Calcaneus

Inferior

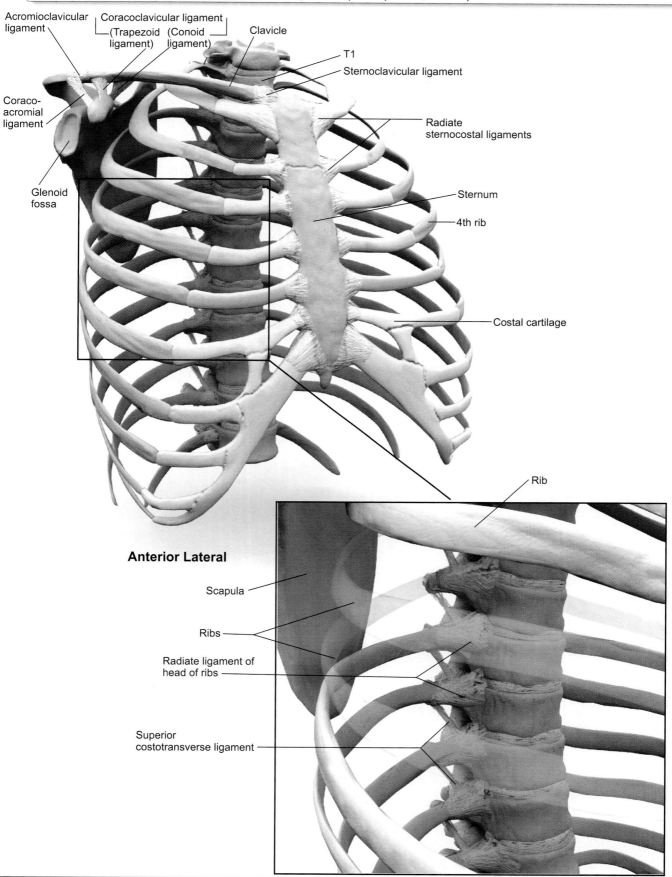

Acromioclavicular ligament

Coracoclavicular ligament
(Trapezoid ligament) (Conoid ligament)

Clavicle

T1

Sternoclavicular ligament

Coraco-acromial ligament

Radiate sternocostal ligaments

Glenoid fossa

Sternum

4th rib

Costal cartilage

Rib

Anterior Lateral

Scapula

Ribs

Radiate ligament of head of ribs

Superior costotransverse ligament

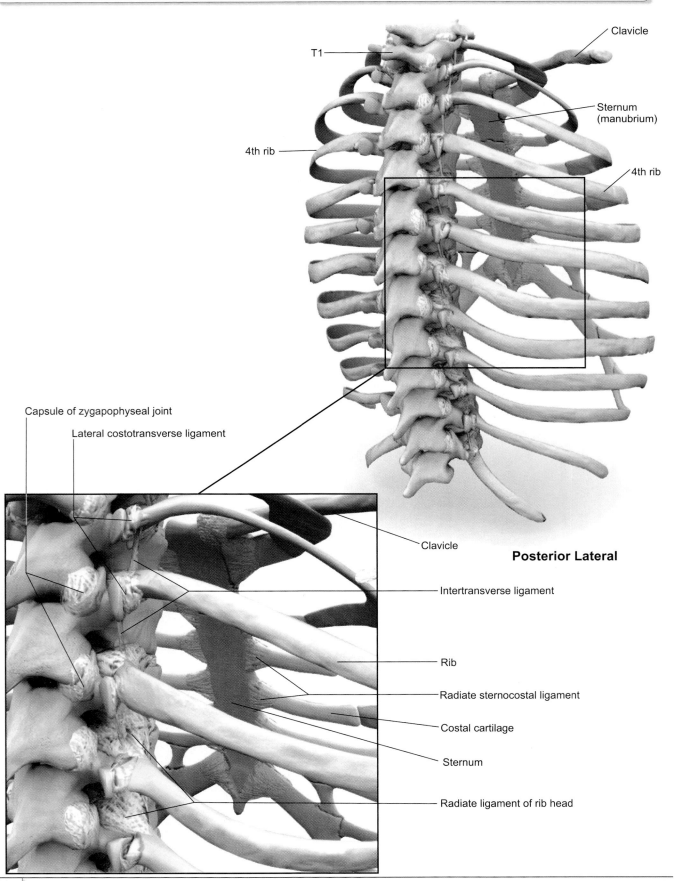

T1

Clavicle

Sternum
(manubrium)

4th rib

4th rib

Capsule of zygapophyseal joint

Lateral costotransverse ligament

Clavicle

Posterior Lateral

Intertransverse ligament

Rib

Radiate sternocostal ligament

Costal cartilage

Sternum

Radiate ligament of rib head

Unit 2 Ligaments

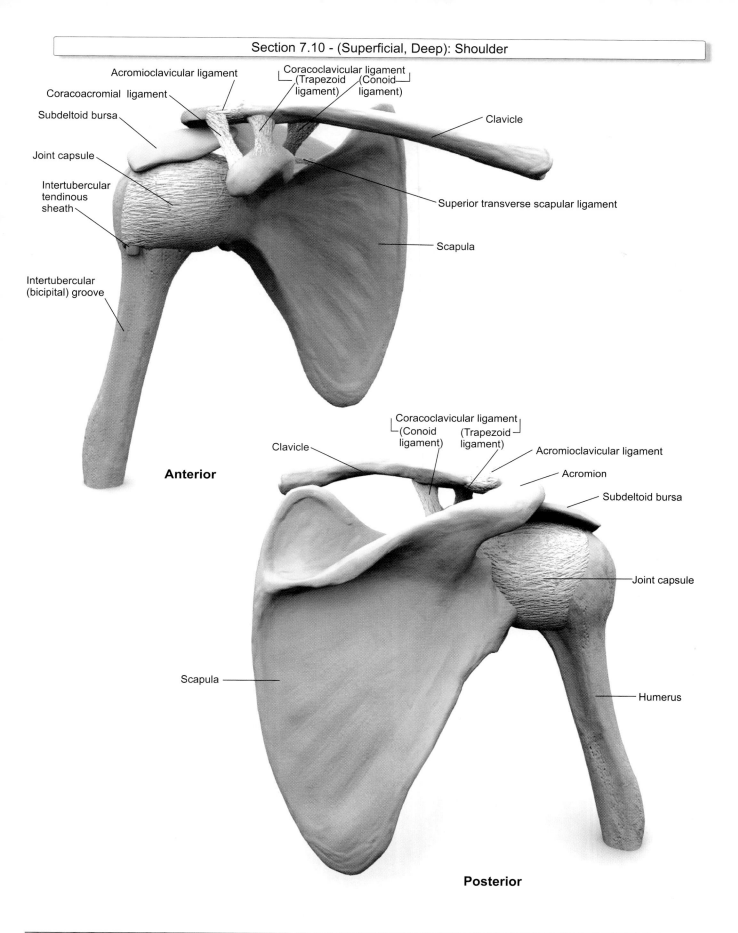

Acromioclavicular ligament

Coracoacromial ligament

Coracoclavicular ligament
(Trapezoid ligament) (Conoid ligament)

Subdeltoid bursa

Clavicle

Joint capsule

Intertubercular tendinous sheath

Superior transverse scapular ligament

Scapula

Intertubercular (bicipital) groove

Anterior

Coracoclavicular ligament
(Conoid ligament) (Trapezoid ligament)

Clavicle

Acromioclavicular ligament

Acromion

Subdeltoid bursa

Joint capsule

Scapula

Humerus

Posterior

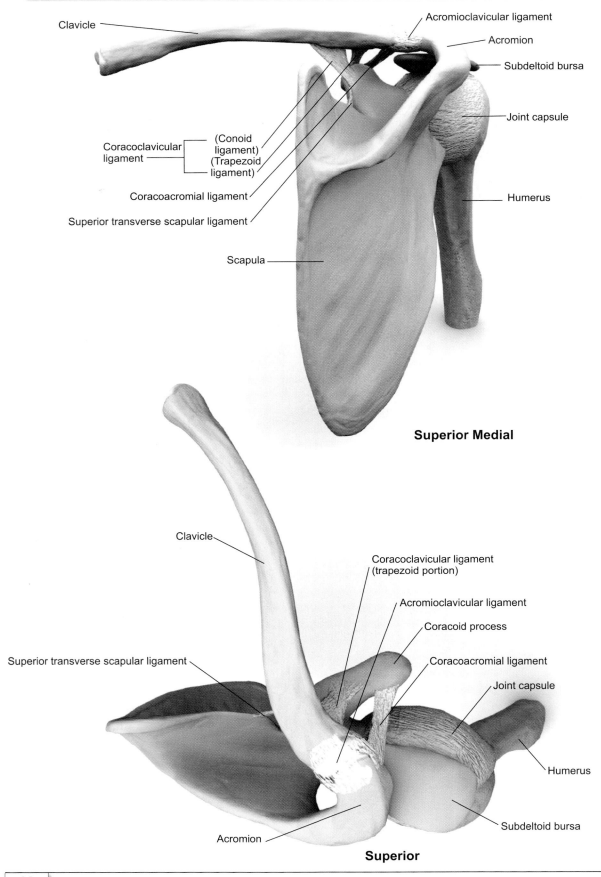

Clavicle

Acromioclavicular ligament

Acromion

Subdeltoid bursa

Joint capsule

Coracoclavicular ligament

(Conoid ligament)

(Trapezoid ligament)

Coracoacromial ligament

Superior transverse scapular ligament

Humerus

Scapula

Superior Medial

Clavicle

Coracoclavicular ligament (trapezoid portion)

Acromioclavicular ligament

Coracoid process

Coracoacromial ligament

Joint capsule

Superior transverse scapular ligament

Humerus

Subdeltoid bursa

Acromion

Superior

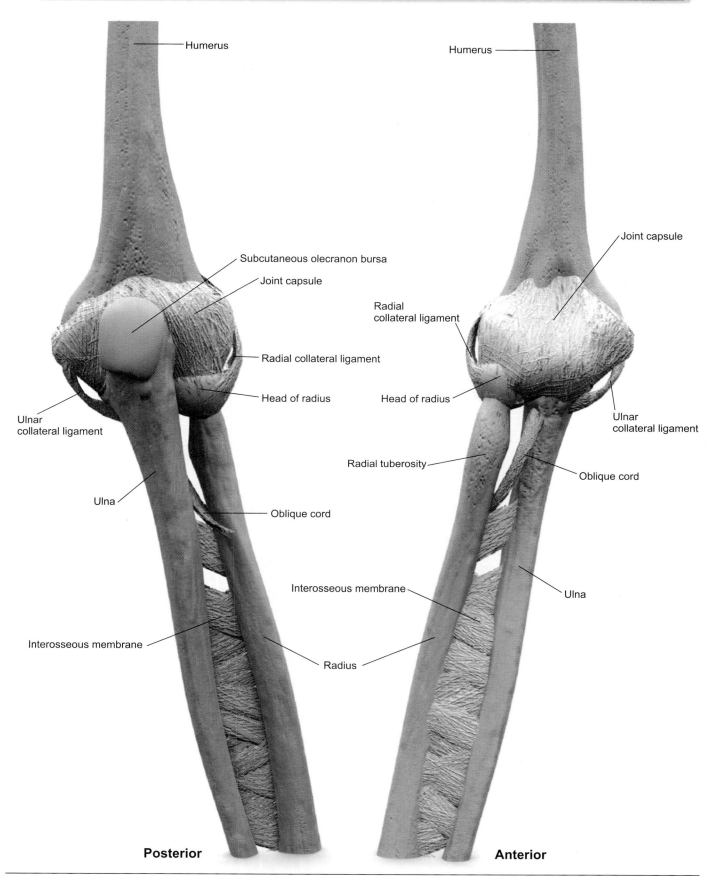

Posterior

Anterior

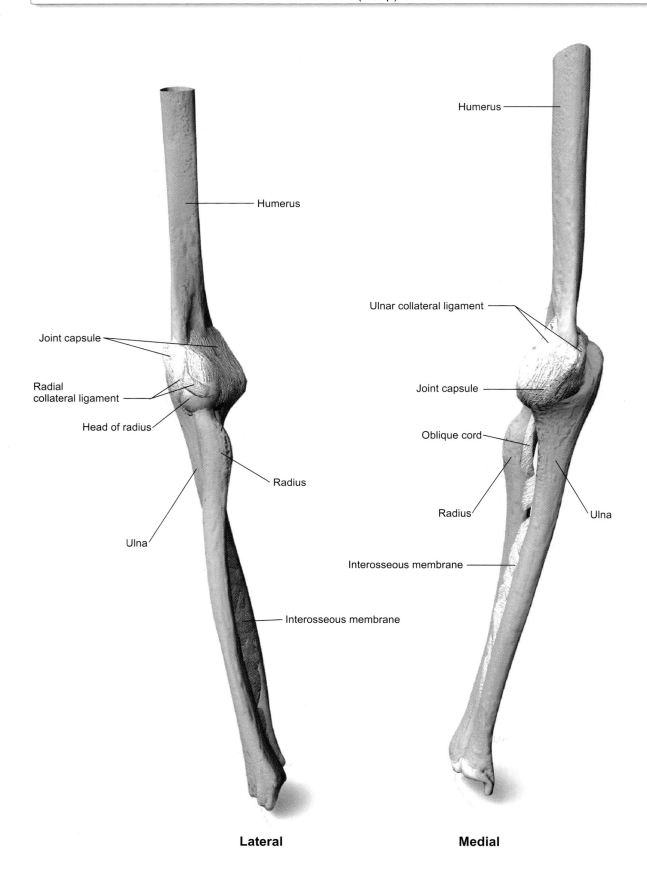

Humerus

Joint capsule

Radial
collateral ligament

Head of radius

Radius

Ulna

Interosseous membrane

Lateral

Humerus

Ulnar collateral ligament

Joint capsule

Oblique cord

Radius

Ulna

Interosseous membrane

Medial

Unit 2 Ligaments

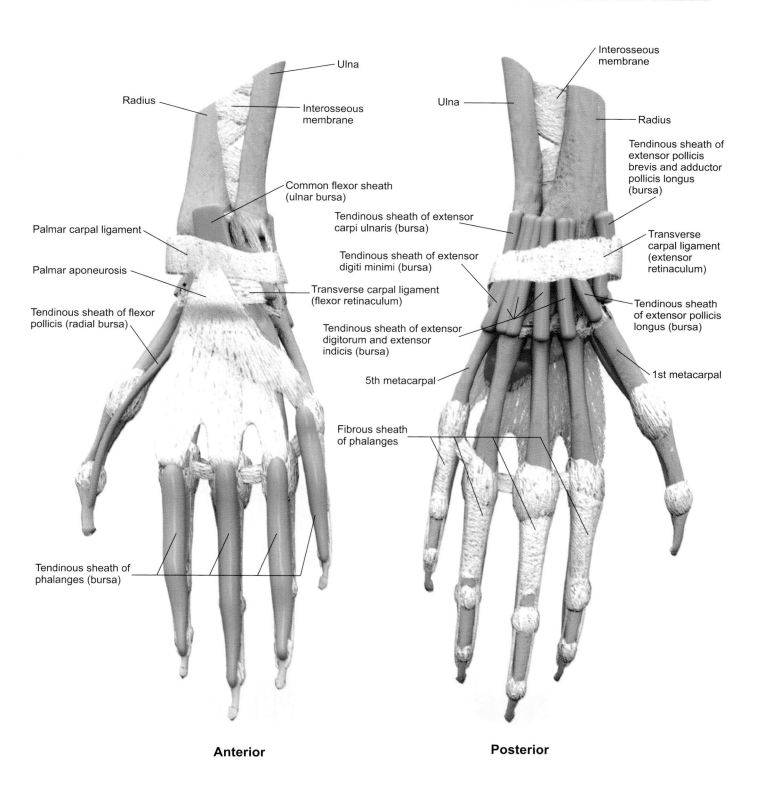

Ulna

Radius

Interosseous
membrane

Common flexor sheath
(ulnar bursa)

Palmar carpal ligament

Palmar aponeurosis

Tendinous sheath of flexor
pollicis (radial bursa)

Tendinous sheath of
phalanges (bursa)

Anterior

Interosseous
membrane

Ulna

Radius

Tendinous sheath of
extensor pollicis
brevis and adductor
pollicis longus
(bursa)

Tendinous sheath of extensor
carpi ulnaris (bursa)

Tendinous sheath of extensor
digiti minimi (bursa)

Transverse carpal ligament
(flexor retinaculum)

Transverse
carpal ligament
(extensor
retinaculum)

Tendinous sheath of extensor
digitorum and extensor
indicis (bursa)

Tendinous sheath
of extensor pollicis
longus (bursa)

5th metacarpal

1st metacarpal

Fibrous sheath
of phalanges

Posterior

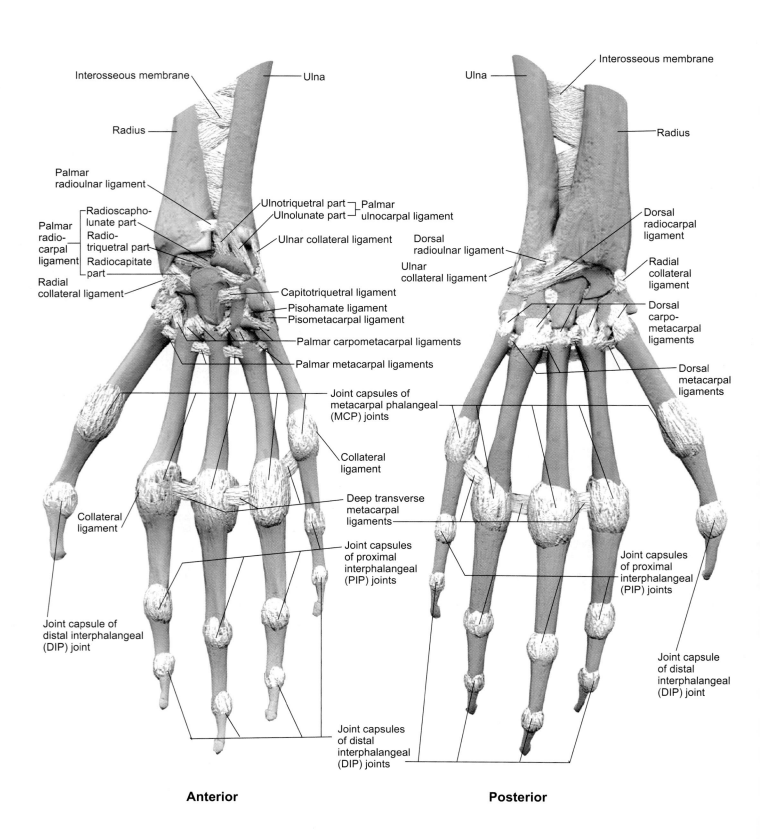

Interosseous membrane

Ulna

Radius

Palmar radioulnar ligament

Radioscapho-lunate part
Radio-triquetral part
Radiocapitate part

Palmar radio-carpal ligament

Radial collateral ligament

Ulnotriquetral part
Ulnolunate part

Palmar ulnocarpal ligament

Ulnar collateral ligament

Capitotriquetral ligament

Pisohamate ligament
Pisometacarpal ligament

Palmar carpometacarpal ligaments

Palmar metacarpal ligaments

Joint capsules of metacarpal phalangeal (MCP) joints

Collateral ligament

Deep transverse metacarpal ligaments

Collateral ligament

Joint capsules of proximal interphalangeal (PIP) joints

Joint capsule of distal interphalangeal (DIP) joint

Joint capsules of distal interphalangeal (DIP) joints

Anterior

Ulna

Interosseous membrane

Radius

Dorsal radioulnar ligament

Ulnar collateral ligament

Dorsal radiocarpal ligament

Radial collateral ligament

Dorsal carpo-metacarpal ligaments

Dorsal metacarpal ligaments

Joint capsules of proximal interphalangeal (PIP) joints

Joint capsule of distal interphalangeal (DIP) joint

Posterior

Unit 2 Ligaments

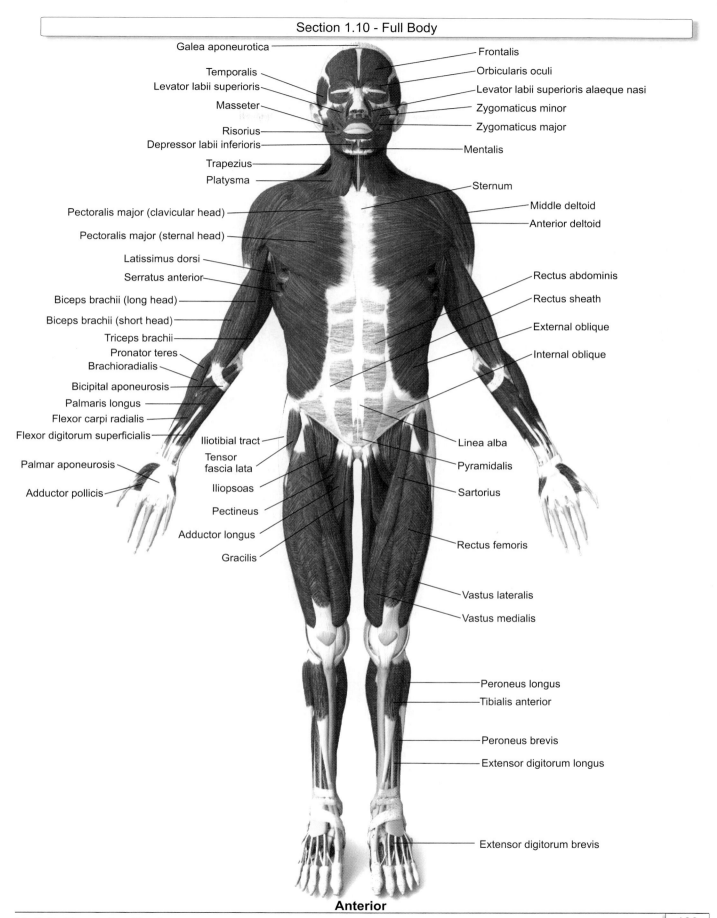

Galea aponeurotica
Temporalis
Levator labii superioris
Masseter
Risorius
Depressor labii inferioris
Trapezius
Platysma
Pectoralis major (clavicular head)
Pectoralis major (sternal head)
Latissimus dorsi
Serratus anterior
Biceps brachii (long head)
Biceps brachii (short head)
Triceps brachii
Pronator teres
Brachioradialis
Bicipital aponeurosis
Palmaris longus
Flexor carpi radialis
Flexor digitorum superficialis
Palmar aponeurosis
Adductor pollicis

Iliotibial tract
Tensor fascia lata
Iliopsoas
Pectineus
Adductor longus
Gracilis

Frontalis
Orbicularis oculi
Levator labii superioris alaeque nasi
Zygomaticus minor
Zygomaticus major
Mentalis
Sternum
Middle deltoid
Anterior deltoid
Rectus abdominis
Rectus sheath
External oblique
Internal oblique

Linea alba
Pyramidalis
Sartorius
Rectus femoris
Vastus lateralis
Vastus medialis
Peroneus longus
Tibialis anterior
Peroneus brevis
Extensor digitorum longus
Extensor digitorum brevis

Anterior

Unit 3 Muscular System

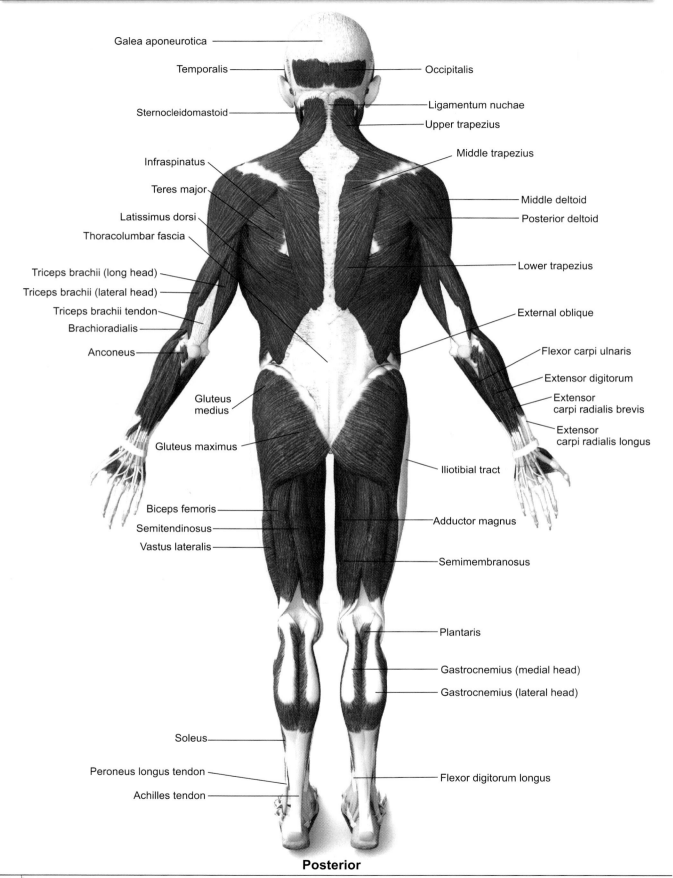

Galea aponeurotica

Temporalis

Occipitalis

Sternocleidomastoid

Ligamentum nuchae

Upper trapezius

Middle trapezius

Infraspinatus

Teres major

Latissimus dorsi

Thoracolumbar fascia

Middle deltoid

Posterior deltoid

Lower trapezius

Triceps brachii (long head)

Triceps brachii (lateral head)

Triceps brachii tendon

Brachioradialis

Anconeus

External oblique

Flexor carpi ulnaris

Extensor digitorum

Extensor
carpi radialis brevis

Extensor
carpi radialis longus

Gluteus
medius

Gluteus maximus

Iliotibial tract

Biceps femoris

Semitendinosus

Vastus lateralis

Adductor magnus

Semimembranosus

Plantaris

Gastrocnemius (medial head)

Gastrocnemius (lateral head)

Soleus

Peroneus longus tendon

Achilles tendon

Flexor digitorum longus

Posterior

Unit 3 Muscular System

Muscles of the head and neck
Section 2

Muscles of the shoulder
Section 6

Muscles of the arm
Section 7

Muscles of the thorax
Section 5

Muscles of the back
Section 3

Muscles of the head and neck
Section 2

Muscles of the shoulder
Section 6

Muscles of the thorax
Section 5

Muscles of the arm
Section 7

Muscles of the head and neck
Section 2

Muscles of the shoulder
Section 6

Muscles of the arm
Section 7

Muscles of the
hip, full leg, foot
Section 4

Muscles of the
hip, full leg, foot
Section 4

Muscles of the back
Section 3

Muscles of the
hip, full leg, foot
Section 4

Anterior Lateral

Lateral

Posterior Lateral

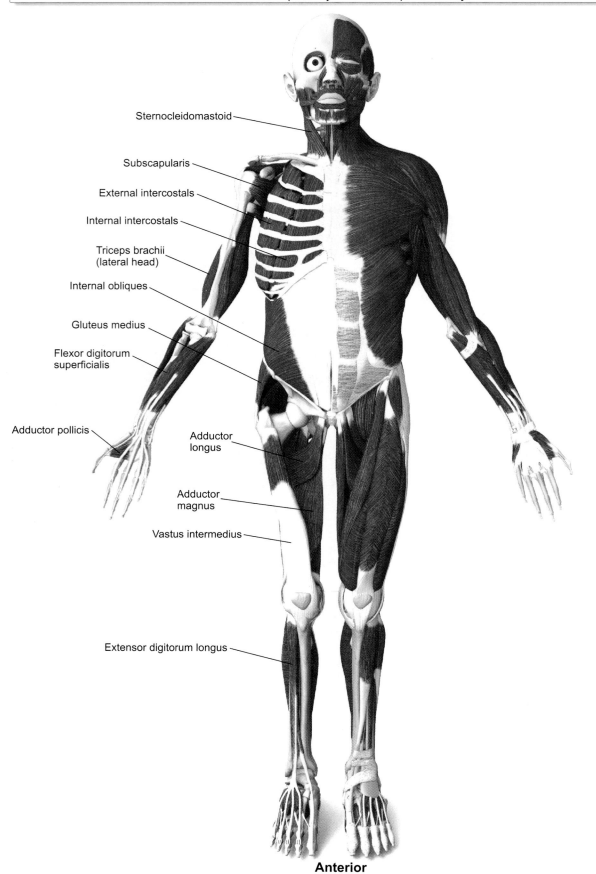

Sternocleidomastoid

Subscapularis

External intercostals

Internal intercostals

Triceps brachii
(lateral head)

Internal obliques

Gluteus medius

Flexor digitorum
superficialis

Adductor pollicis

Adductor
longus

Adductor
magnus

Vastus intermedius

Extensor digitorum longus

Anterior

Unit 3 Muscular System

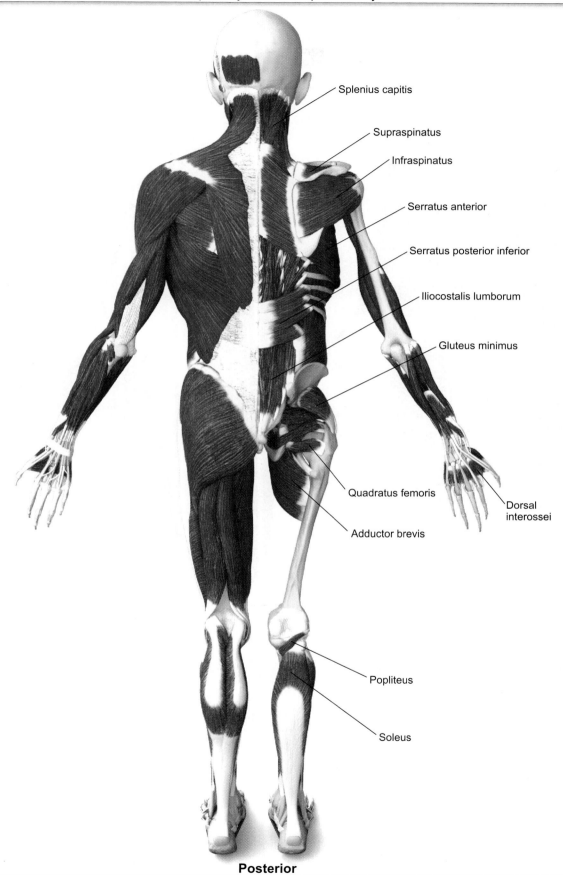

Splenius capitis

Supraspinatus

Infraspinatus

Serratus anterior

Serratus posterior inferior

Iliocostalis lumborum

Gluteus minimus

Quadratus femoris

Adductor brevis

Dorsal interossei

Popliteus

Soleus

Posterior

Unit 3 Muscular System

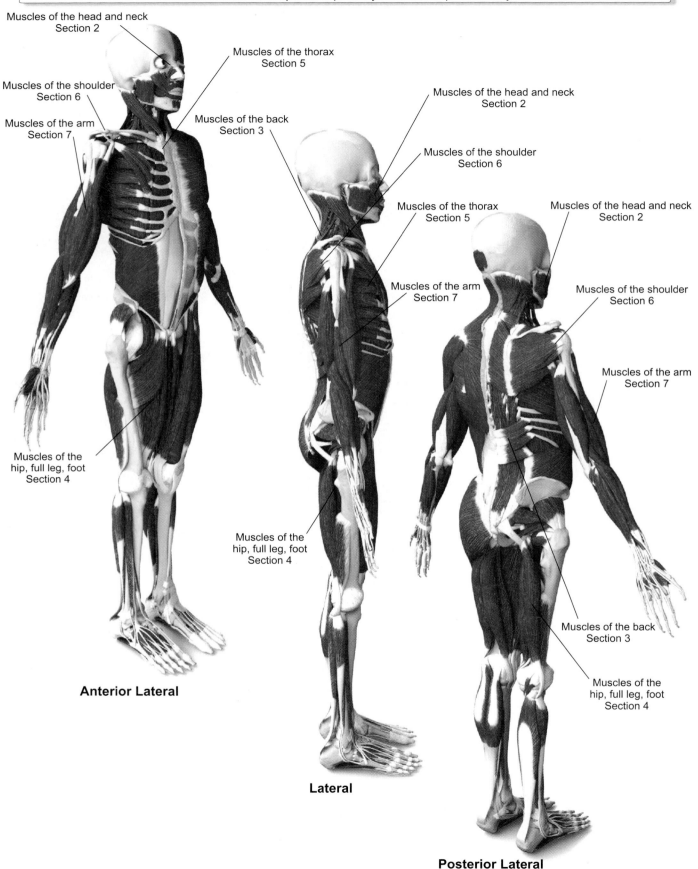

Muscles of the head and neck
Section 2

Muscles of the thorax
Section 5

Muscles of the shoulder
Section 6

Muscles of the back
Section 3

Muscles of the arm
Section 7

Muscles of the head and neck
Section 2

Muscles of the shoulder
Section 6

Muscles of the thorax
Section 5

Muscles of the head and neck
Section 2

Muscles of the arm
Section 7

Muscles of the shoulder
Section 6

Muscles of the arm
Section 7

Muscles of the hip, full leg, foot
Section 4

Muscles of the hip, full leg, foot
Section 4

Muscles of the back
Section 3

Muscles of the hip, full leg, foot
Section 4

Anterior Lateral

Lateral

Posterior Lateral

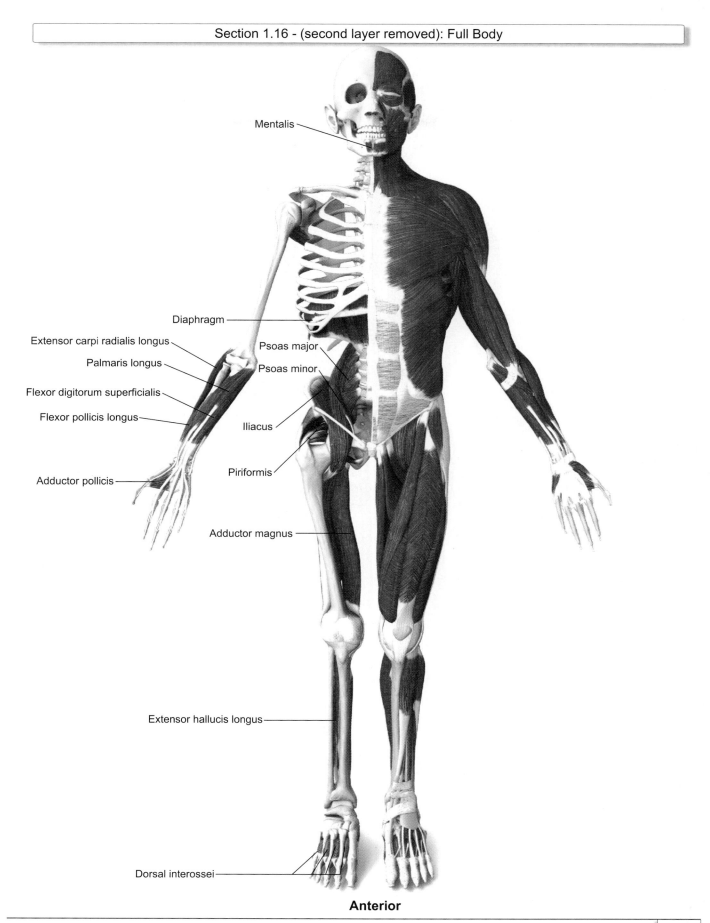

Mentalis

Diaphragm

Extensor carpi radialis longus

Palmaris longus

Flexor digitorum superficialis

Flexor pollicis longus

Psoas major

Psoas minor

Iliacus

Adductor pollicis

Piriformis

Adductor magnus

Extensor hallucis longus

Dorsal interossei

Anterior

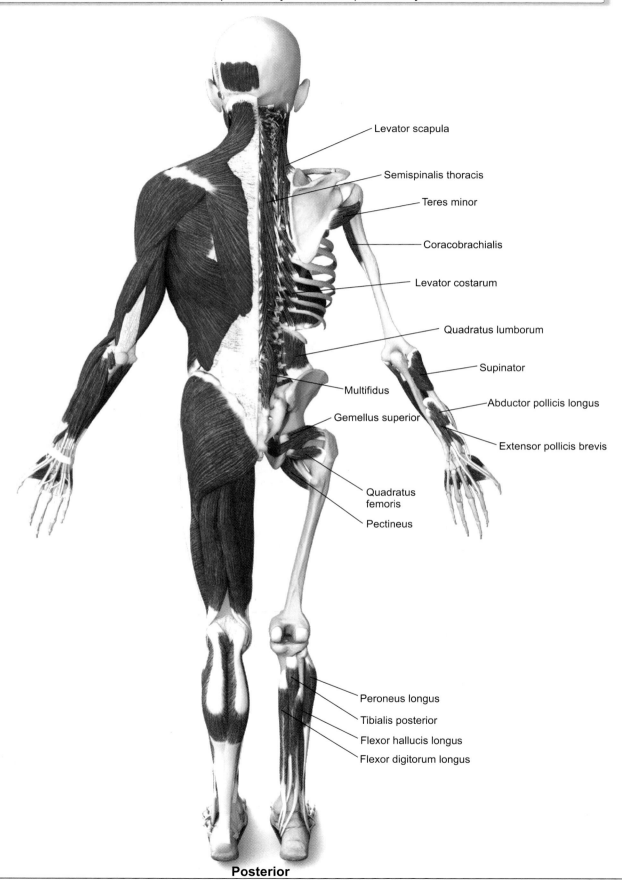

Levator scapula

Semispinalis thoracis

Teres minor

Coracobrachialis

Levator costarum

Quadratus lumborum

Supinator

Abductor pollicis longus

Extensor pollicis brevis

Multifidus

Gemellus superior

Quadratus femoris

Pectineus

Peroneus longus

Tibialis posterior

Flexor hallucis longus

Flexor digitorum longus

Posterior

Unit 3 Muscular System

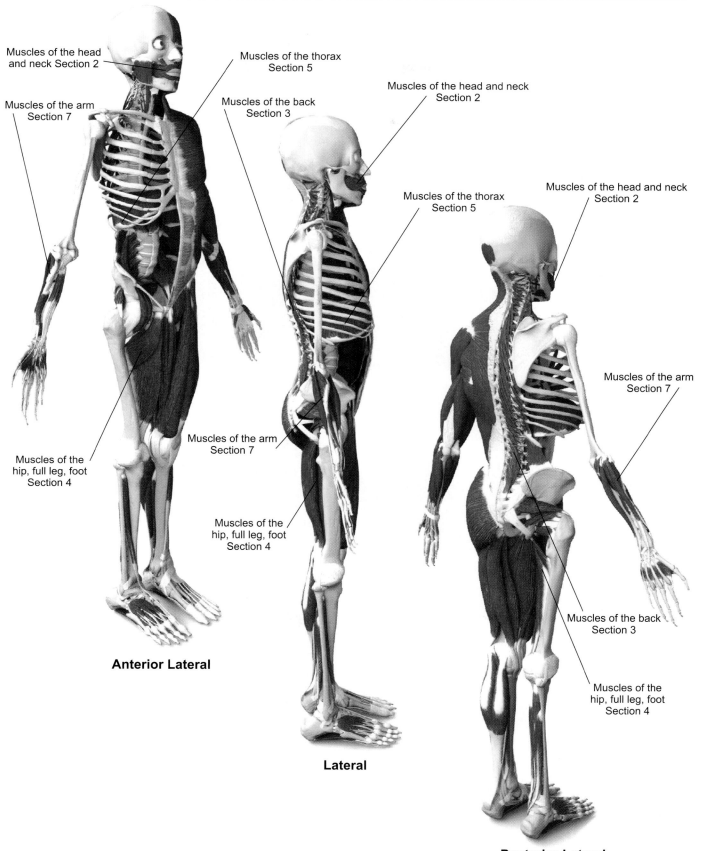

Muscles of the head and neck Section 2

Muscles of the arm Section 7

Muscles of the thorax Section 5

Muscles of the back Section 3

Muscles of the head and neck Section 2

Muscles of the thorax Section 5

Muscles of the head and neck Section 2

Muscles of the hip, full leg, foot Section 4

Muscles of the arm Section 7

Muscles of the arm Section 7

Muscles of the hip, full leg, foot Section 4

Muscles of the back Section 3

Muscles of the hip, full leg, foot Section 4

Anterior Lateral

Lateral

Posterior Lateral

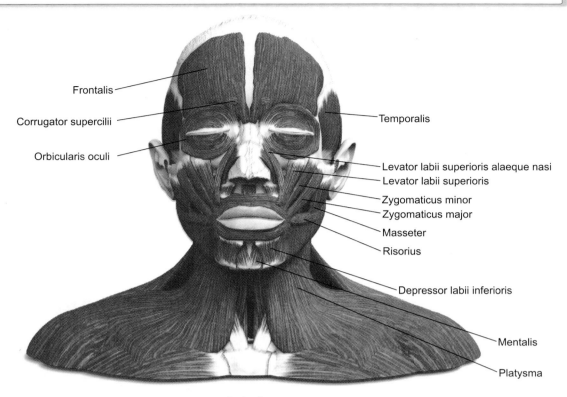

Frontalis

Corrugator supercilii

Orbicularis oculi

Temporalis

Levator labii superioris alaeque nasi
Levator labii superioris
Zygomaticus minor
Zygomaticus major
Masseter
Risorius

Depressor labii inferioris

Mentalis

Platysma

Anterior

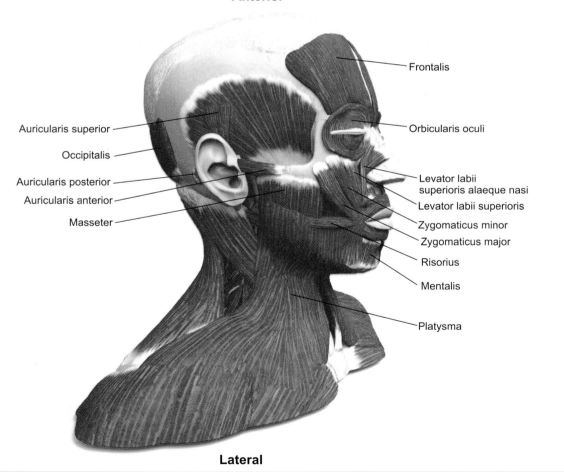

Frontalis

Orbicularis oculi

Auricularis superior

Occipitalis

Auricularis posterior

Auricularis anterior

Masseter

Levator labii
superioris alaeque nasi
Levator labii superioris
Zygomaticus minor
Zygomaticus major
Risorius
Mentalis

Platysma

Lateral

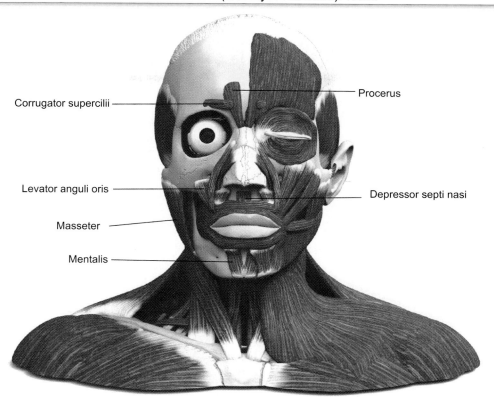

Anterior

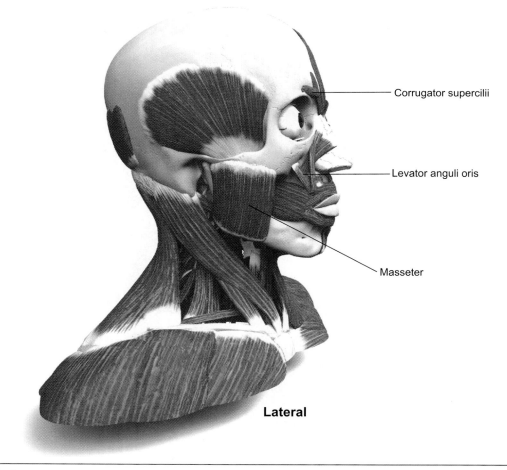

Lateral

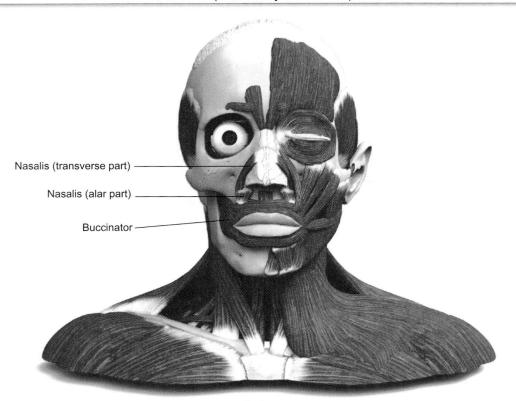

Nasalis (transverse part)

Nasalis (alar part)

Buccinator

Anterior

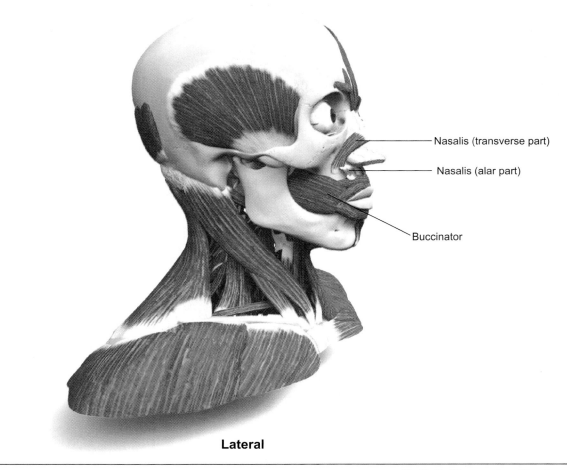

Nasalis (transverse part)

Nasalis (alar part)

Buccinator

Lateral

Unit 3 Muscular System

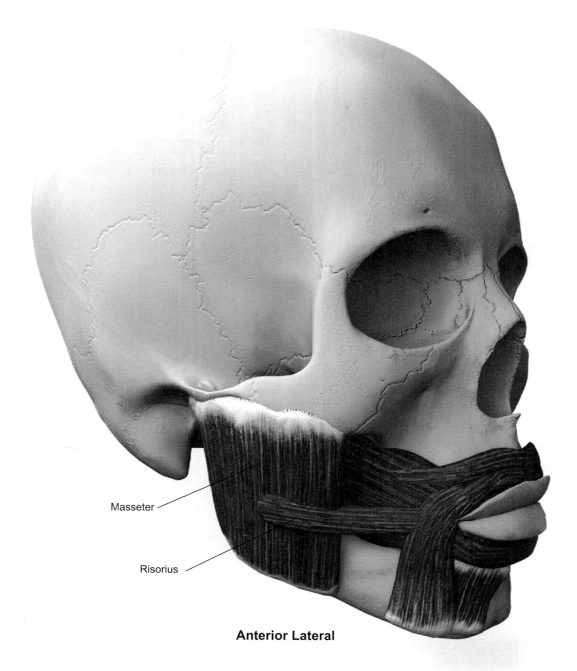

Masseter

Risorius

Anterior Lateral

Masseter

O. Zygomatic process and zygomatic arch of maxilla

I. Angle of mandible, ramus—lateral surface

A. Elevation of mandible, assists protraction of mandible; muscle of mastication

N. Trigeminal nerve (cranial nerve V)

Risorius

O. Lateral fascia of cheek and parotid salivary gland

I. Skin at angle of mouth

A. Retraction of angle of mouth

N. Facial nerve (cranial nerve VII)

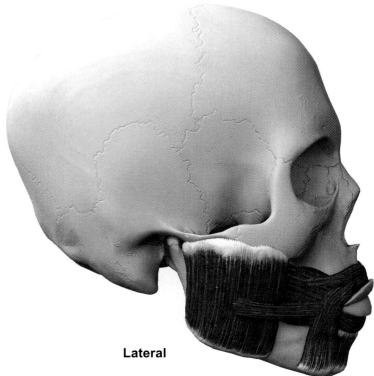

Lateral

Depressor anguli oris

O. Oblique line of mandible

I. Angle of mouth—blending with skin and muscles

A. Draws angle of mouth downward

N. Facial nerve (cranial nerve VII)

Depressor labii inferioris

O. Oblique line of mandible between symphysis and mental foramen

I. Skin of lower lip—blending with fibers of orbicularis oris

A. Draws lower lip downward and laterally

N. Facial nerve (cranial nerve VII)

Depressor anguli oris

Depressor labii inferioris

Anterior

Unit 3 Muscular System

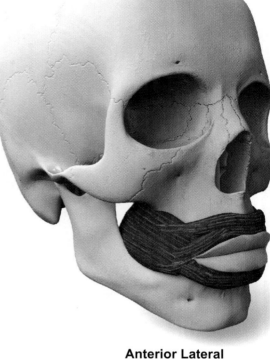

Anterior Lateral

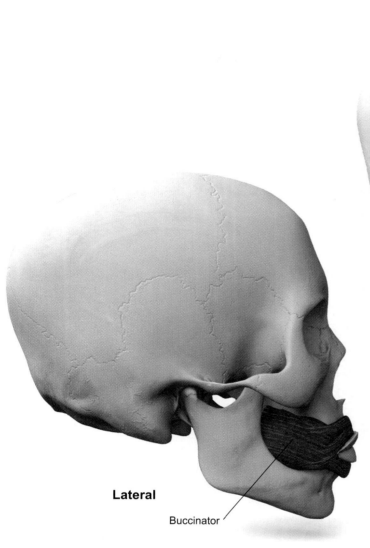

Lateral

Buccinator

Buccinator

O. Alveolar processes of maxilla—external surface, mandible and pterygomandibular raphe

I. Angle of mouth and fibers of orbicularis oris muscle

A. Compression of cheeks, retraction of corners of mouth, assists in mastication

N. Facial nerve (cranial nerve VII)

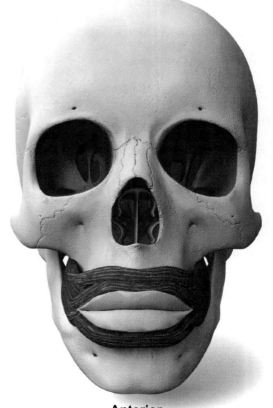

Anterior

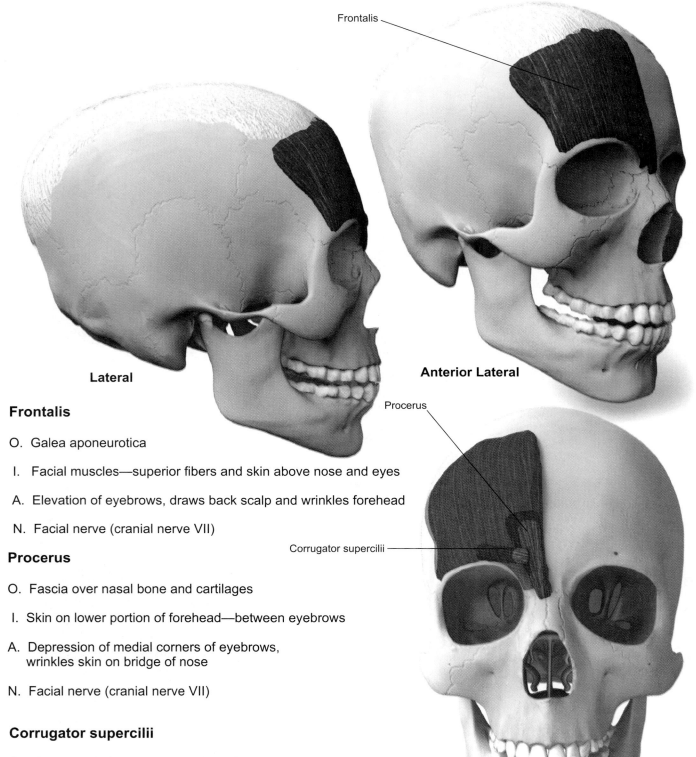

Frontalis

Lateral

Anterior Lateral

Procerus

Corrugator supercilii

Anterior

Frontalis

O. Galea aponeurotica

I. Facial muscles—superior fibers and skin above nose and eyes

A. Elevation of eyebrows, draws back scalp and wrinkles forehead

N. Facial nerve (cranial nerve VII)

Procerus

O. Fascia over nasal bone and cartilages

I. Skin on lower portion of forehead—between eyebrows

A. Depression of medial corners of eyebrows, wrinkles skin on bridge of nose

N. Facial nerve (cranial nerve VII)

Corrugator supercilii

O. Medial end of superciliary arch on frontal bone

I. Surface of skin above middle of orbital arch

A. Draws eyebrows inferiorly and medially

N. Facial nerve (cranial nerve VII)

Unit 3 Muscular System

Levator labii superioris

O. Maxilla—superior to infraorbital foramen

I. Orbicularis oris and skin at angle of mouth

A. Elevation of upper lip

N. Facial nerve (cranial nerve VII)

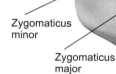

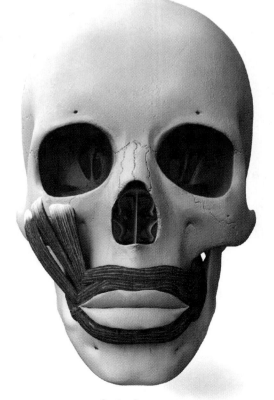

Levator
labii superioris

Zygomaticus
minor

Zygomaticus
major

Anterior Lateral

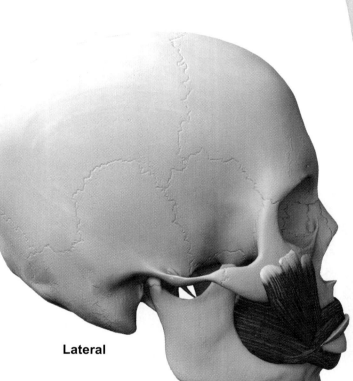

Lateral

Zygomaticus major

O. Zygomatic bone—anterior to temporal process

I. Angle of mouth—blending with adjacent muscles

A. Elevation and retraction of angle of mouth

N. Facial nerve (cranial nerve VII)

Zygomaticus minor

O. Zygomatic bone—posterior to maxillary zygomatic suture

I. Angle of mouth and orbicularis oris

A. Retraction and elevation of upper lip (forms nasolabial furrow)

N. Facial nerve (cranial nerve VII)

Anterior

Unit 3 Muscular System

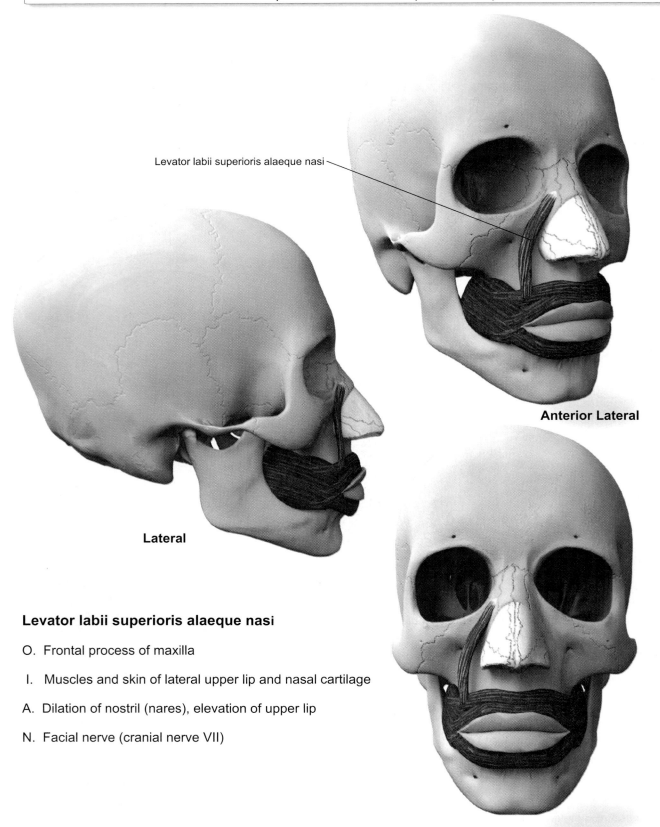

Levator labii superioris alaeque nasi

Anterior Lateral

Lateral

Anterior

Levator labii superioris alaeque nasi

O. Frontal process of maxilla

I. Muscles and skin of lateral upper lip and nasal cartilage

A. Dilation of nostril (nares), elevation of upper lip

N. Facial nerve (cranial nerve VII)

Orbicularis oris

O. Maxilla, mandible, and fascia surrounding lips

I. Mucous membrane of lips

A. Closure of lips, purses lips, and puckers lip edges, assists in mastication

N. Facial nerve (cranial nerve VII)

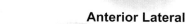

Orbicularis oris

Mentalis

Anterior Lateral

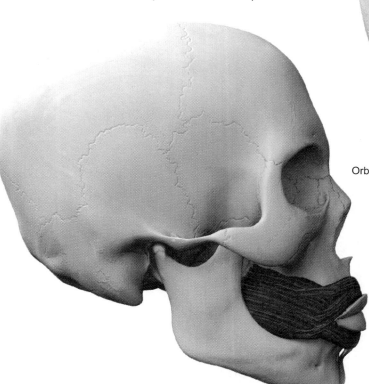

Lateral

Mentalis

O. Mandible—superior medial surface

I. Skin of chin

A. Elevation and protrusion of lower lip, wrinkles skin over chin

N. Facial nerve (cranial VII)

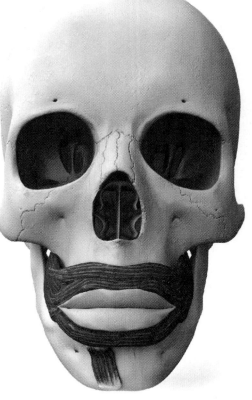

Anterior

Unit 3 Muscular System

Nasalis

O. **Alar portion:** maxilla—frontal portion, alar cartilage of nose
Transverse portion: maxilla—below infraorbital foramen

I. **Alar portion:** ipsilateral alar cartilages and skin of nostril (nares)
Transverse portion: aponeurosis of nasalis on opposite side

A. **Alar portion:** opens aperture of nostril (nares)
Transverse portion: closes aperture of nostril (nares)

N. Buccal branch of facial nerve (cranial nerve VII)

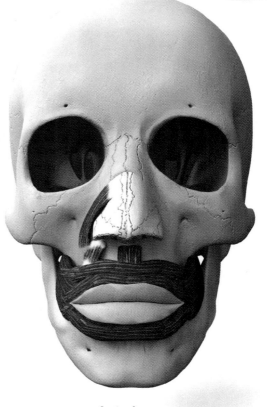

Nasalis (transverse portion)

Nasalis (alar portion)

Depressor septi nasi

Anterior Lateral

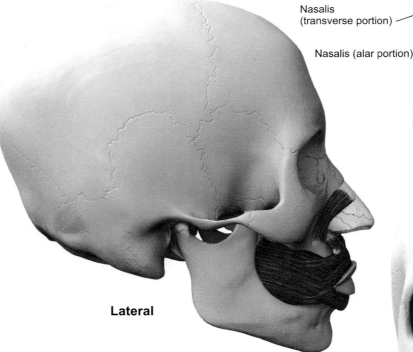

Lateral

Depressor septi nasi

O. Incisive fossa of maxilla

I. Ala and nasal septum

A. Depression and restriction of nostrils (nares)

N. Buccal branch of facial nerve (cranial nerve VII)

Anterior

Unit 3 Muscular System

Levator anguli oris

O. Canine fossa of maxilla immediately below infraorbital foramen

I. Angle of mouth blending with adjacent muscles

A. Elevation of angle of mouth

N. Facial nerve (cranial nerve VII)

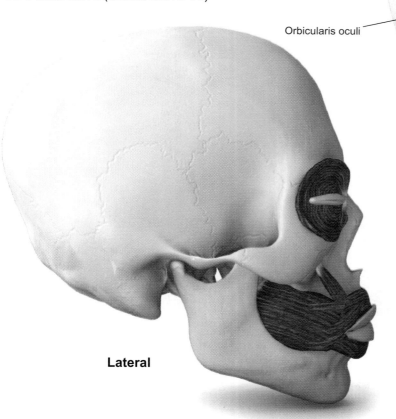

Orbicularis oculi

Lateral

Anterior Lateral

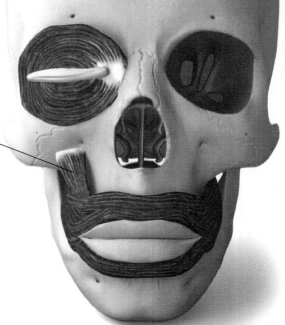

Levator anguli oris

Anterior

Orbicularis oculi

O. *Orbital part:* frontal bone and maxilla at medial orbital margin and palpebral ligament
Palpebral part: medial palpebral ligament
Lacrimal part: lacrimal bone

I. Circumferentially around orbit, merging into palpebral raphe

A. Closure of eyelids

N. Facial nerve (cranial nerve VII)

Unit 3 Muscular System

123

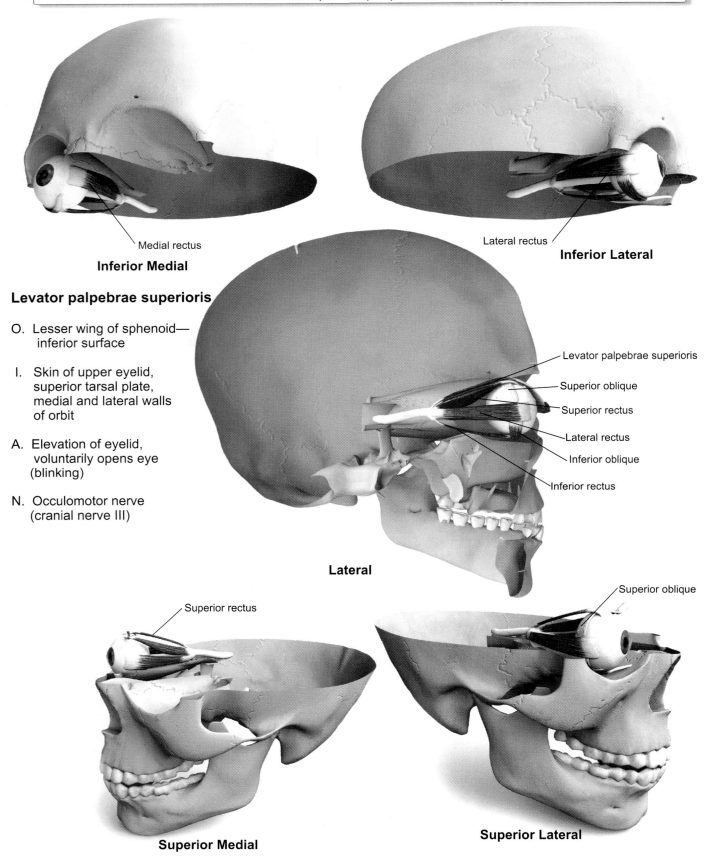

Medial rectus

Inferior Medial

Lateral rectus

Inferior Lateral

Levator palpebrae superioris

O. Lesser wing of sphenoid—
    inferior surface

I. Skin of upper eyelid,
    superior tarsal plate,
    medial and lateral walls
    of orbit

A. Elevation of eyelid,
    voluntarily opens eye
    (blinking)

N. Occulomotor nerve
    (cranial nerve III)

Levator palpebrae superioris

Superior oblique

Superior rectus

Lateral rectus

Inferior oblique

Inferior rectus

Lateral

Superior rectus

Superior Medial

Superior oblique

Superior Lateral

Unit 3 Muscular System

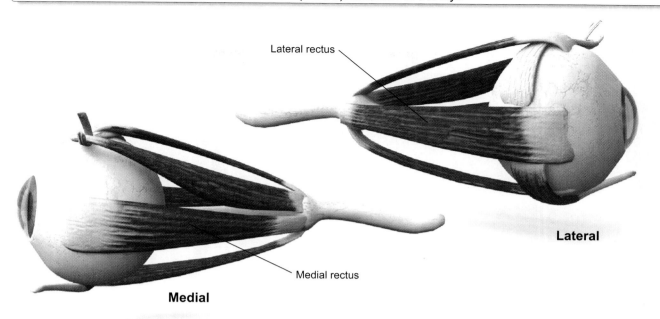

Lateral rectus

Lateral

Medial rectus

Medial

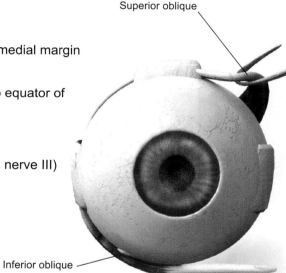

Superior oblique

Inferior oblique

Anterior

Medial rectus

O. Fibrous ring surrounding medial margin of optic foramen

I. Medial sclera—anterior to equator of eyeball

A. Medial rotation of eyeball

N. Oculomotor nerve (cranial nerve III)

Lateral rectus

O. Fibrous ring surrounding lateral margin of optic foramen

I. Lateral sclera—anterior to equator of eyeball

A. Lateral rotation of eyeball

N. Abducens nerve (cranial nerve VI)

Inferior oblique

O. Orbital plate of maxilla

I. External portion of sclera—between inferior and lateral rectus muscles—posterior to equator of eyeball

A. Rotation of eyeball upward and laterally

N. Oculomotor nerve (cranial nerve III)

Superior oblique

O. Above medial margin of optic foramen

I. Sclera—between superior and lateral rectus muscles—posterior to equator of eyeball

A. Rotation of eyeball downward and laterally

N. Trochlear nerve (cranial nerve IV)

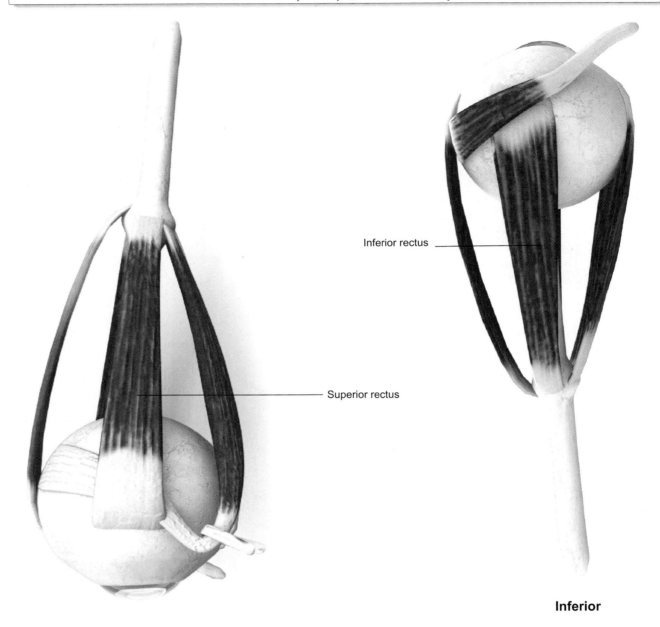

Inferior rectus

Superior rectus

Superior

Inferior

Superior rectus

O. Fibrous ring surrounding superior margin of optic foramen

I. Superior sclera—anterior to equator of eyeball

A. Elevation of eye

N. Oculomotor nerve (cranial nerve III)

Inferior rectus

O. Fibrous ring surrounding inferior margin of optic foramen

I. Inferior sclera—anterior to equator of eyeball

A. Depression of eyeball

N. Oculomotor nerve (cranial nerve III)

Auricularis anterior

O. Fascia in temporal region

I. Cartilage of auricle—anterior surface

A. Protraction of ear

N. Facial nerve temporal branch
    (cranial nerve VII)

Auricularis superior

O. Fascia in temporal region

I. Cartilage of auricle—superior surface

A. Elevation of ear

N. Facial nerve temporal branch (cranial nerve VII)

Auricularis superior

Auricularis posterior

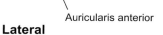

Auricularis anterior

Lateral

Auricularis posterior

O. Mastoid region of temporal bone

I. Root of auricle

A. Retraction and depression of ear

N. Facial nerve, posterior auricular branch
    (cranial nerve VII)

Posterior Lateral

Temporalis

O. Temporal fossa and fascia

I. Coronoid process and ramus of mandible

A. Elevation and retraction of mandible, assists in mastication

N. Trigeminal nerve (cranial nerve V)

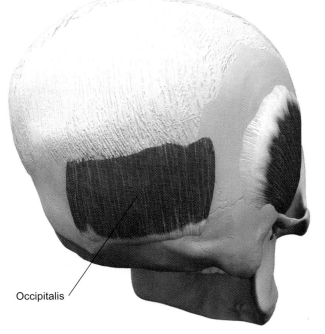

Temporalis

Lateral

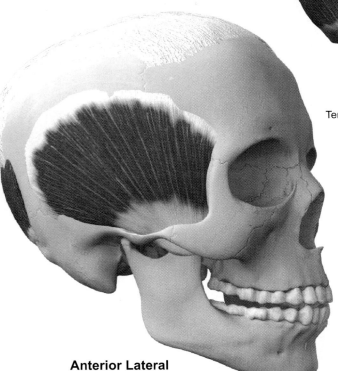

Anterior Lateral

Occipitalis

O. Superior nuchal line of occiput, mastoid process of temporal bone via fascial attachments

I. Galea aponeurotica over occipital bone

A. Elevation of eyebrows, draws scalp backward and wrinkles forehead (by means of tightening galea aponeurotica, affecting anterior musculature)

N. Facial nerve (cranial nerve VII)

Occipitalis

Posterior Lateral

Unit 3 Muscular System

Medial pterygoid

O. Lateral pterygoid plate and fossa—medial surface, palatine bone—lateral surface

I. Ramus—medial surface, angle of mandible

A. *Bilaterally:* elevation of mandible, assists protraction of mandible, assists mastication
Unilaterally: deviation of mandible toward opposite side

N. Trigeminal nerve (cranial nerve V)

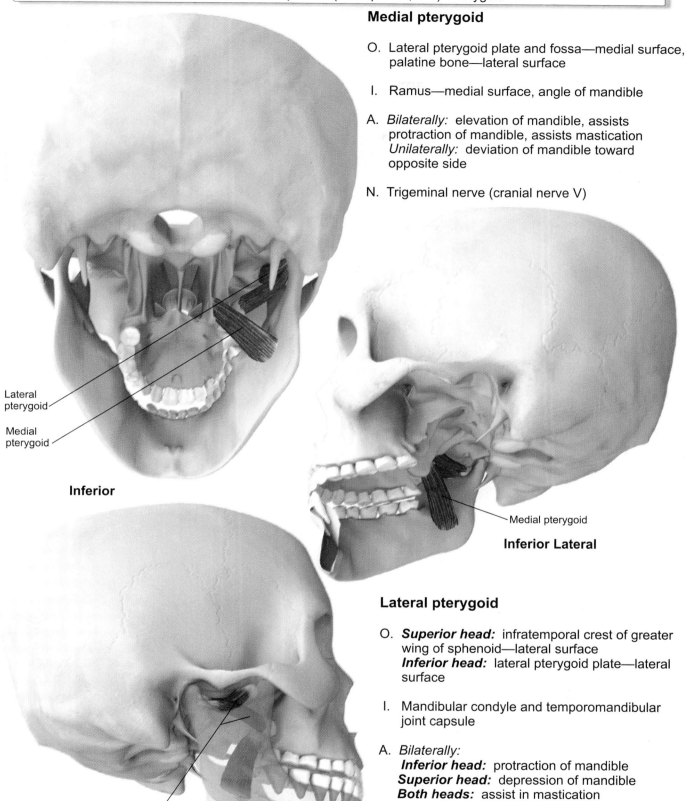

Lateral pterygoid

Medial pterygoid

Inferior

Medial pterygoid

Inferior Lateral

Lateral pterygoid

Lateral

Lateral pterygoid

O. **Superior head:** infratemporal crest of greater wing of sphenoid—lateral surface
Inferior head: lateral pterygoid plate—lateral surface

I. Mandibular condyle and temporomandibular joint capsule

A. *Bilaterally:*
Inferior head: protraction of mandible
Superior head: depression of mandible
Both heads: assist in mastication
Unilaterally: deviation of mandible to opposite side

N. Trigeminal nerve (cranial nerve V)

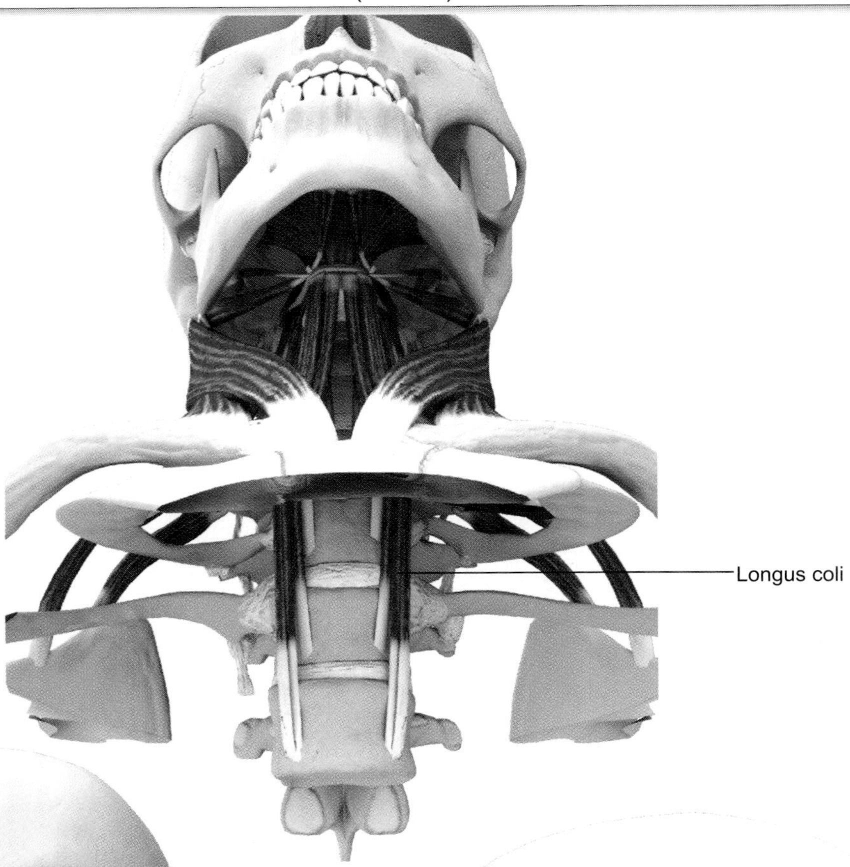

Longus coli

Inferior

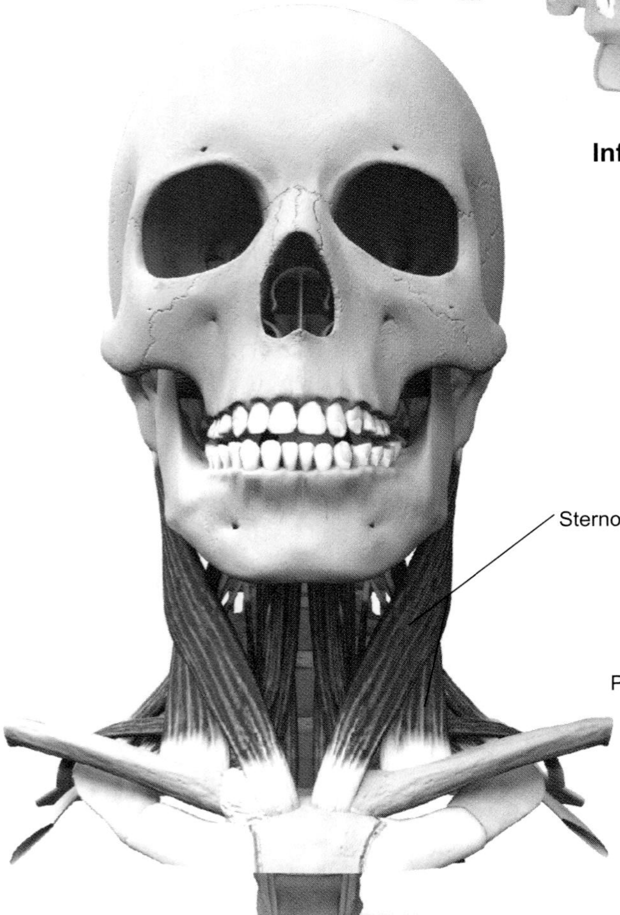

Sternocleidomastoid

Middle scalene

Posterior scalene

Anterior

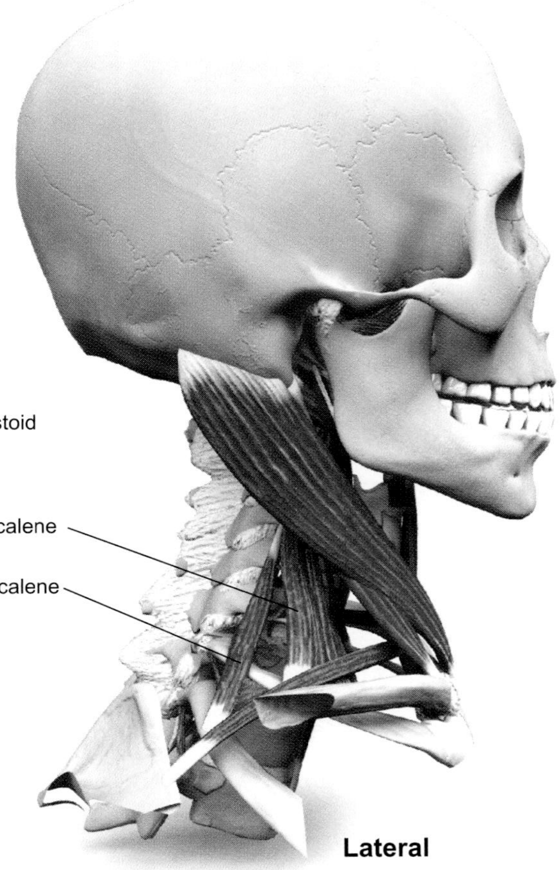

Lateral

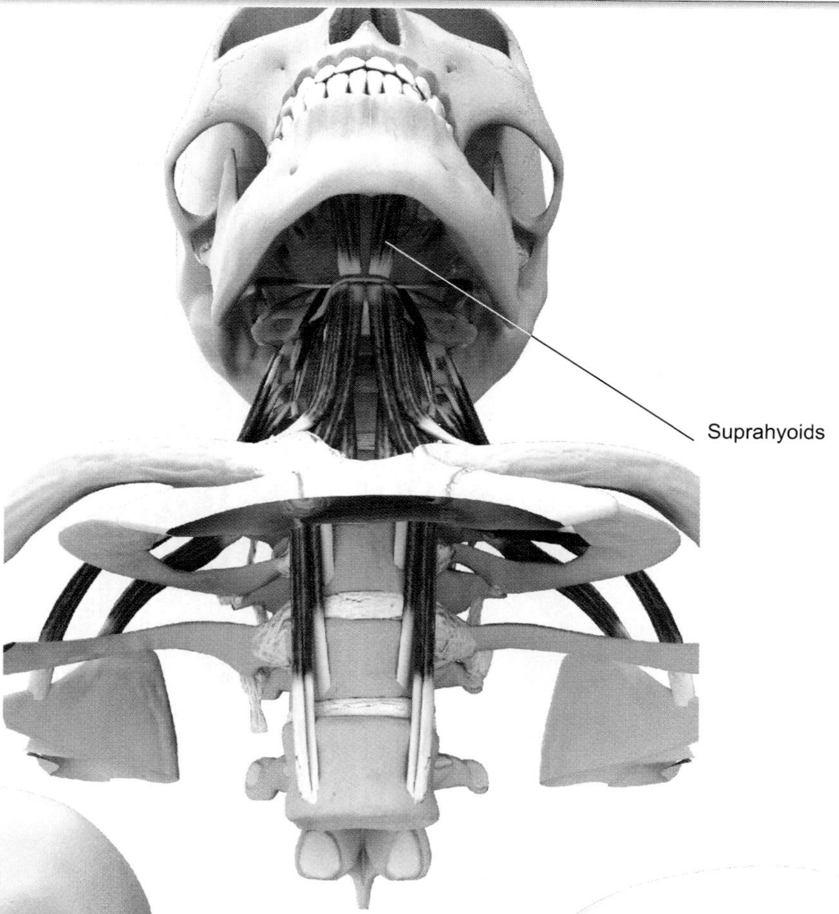

Suprahyoids

Inferior

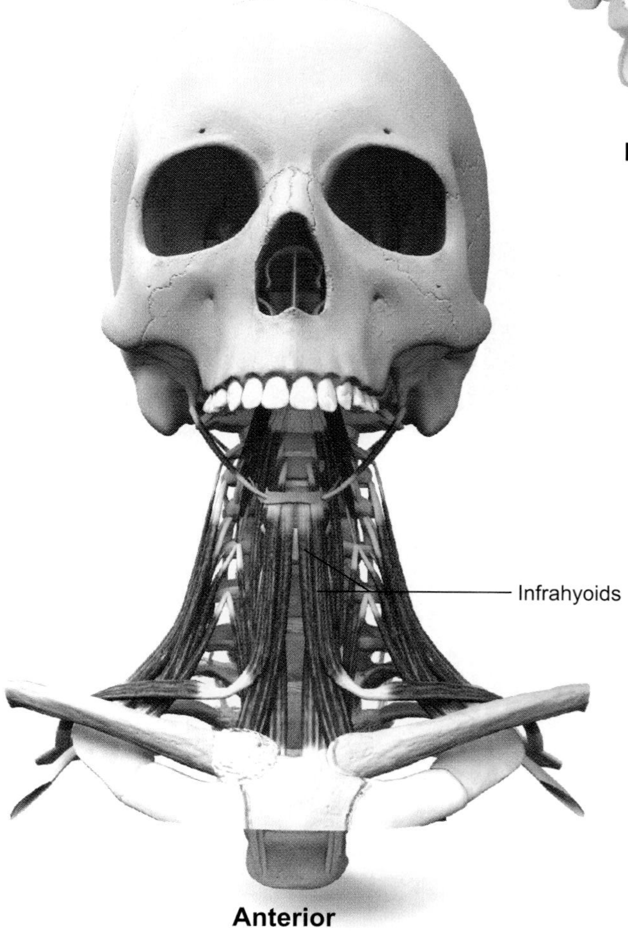

Infrahyoids

Anterior

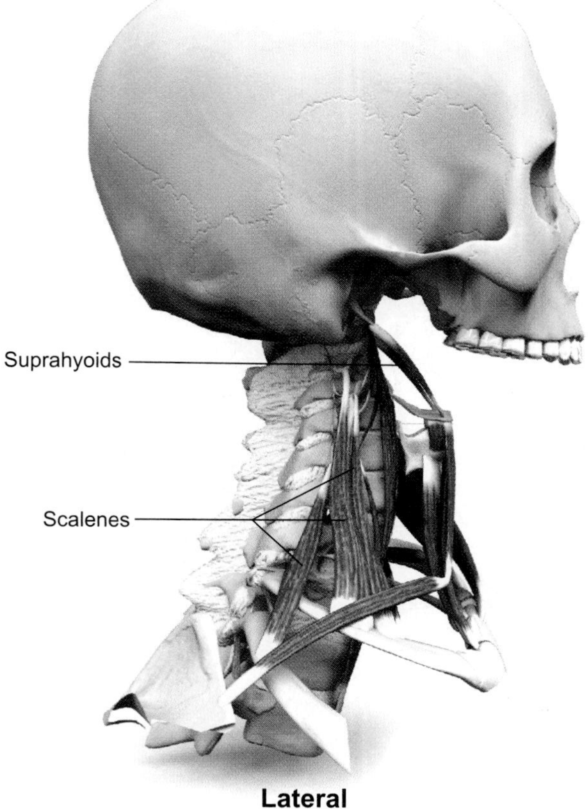

Suprahyoids

Scalenes

Lateral

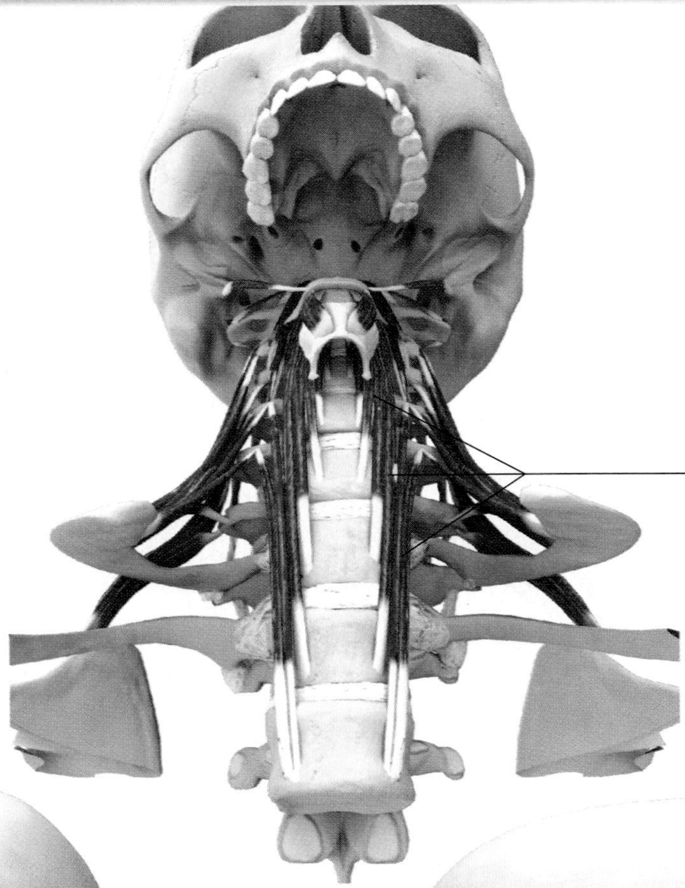

Longus coli

Inferior

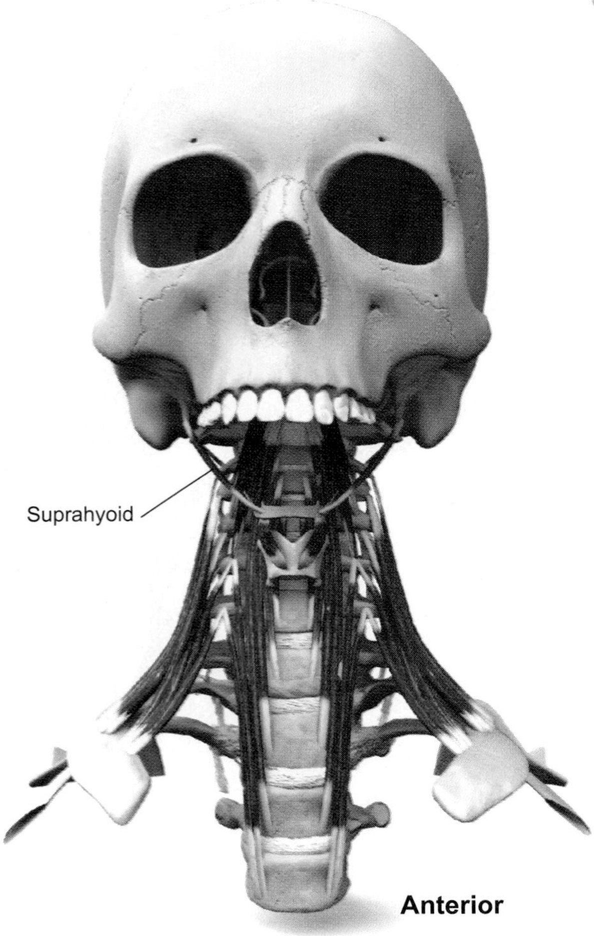

Suprahyoid

Anterior

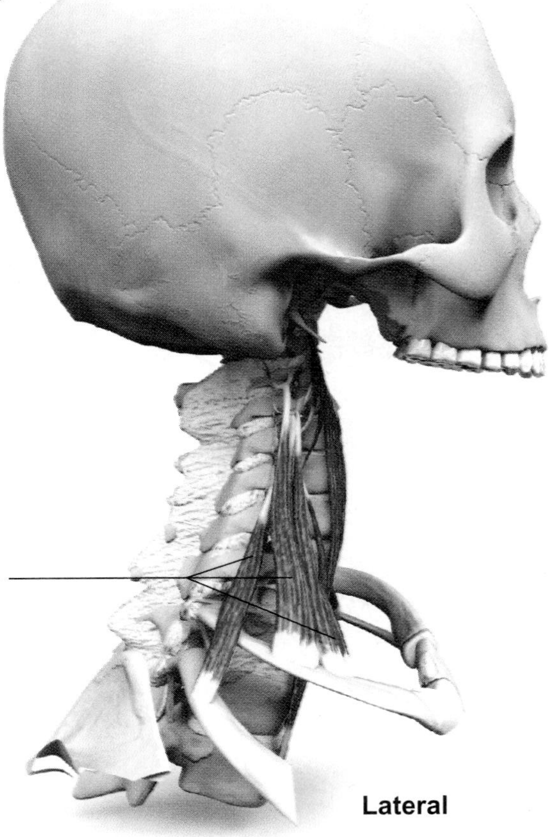

Scalenes

Lateral

Unit 3 Muscular System

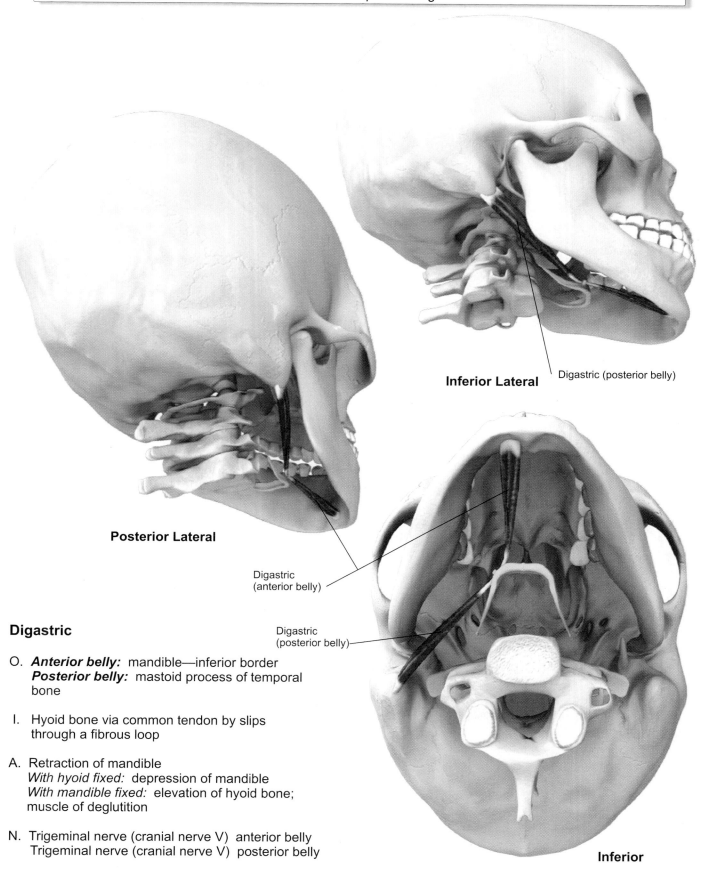

Inferior Lateral

Digastric (posterior belly)

Posterior Lateral

Digastric
(anterior belly)

Digastric
(posterior belly)

Inferior

Digastric

O. ***Anterior belly:*** mandible—inferior border
Posterior belly: mastoid process of temporal
bone

I. Hyoid bone via common tendon by slips
through a fibrous loop

A. Retraction of mandible
With hyoid fixed: depression of mandible
With mandible fixed: elevation of hyoid bone;
muscle of deglutition

N. Trigeminal nerve (cranial nerve V) anterior belly
Trigeminal nerve (cranial nerve V) posterior belly

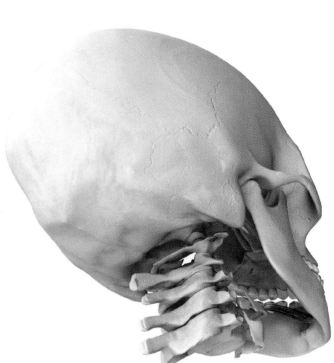

Posterior Lateral

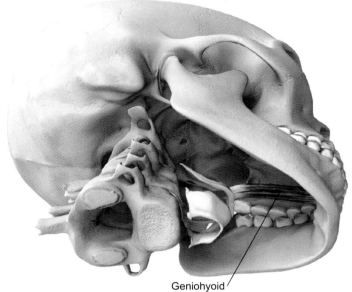

Geniohyoid

Inferior Lateral

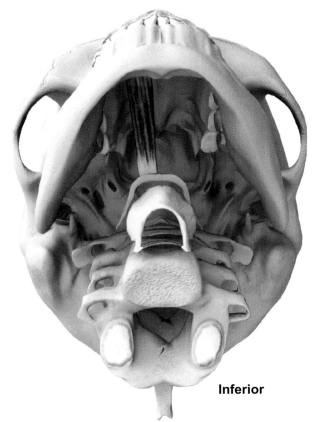

Inferior

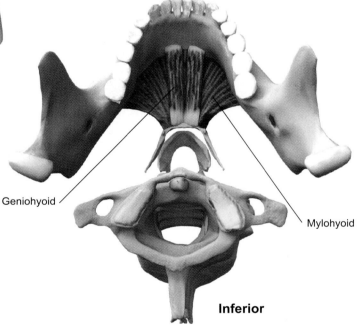

Geniohyoid

Mylohyoid

Inferior

Geniohyoid

O. Inner surface of mandible—inferior mental spines

I. Body of hyoid

A. Elevation and protraction of hyoid, depression of mandible
    Muscle of deglutition

N. Hypoglossal nerve (cranial nerve XII)

Unit 3 Muscular System

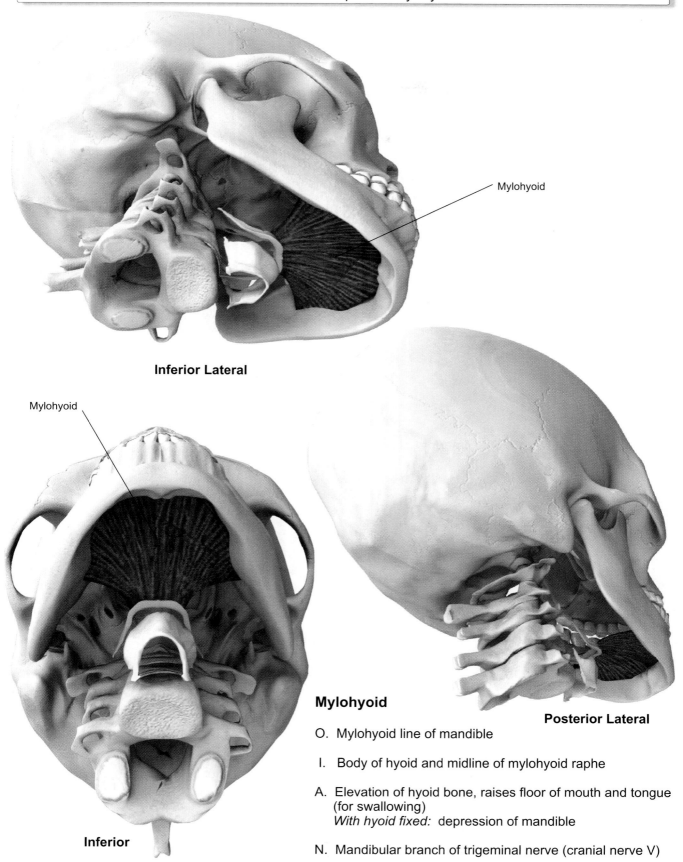

Inferior Lateral

Mylohyoid

Inferior

Mylohyoid

Posterior Lateral

O. Mylohyoid line of mandible

I. Body of hyoid and midline of mylohyoid raphe

A. Elevation of hyoid bone, raises floor of mouth and tongue
    (for swallowing)
    With hyoid fixed: depression of mandible

N. Mandibular branch of trigeminal nerve (cranial nerve V)

Unit 3 Muscular System

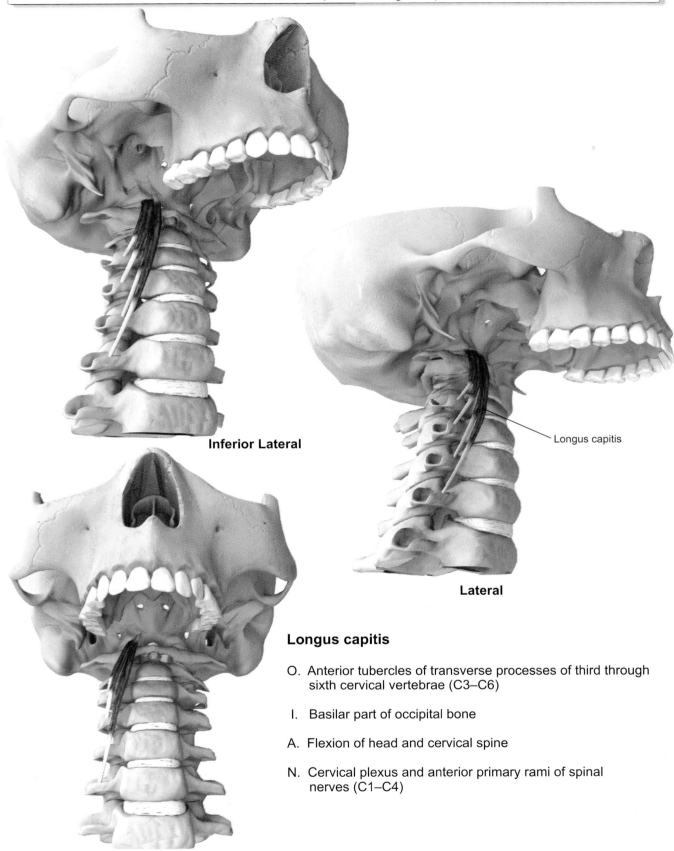

Inferior Lateral

Lateral

Longus capitis

Anterior

Longus capitis

O. Anterior tubercles of transverse processes of third through sixth cervical vertebrae (C3–C6)

I. Basilar part of occipital bone

A. Flexion of head and cervical spine

N. Cervical plexus and anterior primary rami of spinal nerves (C1–C4)

Unit 3 Muscular System

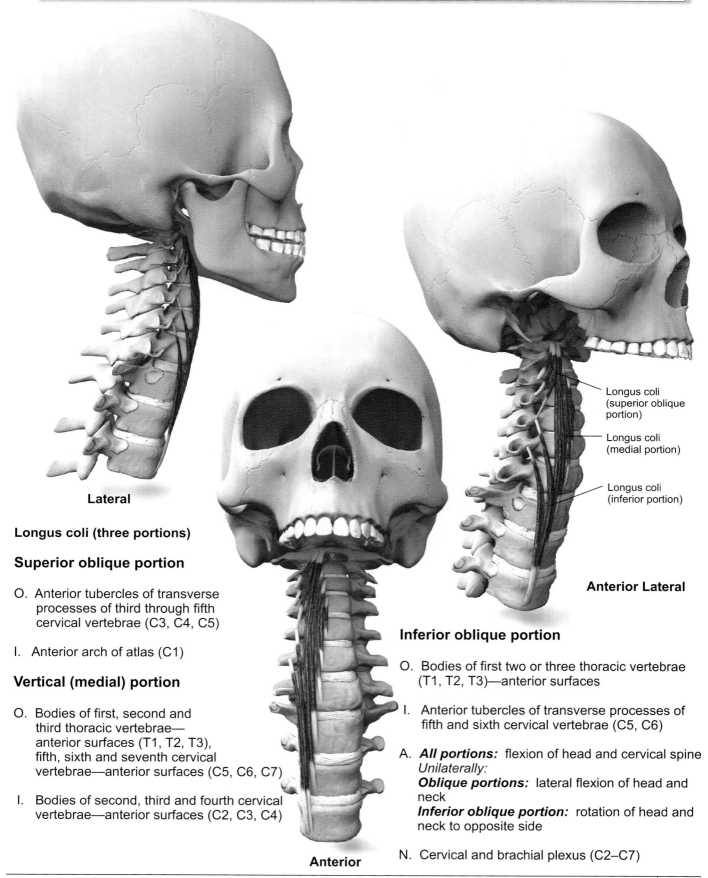

Longus coli
(superior oblique
portion)

Longus coli
(medial portion)

Longus coli
(inferior portion)

Lateral

Anterior Lateral

Longus coli (three portions)

Superior oblique portion

O. Anterior tubercles of transverse
processes of third through fifth
cervical vertebrae (C3, C4, C5)

I. Anterior arch of atlas (C1)

Vertical (medial) portion

O. Bodies of first, second and
third thoracic vertebrae—
anterior surfaces (T1, T2, T3),
fifth, sixth and seventh cervical
vertebrae—anterior surfaces (C5, C6, C7)

I. Bodies of second, third and fourth cervical
vertebrae—anterior surfaces (C2, C3, C4)

Inferior oblique portion

O. Bodies of first two or three thoracic vertebrae
(T1, T2, T3)—anterior surfaces

I. Anterior tubercles of transverse processes of
fifth and sixth cervical vertebrae (C5, C6)

A. ***All portions:*** flexion of head and cervical spine
Unilaterally:
Oblique portions: lateral flexion of head and
neck
Inferior oblique portion: rotation of head and
neck to opposite side

N. Cervical and brachial plexus (C2–C7)

Anterior

Unit 3 Muscular System

137

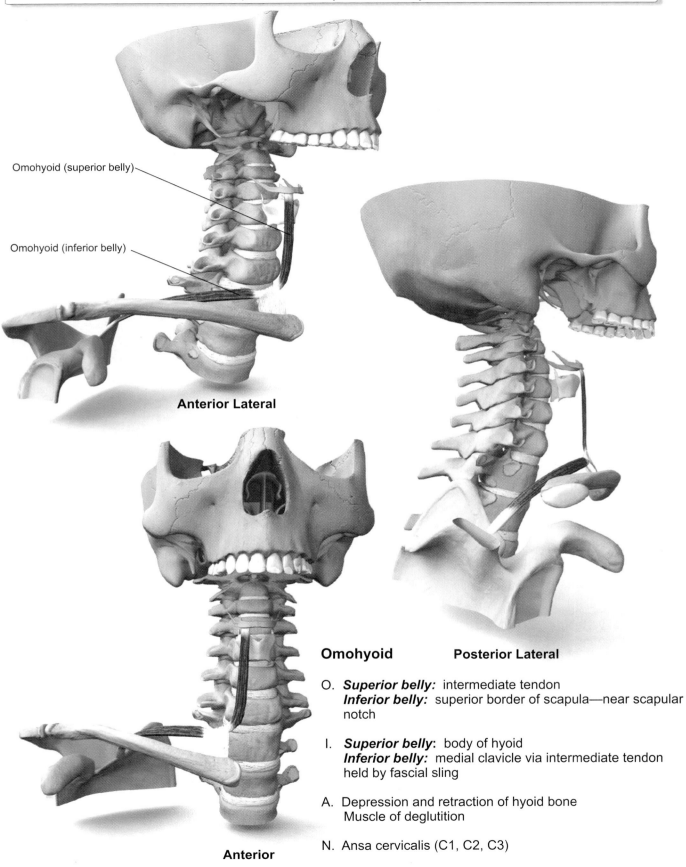

Omohyoid (superior belly)

Omohyoid (inferior belly)

Anterior Lateral

Anterior

Omohyoid

Posterior Lateral

O. *Superior belly:* intermediate tendon
Inferior belly: superior border of scapula—near scapular notch

I. *Superior belly:* body of hyoid
Inferior belly: medial clavicle via intermediate tendon held by fascial sling

A. Depression and retraction of hyoid bone
Muscle of deglutition

N. Ansa cervicalis (C1, C2, C3)

Unit 3 Muscular System

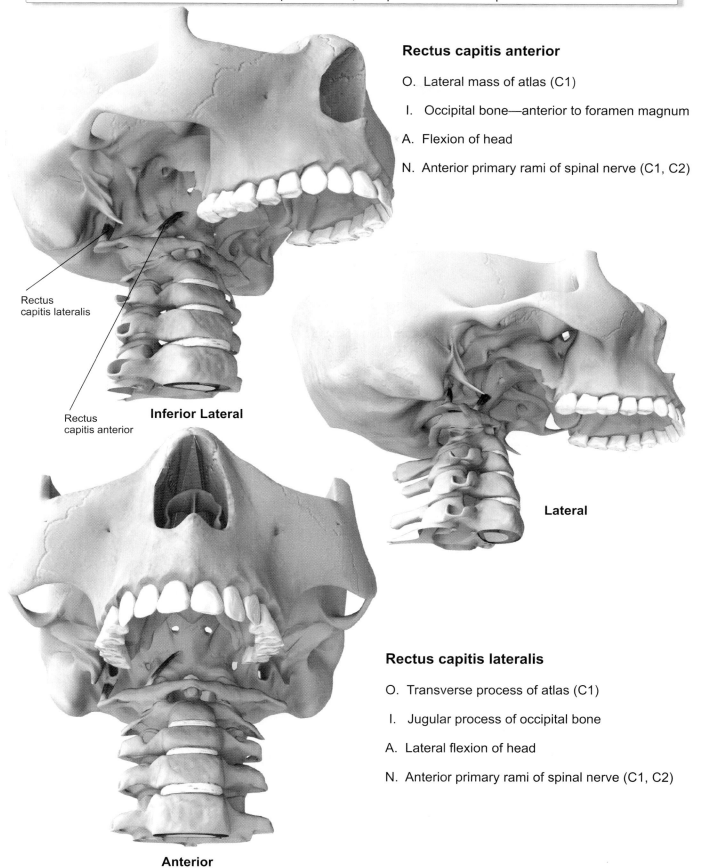

Rectus capitis anterior

O. Lateral mass of atlas (C1)

I. Occipital bone—anterior to foramen magnum

A. Flexion of head

N. Anterior primary rami of spinal nerve (C1, C2)

Rectus
capitis lateralis

Rectus
capitis anterior

Inferior Lateral

Lateral

Anterior

Rectus capitis lateralis

O. Transverse process of atlas (C1)

I. Jugular process of occipital bone

A. Lateral flexion of head

N. Anterior primary rami of spinal nerve (C1, C2)

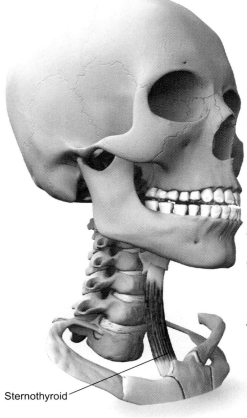

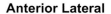

Sternothyroid

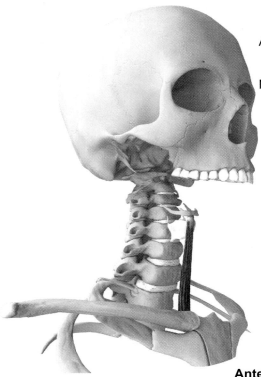

Anterior Lateral

Sternothyroid

O. Manubrium of sternum—posterior surface

I. Oblique line of thyroid cartilage

A. Depression of thyroid cartilage; muscle of deglutition

N. Hypoglossal nerve (cranial nerve XII)

Sternohyoid

O. Manubrium of sternum and sternal end of clavicle

I. Body of hyoid—inferior border

A. Depression of hyoid; muscle of deglutition

N. Ansa cervicalis (C1, C2, C3)

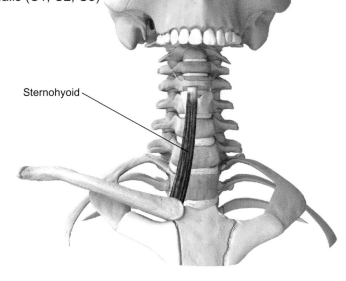

Sternohyoid

Anterior Lateral

Anterior

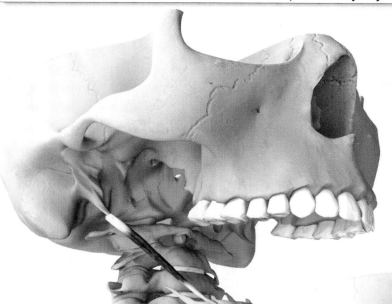

Stylohyoid

O. Styloid process of temporal bone

I. Body of hyoid

A. Elevation and retraction of hyoid, assists in deglutition

N. Facial nerve (cranial nerve VII)

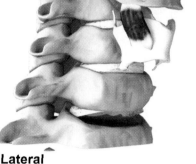

Anterior Lateral

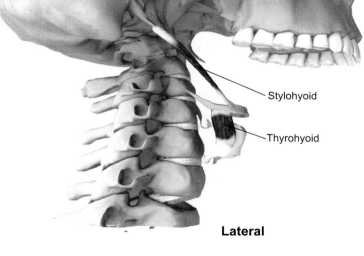

Stylohyoid

Thyrohyoid

Lateral

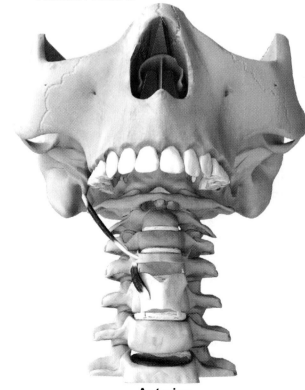

Anterior

Thyrohyoid

O. Oblique line of thyroid cartilage

I. Greater cornu of hyoid bone

A. Depression of hyoid bone, elevation of thyroid cartilage; muscle of deglutition

N. Hypoglossal nerve (cranial nerve XII)

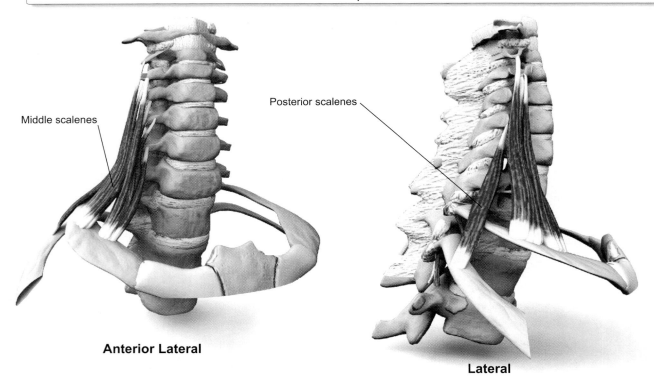

Middle scalenes

Anterior Lateral

Posterior scalenes

Lateral

Anterior scalenes

Anterior

Scalenes

O. **Anterior fibers:** anterior tubercles of transverse processes of third through sixth cervical vertebrae (C3–C6)
Middle fibers: posterior tubercles of transverse processes of second through seventh cervical vertebrae (C2–C7)
Posterior: posterior tubercles of transverse processes of fourth through sixth cervical vertebrae (C4–C6)

I. **Anterior fibers:** crest of first rib—medial border, scalene tubercle
Middle fibers: first rib—superior border
Posterior fibers: second rib—lateral surface

A. *Bilaterally:*
All fibers: assist respiration (by elevating ribs)
Anterior fibers: assist flexion of neck, assist elevation of first rib
Middle fibers: assist elevation of first rib
Posterior fibers: elevation of second rib, stabilizes base of neck
Unilaterally:
All fibers: lateral flexion of neck, rotation of head and neck to opposite side

N. Ventral rami of cervical nerves
(C4, C5, C6) anterior
Ventral rami of cervical nerves
(C4, C5, C6, C7, C8) middle
Ventral rami of cervical nerves
(C6, C7, C8) posterior

Unit 3 Muscular System

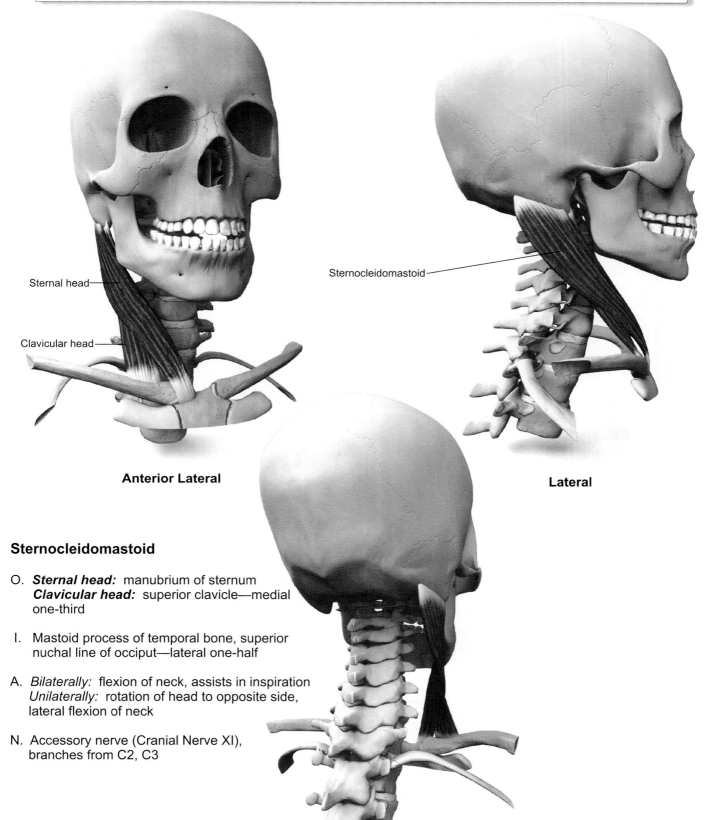

Sternal head

Clavicular head

Anterior Lateral

Sternocleidomastoid

Lateral

Posterior Lateral

Sternocleidomastoid

O. ***Sternal head:*** manubrium of sternum
Clavicular head: superior clavicle—medial one-third

I. Mastoid process of temporal bone, superior nuchal line of occiput—lateral one-half

A. *Bilaterally:* flexion of neck, assists in inspiration
Unilaterally: rotation of head to opposite side, lateral flexion of neck

N. Accessory nerve (Cranial Nerve XI), branches from C2, C3

Unit 3 Muscular System

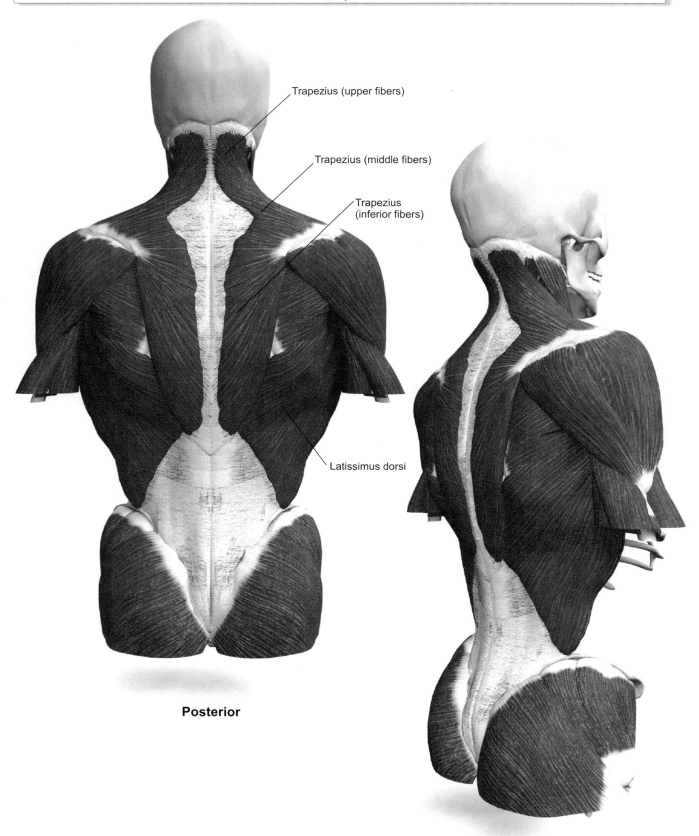

Trapezius (upper fibers)

Trapezius (middle fibers)

Trapezius (inferior fibers)

Latissimus dorsi

Posterior

Posterior Lateral

Unit 3 Muscular System

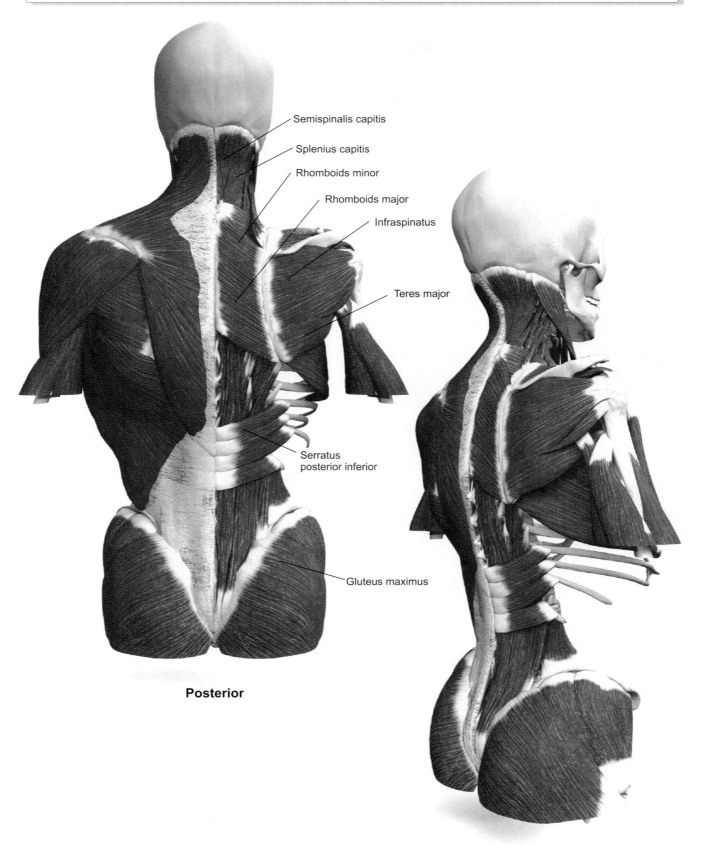

Semispinalis capitis

Splenius capitis

Rhomboids minor

Rhomboids major

Infraspinatus

Teres major

Serratus
posterior inferior

Gluteus maximus

Posterior

Posterior Lateral

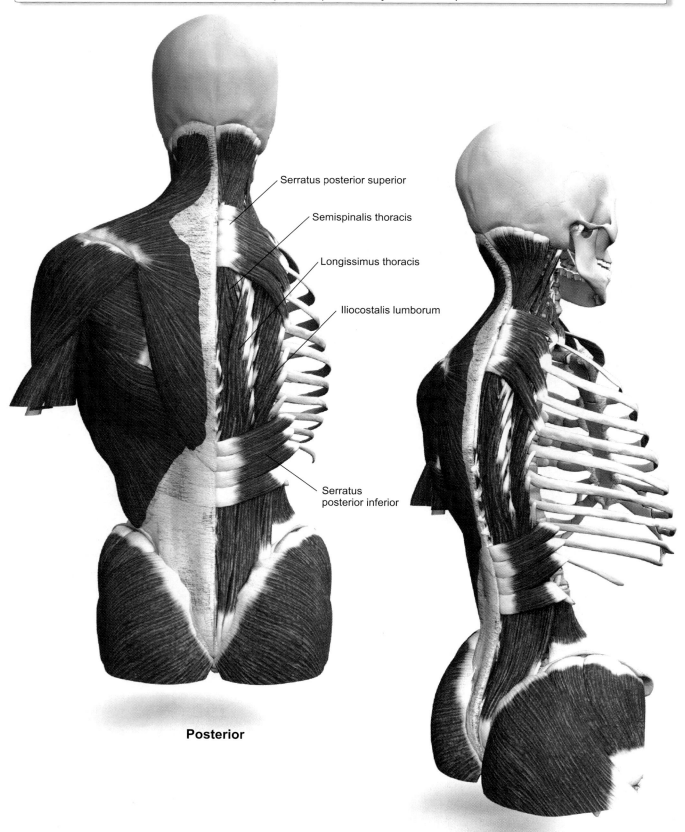

Serratus posterior superior

Semispinalis thoracis

Longissimus thoracis

Iliocostalis lumborum

Serratus
posterior inferior

Posterior

Posterior Lateral

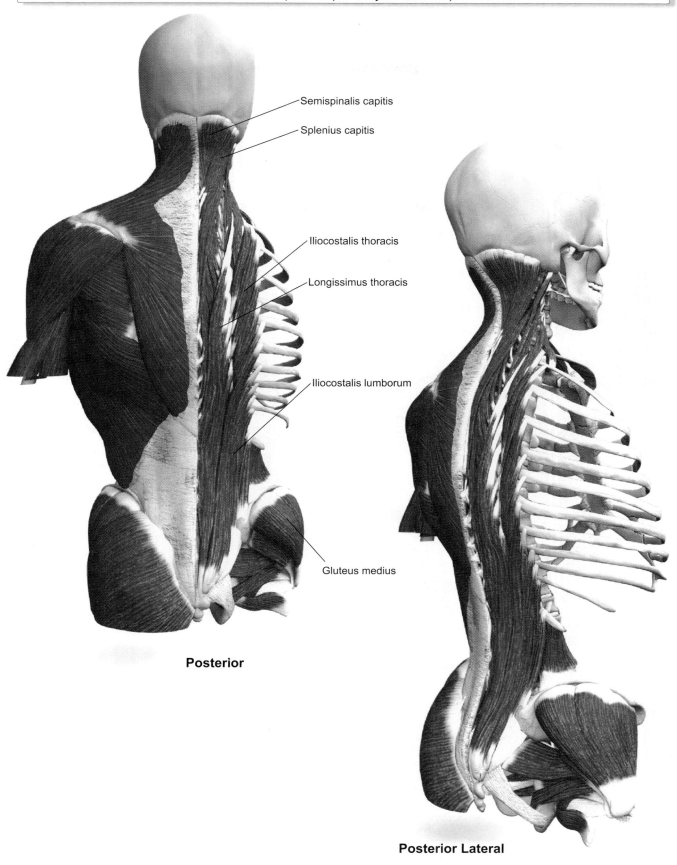

Semispinalis capitis

Splenius capitis

Iliocostalis thoracis

Longissimus thoracis

Iliocostalis lumborum

Gluteus medius

Posterior

Posterior Lateral

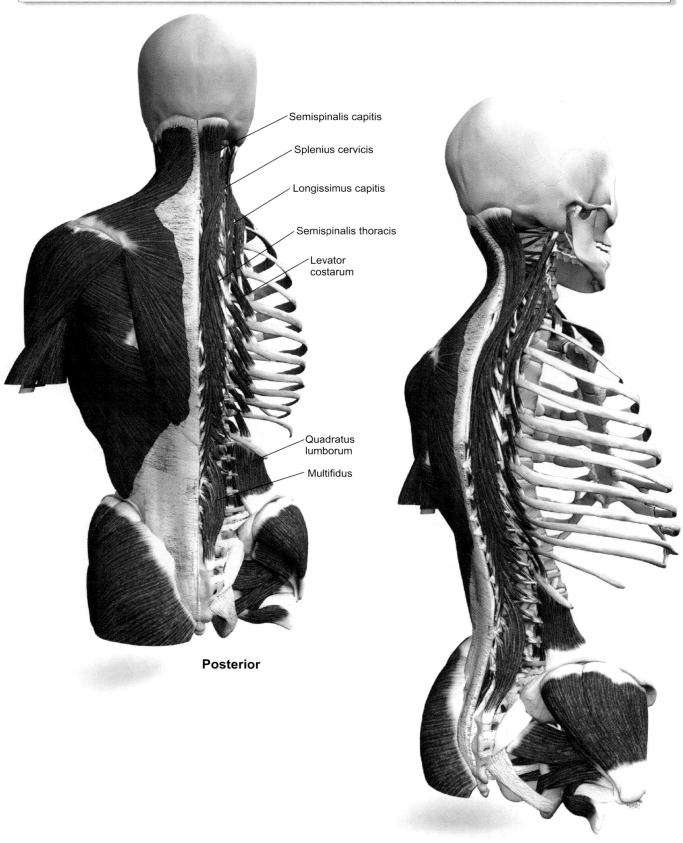

Semispinalis capitis

Splenius cervicis

Longissimus capitis

Semispinalis thoracis

Levator costarum

Quadratus lumborum

Multifidus

Posterior

Posterior Lateral

Unit 3 Muscular System

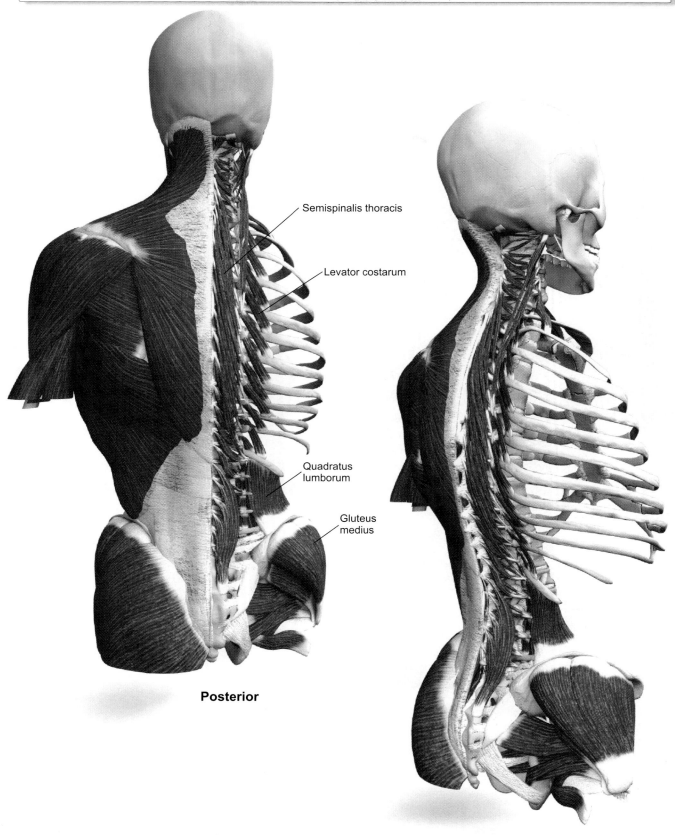

Semispinalis thoracis

Levator costarum

Quadratus
lumborum

Gluteus
medius

Posterior

Posterior Lateral

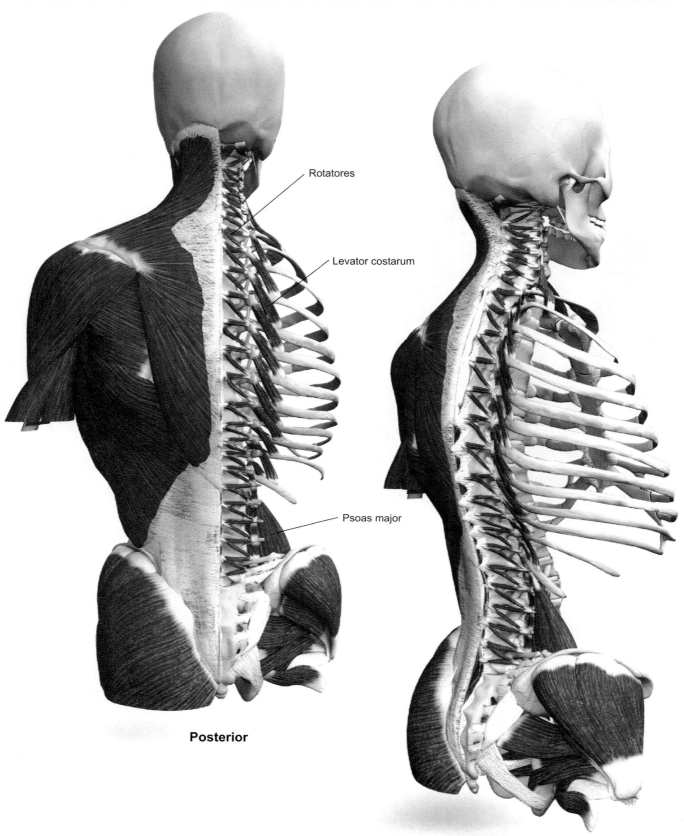

Rotatores

Levator costarum

Psoas major

Posterior

Posterior Lateral

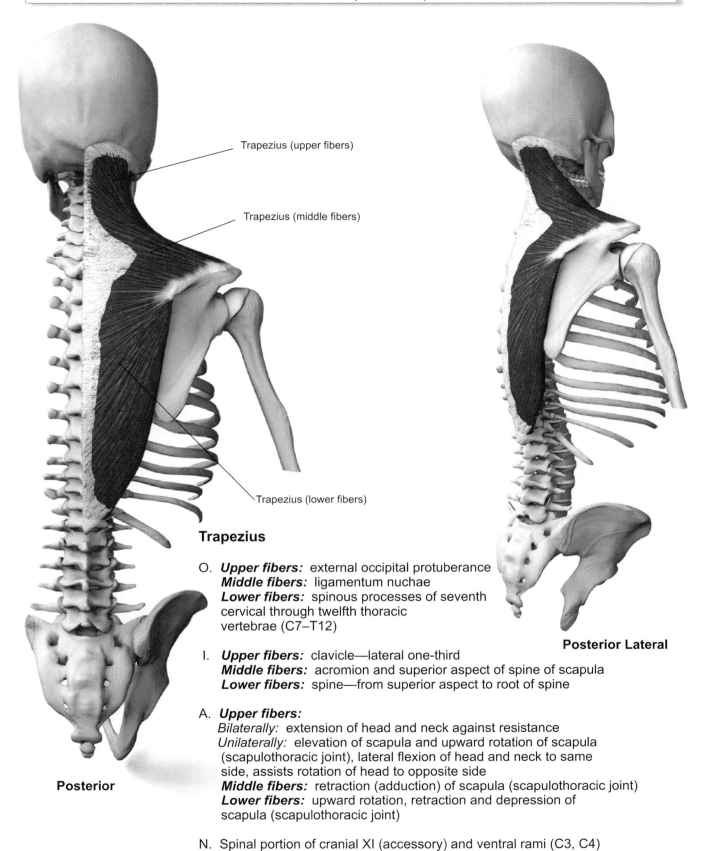

Trapezius (upper fibers)

Trapezius (middle fibers)

Trapezius (lower fibers)

Posterior Lateral

Posterior

Trapezius

O. ***Upper fibers:*** external occipital protuberance
Middle fibers: ligamentum nuchae
Lower fibers: spinous processes of seventh
cervical through twelfth thoracic
vertebrae (C7–T12)

I. ***Upper fibers:*** clavicle—lateral one-third
Middle fibers: acromion and superior aspect of spine of scapula
Lower fibers: spine—from superior aspect to root of spine

A. ***Upper fibers:***
Bilaterally: extension of head and neck against resistance
Unilaterally: elevation of scapula and upward rotation of scapula
(scapulothoracic joint), lateral flexion of head and neck to same
side, assists rotation of head to opposite side
Middle fibers: retraction (adduction) of scapula (scapulothoracic joint)
Lower fibers: upward rotation, retraction and depression of
scapula (scapulothoracic joint)

N. Spinal portion of cranial XI (accessory) and ventral rami (C3, C4)

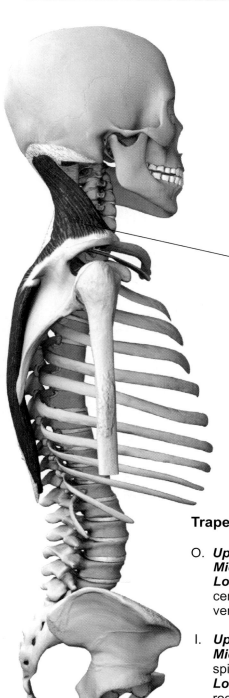

Trapezius (upper fibers)

Lateral

Anterior Lateral

Trapezius

O. ***Upper fibers:*** external occipital protuberance
Middle fibers: ligamentum nuchae
Lower fibers: spinous processes of seventh cervical through twelfth thoracic vertebrae (C7–T12)

I. ***Upper fibers:*** clavicle—lateral one-third
Middle fibers: acromion and superior aspect of spine of scapula
Lower fibers: spine—from superior aspect to root of spine

A. ***Upper fibers:***
Bilaterally: extension of head and neck against resistance
Unilaterally: elevation of scapula and upward rotation of scapula (scapulothoracic joint), lateral flexion of head and neck to same side, assists rotation of head to opposite side
Middle fibers: retraction (adduction) of scapula (scapulothoracic joint)
Lower fibers: upward rotation, retraction and depression of scapula (scapulothoracic joint)

N. Spinal portion of cranial XI (accessory) and ventral rami (C3, C4)

Unit 3 Muscular System

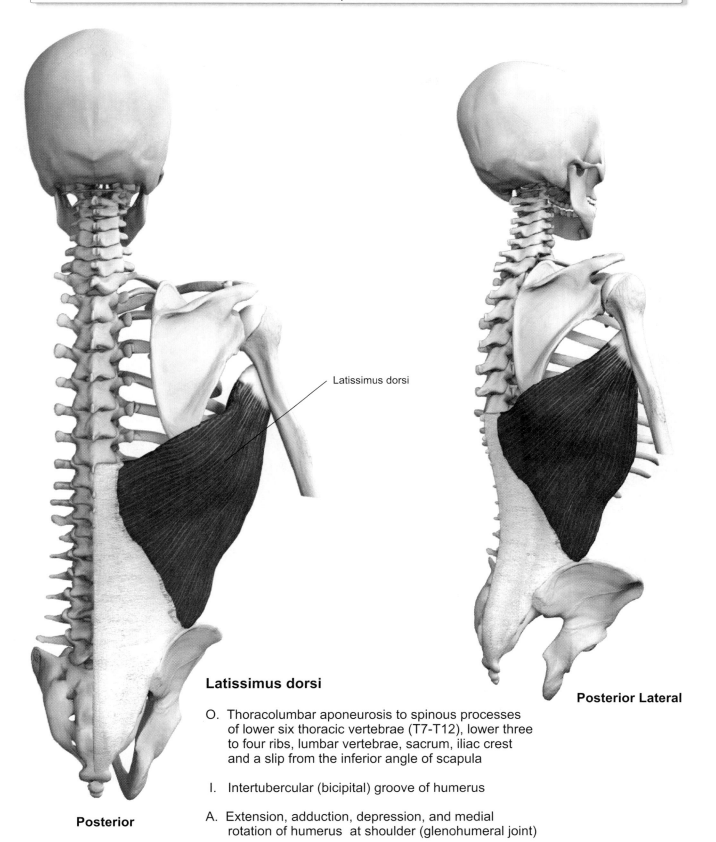

Latissimus dorsi

Posterior

Posterior Lateral

Latissimus dorsi

O. Thoracolumbar aponeurosis to spinous processes of lower six thoracic vertebrae (T7-T12), lower three to four ribs, lumbar vertebrae, sacrum, iliac crest and a slip from the inferior angle of scapula

I. Intertubercular (bicipital) groove of humerus

A. Extension, adduction, depression, and medial rotation of humerus at shoulder (glenohumeral joint)

N. Thoracodorsal nerve (C6, C7, C8)

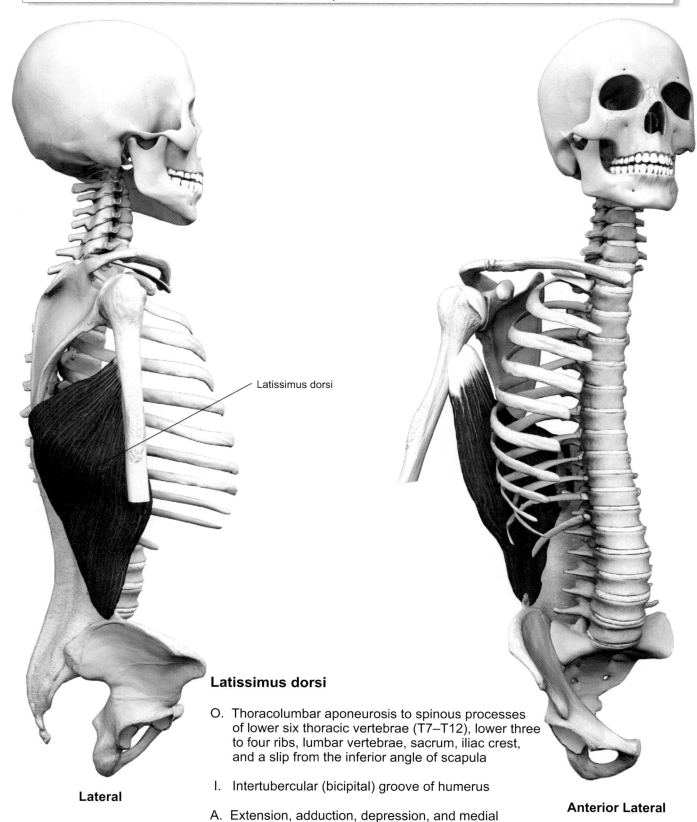

Latissimus dorsi

Lateral

Anterior Lateral

Latissimus dorsi

O. Thoracolumbar aponeurosis to spinous processes
of lower six thoracic vertebrae (T7–T12), lower three
to four ribs, lumbar vertebrae, sacrum, iliac crest,
and a slip from the inferior angle of scapula

I. Intertubercular (bicipital) groove of humerus

A. Extension, adduction, depression, and medial
rotation of humerus at shoulder (glenohumeral joint)

N. Thoracodorsal nerve (C6, C7, C8)

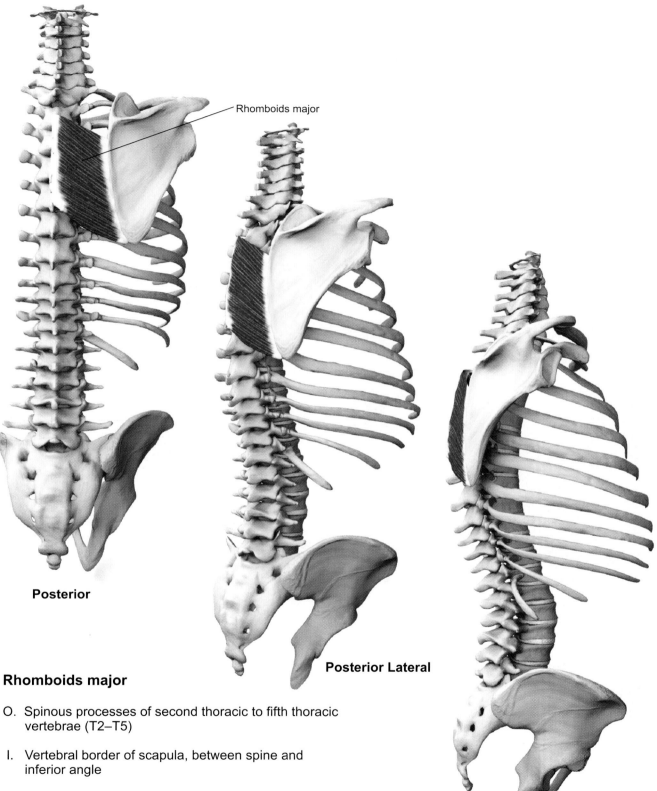

Rhomboids major

Posterior

Posterior Lateral

Lateral

Rhomboids major

O. Spinous processes of second thoracic to fifth thoracic vertebrae (T2–T5)

I. Vertebral border of scapula, between spine and inferior angle

A. Retraction, downward rotation and elevation of vertebral border of scapula (scapulothoracic joint)

N. Dorsal scapular nerve (C5)

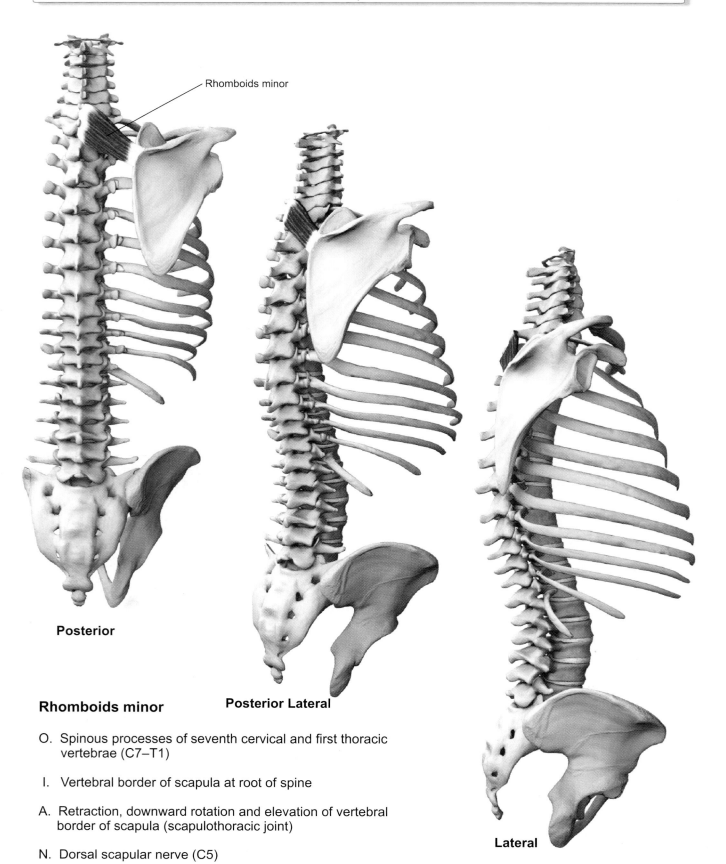

Posterior

Posterior Lateral

Lateral

Rhomboids minor

Rhomboids minor

O. Spinous processes of seventh cervical and first thoracic vertebrae (C7–T1)

I. Vertebral border of scapula at root of spine

A. Retraction, downward rotation and elevation of vertebral border of scapula (scapulothoracic joint)

N. Dorsal scapular nerve (C5)

Unit 3 Muscular System

Levator scapula

O. Transverse processes of upper four cervical vertebrae (C1–C4)

I. Vertebral border of scapula—between superior angle and root of spine

A. *Unilaterally:*
With origin fixed: elevation of scapula, assists downward rotation of scapula (scapulothoracic joint)
With insertion fixed: lateral flexion of neck and rotation of neck and head to same side
Bilaterally: assists in extension of the neck

N. Dorsal scapular nerve (C5) and branches of cervical nerves (C3, C4)

Levator scapula

Posterior Lateral

Posterior

Anterior Lateral

Serratus posterior superior

O. Lower portion of ligamentum nuchae, spinous processes of seventh cervical vertebrae, first and second thoracic vertebrae (C7–T2)

I. Superior borders of second through fifth ribs—posterior aspect

A. Assists in forced inspiration by elevation of ribs

N. Intercostal nerves (T1–T4)

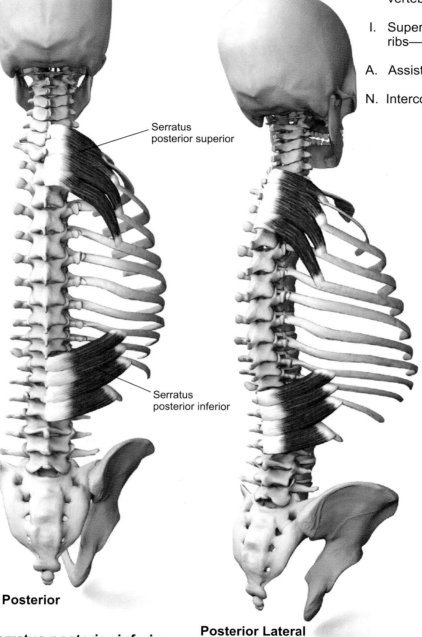

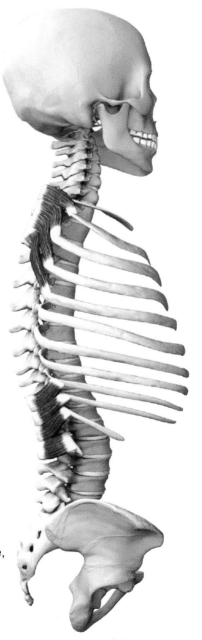

Serratus posterior superior

Serratus posterior inferior

Posterior

Posterior Lateral

Lateral

Serratus posterior inferior

O. Spinous processes and supraspinous ligaments of lower two thoracic vertebrae, upper two lumbar vertebrae (T11–L2)

I. Inferior borders of ninth through twelfth ribs—posterior aspect

A. Depression of lower four ribs

N. Intercostal nerves (T9–T12)

Unit 3 Muscular System

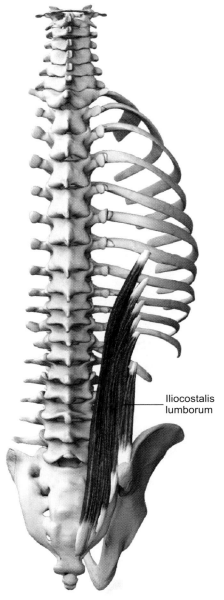

Posterior

Iliocostalis
lumborum

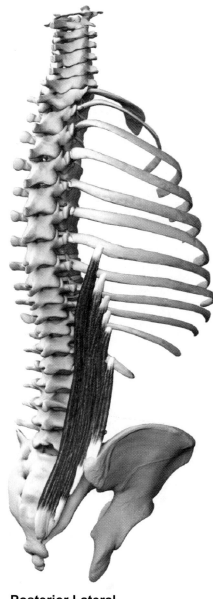

Posterior Lateral

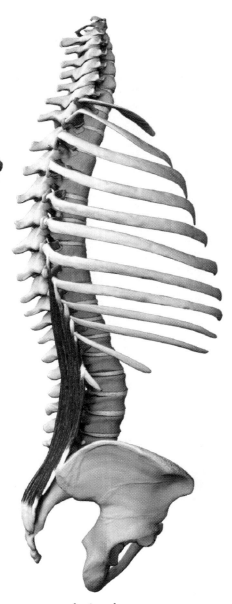

Lateral

Iliocostalis lumborum

O. Medial and lateral sacral crests, posterior iliac crest—medial portion

I. Angles of lower six ribs

A. *Bilaterally:* extension of vertebral column
Unilaterally: lateral flexion of vertebral column

N. Dorsal rami of thoracic and lumbar spinal nerves

Longissimus thoracis

O. Thoracolumbar aponeurosis and transverse processes of lumbar vertebrae

I. Transverse processes of all thoracic vertebrae— between tubercles and angles of lower ten ribs

A. *Bilaterally:* extension of vertebral column
Unilaterally: lateral flexion of vertebral column

N. Dorsal rami of thoracic and lumbar spinal nerves

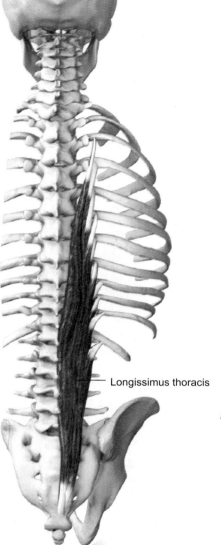

Longissimus thoracis

Posterior

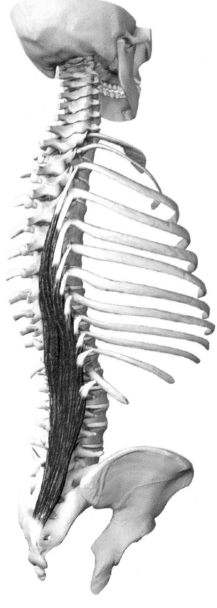

Posterior Lateral

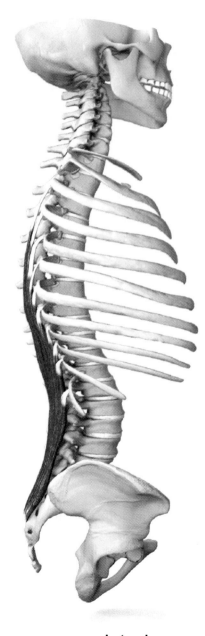

Lateral

Unit 3 Muscular System

Splenius capitis

O. Ligamentum nuchae—lower half, spinous processes of seventh cervical vertebrae, first three or four thoracic vertebrae (C7–T3 or T4)

I. Mastoid process of temporal bone, occipital bone—just inferior to lateral one-third of superior nuchal line

A. Bilaterally: extension of head and neck
Unilaterally: rotation of head to same side
With head rotated to one side and chin tilted upward: same side rotates head and neck, opposite side extends head and neck

N. Dorsal rami of cervical nerves (C2–C6)

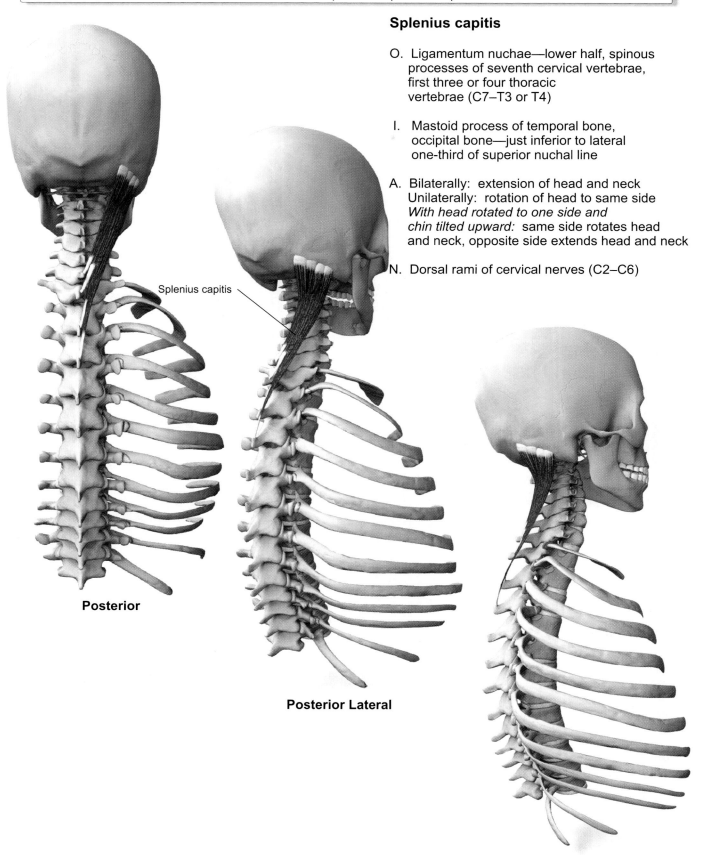

Splenius capitis

Posterior

Posterior Lateral

Lateral

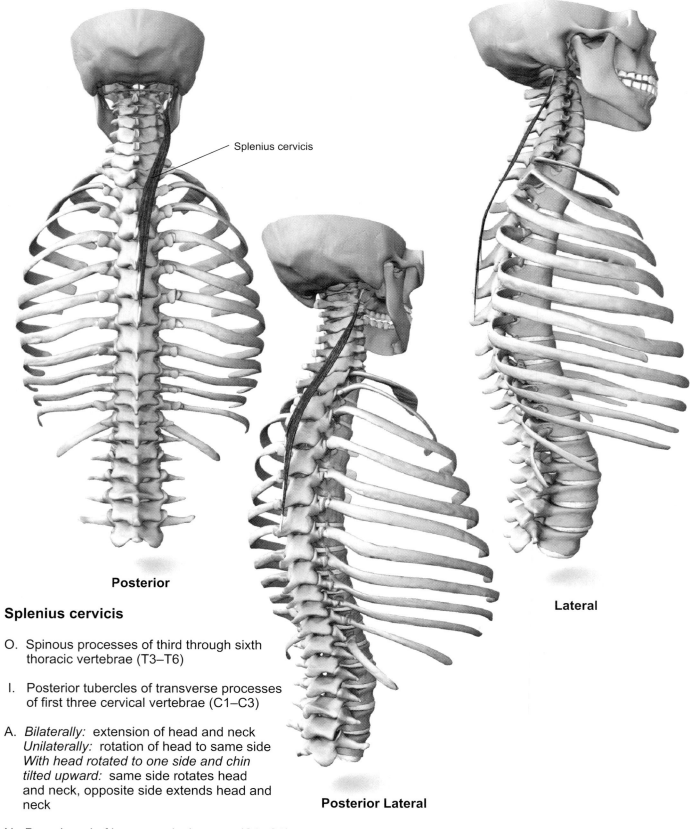

Splenius cervicis

Posterior

Posterior Lateral

Lateral

Splenius cervicis

O. Spinous processes of third through sixth
thoracic vertebrae (T3–T6)

I. Posterior tubercles of transverse processes
of first three cervical vertebrae (C1–C3)

A. *Bilaterally:* extension of head and neck
Unilaterally: rotation of head to same side
*With head rotated to one side and chin
tilted upward:* same side rotates head
and neck, opposite side extends head and
neck

N. Dorsal rami of lower cervical nerves (C2–C6)

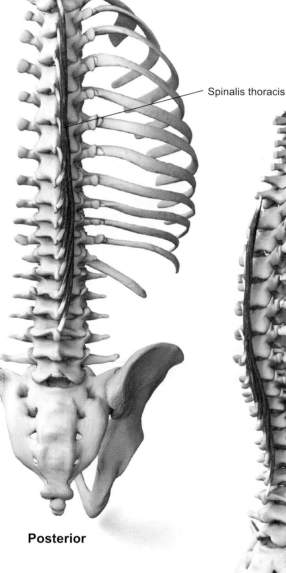

Spinalis thoracis

O. Spinous processes of lower two thoracic and upper two lumbar vertebrae (T11–L2)

I. Spinous processes of upper four or possibly upper eight thoracic vertebrae (T1–T4 up to T8)

A. Extension of vertebral column

N. Dorsal rami of thoracic and lumbar spinal nerves

Spinalis thoracis

Posterior

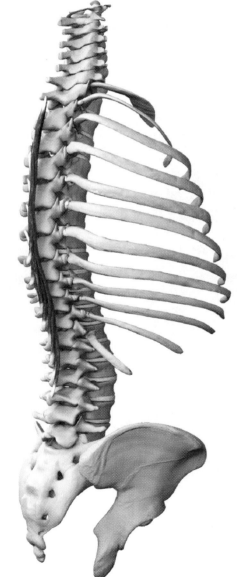

Posterior Lateral

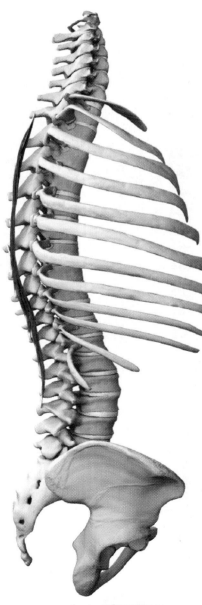

Lateral

Spinalis capitis

O. Transverse processes of seventh cervical and upper seven thoracic vertebrae (C7–T7)

I. Occipital bone—between superior and inferior nuchal lines

A. Extension of vertebral column

N. Dorsal rami of lower cervical and thoracic spinal nerves

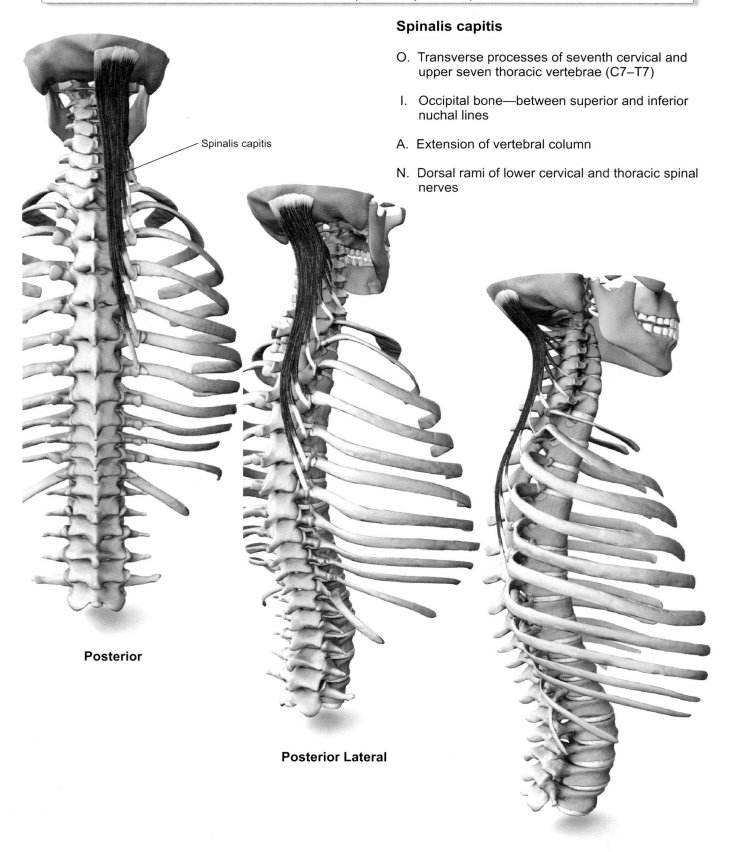

Spinalis capitis

Posterior

Posterior Lateral

Lateral

Unit 3 Muscular System

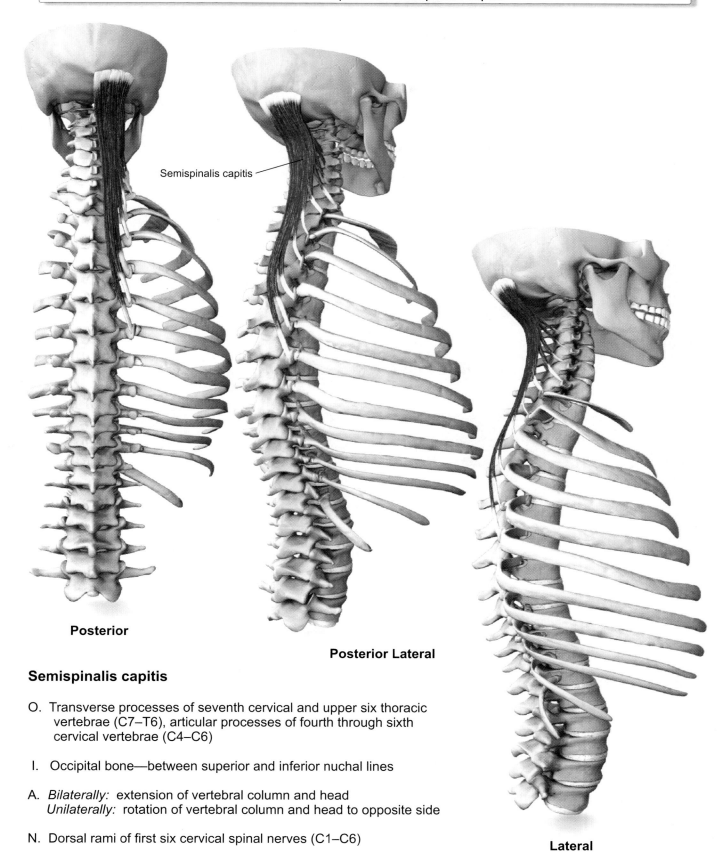

Semispinalis capitis

Posterior

Posterior Lateral

Lateral

Semispinalis capitis

O. Transverse processes of seventh cervical and upper six thoracic vertebrae (C7–T6), articular processes of fourth through sixth cervical vertebrae (C4–C6)

I. Occipital bone—between superior and inferior nuchal lines

A. *Bilaterally:* extension of vertebral column and head
Unilaterally: rotation of vertebral column and head to opposite side

N. Dorsal rami of first six cervical spinal nerves (C1–C6)

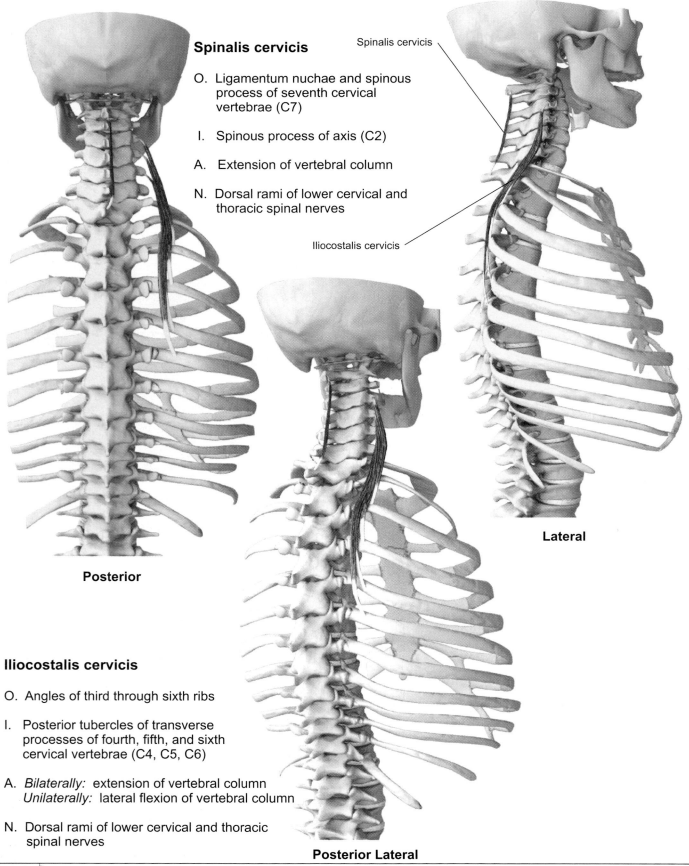

Spinalis cervicis

O. Ligamentum nuchae and spinous process of seventh cervical vertebrae (C7)

I. Spinous process of axis (C2)

A. Extension of vertebral column

N. Dorsal rami of lower cervical and thoracic spinal nerves

Spinalis cervicis

Iliocostalis cervicis

Lateral

Posterior

Iliocostalis cervicis

O. Angles of third through sixth ribs

I. Posterior tubercles of transverse processes of fourth, fifth, and sixth cervical vertebrae (C4, C5, C6)

A. *Bilaterally:* extension of vertebral column
   Unilaterally: lateral flexion of vertebral column

N. Dorsal rami of lower cervical and thoracic spinal nerves

Posterior Lateral

Unit 3 Muscular System

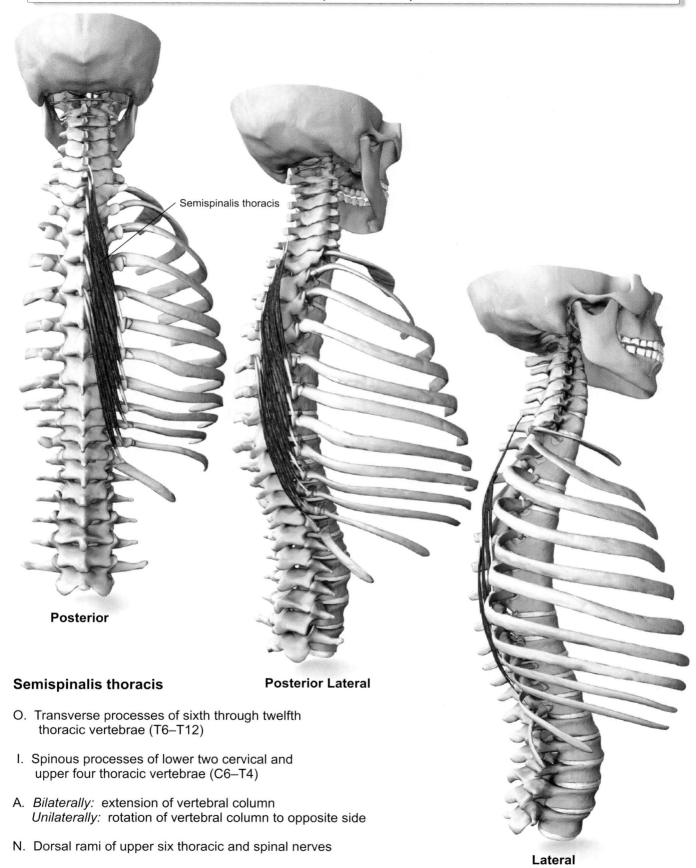

Semispinalis thoracis

Posterior

Posterior Lateral

Lateral

Semispinalis thoracis

O. Transverse processes of sixth through twelfth thoracic vertebrae (T6–T12)

I. Spinous processes of lower two cervical and upper four thoracic vertebrae (C6–T4)

A. *Bilaterally:* extension of vertebral column
Unilaterally: rotation of vertebral column to opposite side

N. Dorsal rami of upper six thoracic and spinal nerves

Unit 3 Muscular System

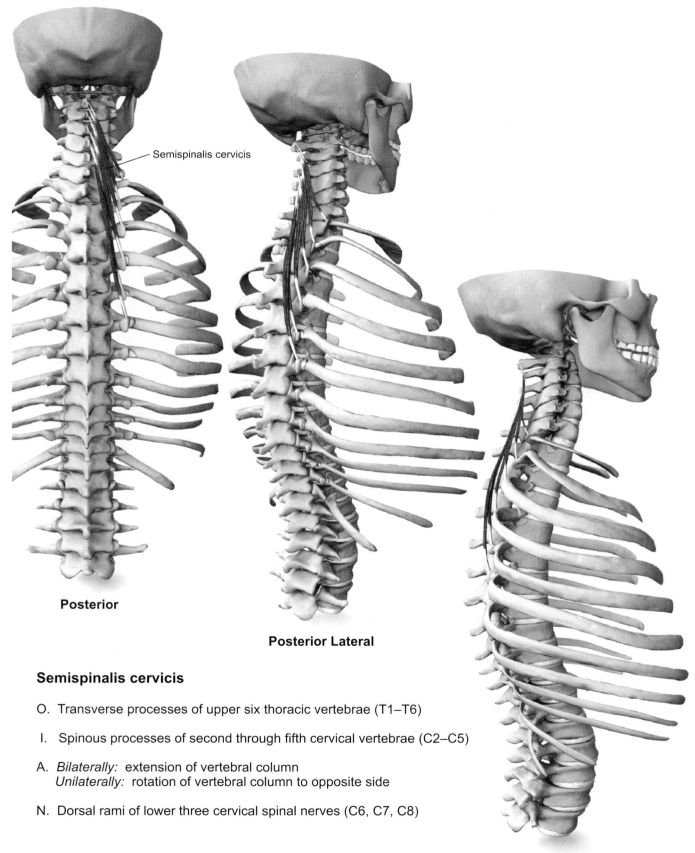

Semispinalis cervicis

Posterior

Posterior Lateral

Lateral

Semispinalis cervicis

O. Transverse processes of upper six thoracic vertebrae (T1–T6)

I. Spinous processes of second through fifth cervical vertebrae (C2–C5)

A. *Bilaterally:* extension of vertebral column
    Unilaterally: rotation of vertebral column to opposite side

N. Dorsal rami of lower three cervical spinal nerves (C6, C7, C8)

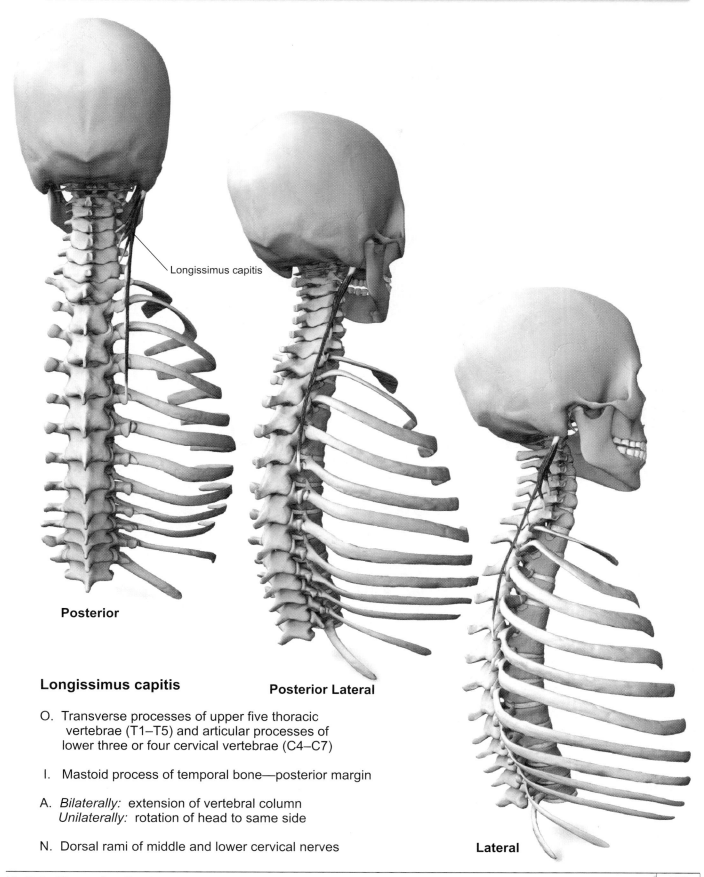

Longissimus capitis

Posterior

Posterior Lateral

Lateral

Longissimus capitis

O. Transverse processes of upper five thoracic
   vertebrae (T1–T5) and articular processes of
   lower three or four cervical vertebrae (C4–C7)

I. Mastoid process of temporal bone—posterior margin

A. *Bilaterally:* extension of vertebral column
   Unilaterally: rotation of head to same side

N. Dorsal rami of middle and lower cervical nerves

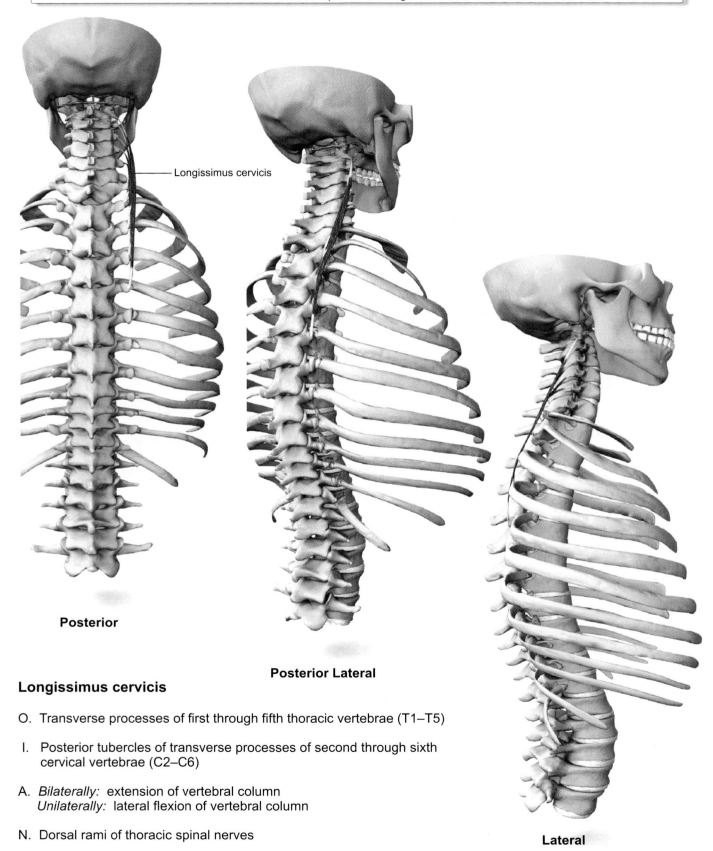

Longissimus cervicis

Posterior

Posterior Lateral

Lateral

Longissimus cervicis

O. Transverse processes of first through fifth thoracic vertebrae (T1–T5)

I. Posterior tubercles of transverse processes of second through sixth cervical vertebrae (C2–C6)

A. *Bilaterally:* extension of vertebral column
    Unilaterally: lateral flexion of vertebral column

N. Dorsal rami of thoracic spinal nerves

Unit 3 Muscular System

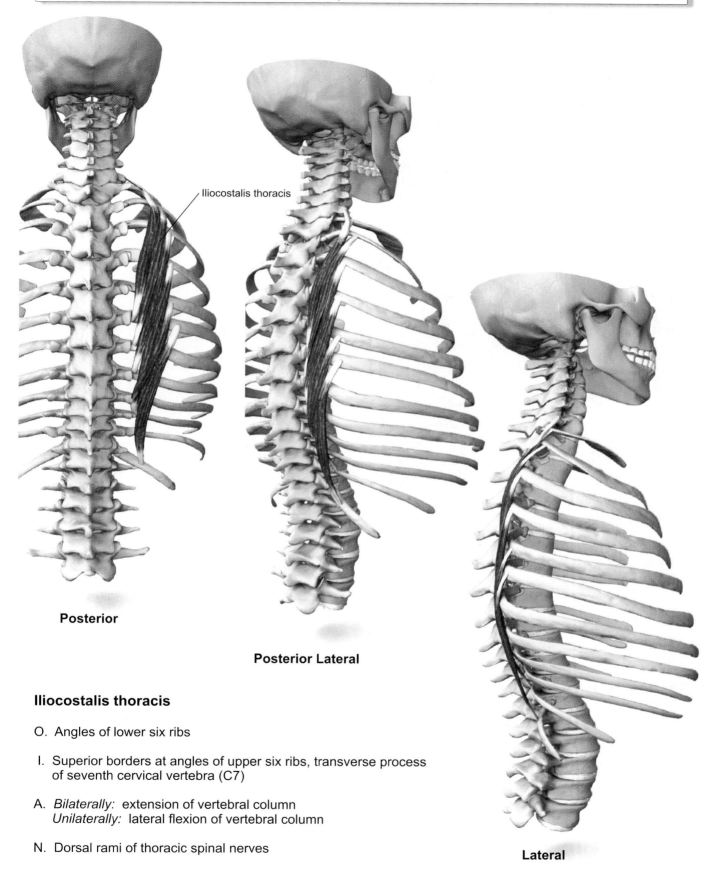

Iliocostalis thoracis

Posterior

Posterior Lateral

Lateral

Iliocostalis thoracis

O. Angles of lower six ribs

I. Superior borders at angles of upper six ribs, transverse process of seventh cervical vertebra (C7)

A. *Bilaterally:* extension of vertebral column
Unilaterally: lateral flexion of vertebral column

N. Dorsal rami of thoracic spinal nerves

Unit 3 Muscular System

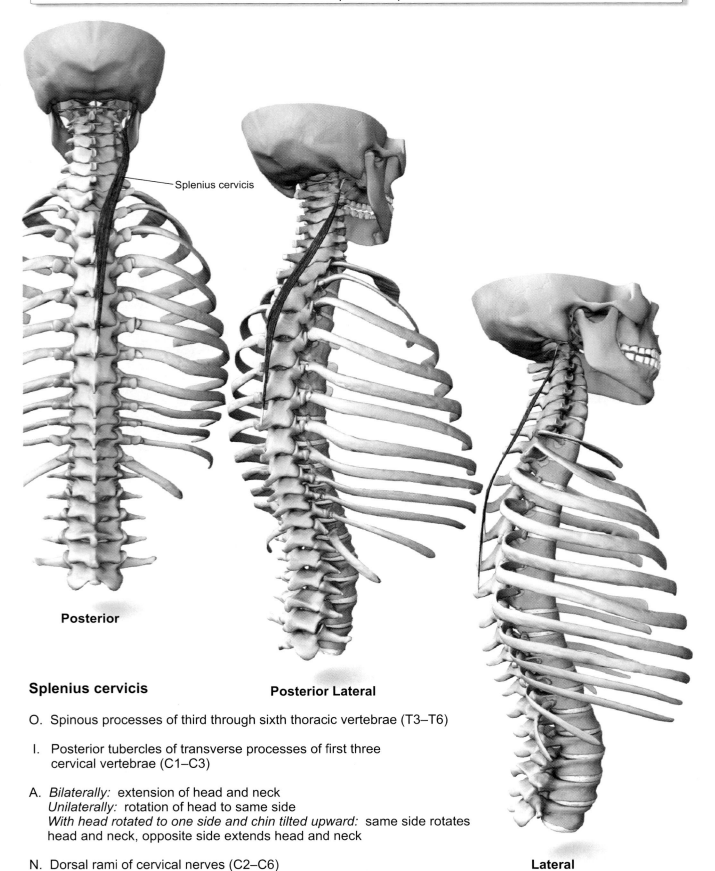

Posterior

Posterior Lateral

Lateral

Splenius cervicis

O. Spinous processes of third through sixth thoracic vertebrae (T3–T6)

I. Posterior tubercles of transverse processes of first three
cervical vertebrae (C1–C3)

A. *Bilaterally:* extension of head and neck
Unilaterally: rotation of head to same side
With head rotated to one side and chin tilted upward: same side rotates
head and neck, opposite side extends head and neck

N. Dorsal rami of cervical nerves (C2–C6)

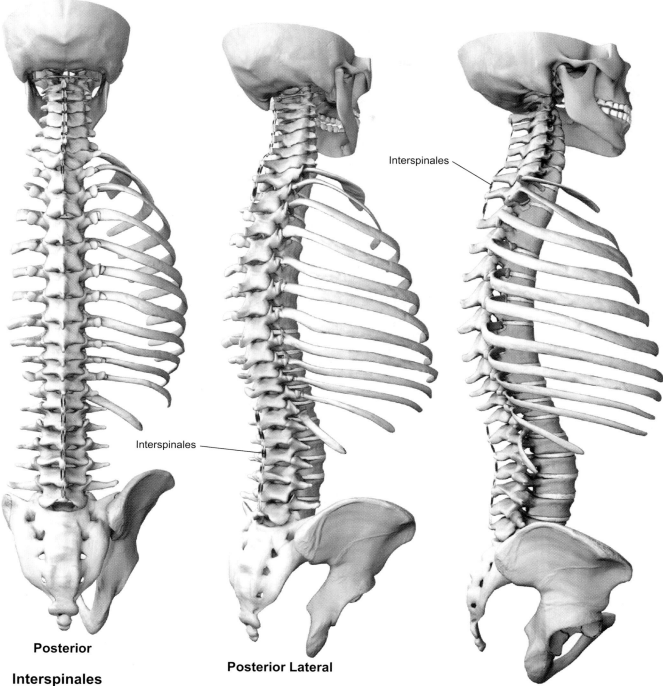

Posterior

Posterior Lateral

Lateral

Interspinales

O. Spinous processes of second to seventh cervical vertebrae (C2–C7), spinous processes of first and second (T1–T2), eleventh and twelfth (T11–T12) thoracic vertebrae, spinous processes of first through fifth lumbar vertebrae (L1–L5)

I. Spinous processes of vertebrae directly above origin

A. Extension of vertebral column

N. Dorsal rami of spinal nerves

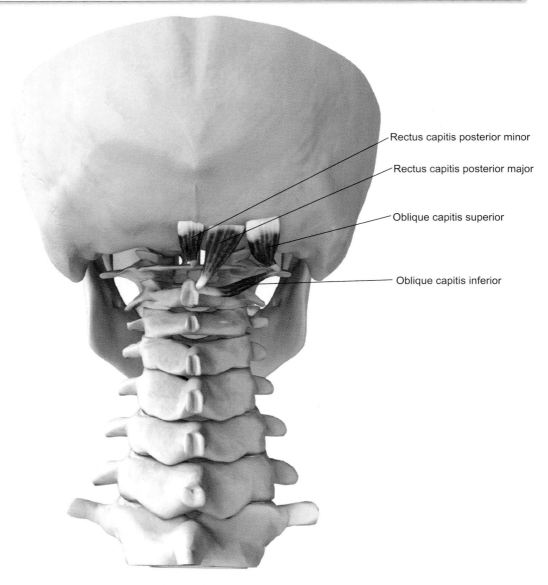

Rectus capitis posterior minor

Rectus capitis posterior major

Oblique capitis superior

Oblique capitis inferior

Posterior

Rectus capitis posterior minor

O. Posterior tubercle of atlas (C1)

I. Inferior nuchal line of occipital bone—adjacent to midline

A. Extension of head

N. Suboccipital nerve (dorsal rami of C1)

Rectus capitis posterior major

O. Spinous process of axis (C2)

I. Inferior nuchal line of occipital bone—lateral aspect

A. Extension of head, rotation of head to same side

N. Suboccipital nerve (dorsal rami of C1)

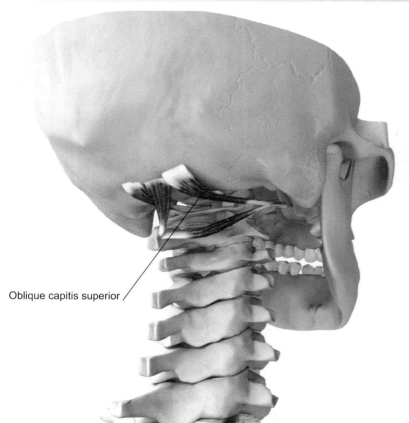

Oblique capitis superior

Posterior Lateral

Oblique capitis superior

O. Transverse process of atlas (C1)

I. Occipital bone—between superior and inferior nuchal lines

A. Extension and lateral flexion of head

N. Suboccipital nerve (dorsal rami of C1)

Oblique capitis inferior

O. Spinous process of axis (C2)

I. Transverse process of atlas (C1)

A. Rotation of head to same side

N. Suboccipital nerve (dorsal rami of C1)

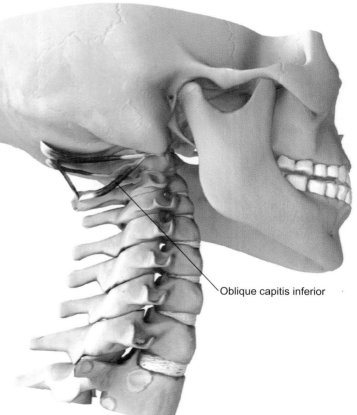

Oblique capitis inferior

Lateral

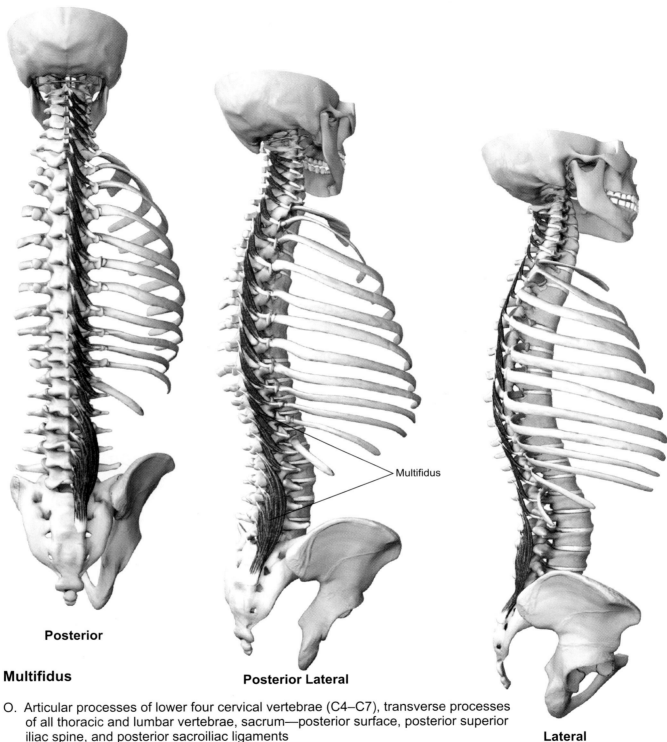

Multifidus

Posterior

Posterior Lateral

Lateral

Multifidus

O. Articular processes of lower four cervical vertebrae (C4–C7), transverse processes of all thoracic and lumbar vertebrae, sacrum—posterior surface, posterior superior iliac spine, and posterior sacroiliac ligaments

I. Spinous processes of two to three vertebrae above vertebrae of origin

A. *Bilaterally:* extension of vertebral column
   Unilaterally: rotation of vertebral column to opposite side

N. Dorsal rami of spinal nerves

Unit 3 Muscular System

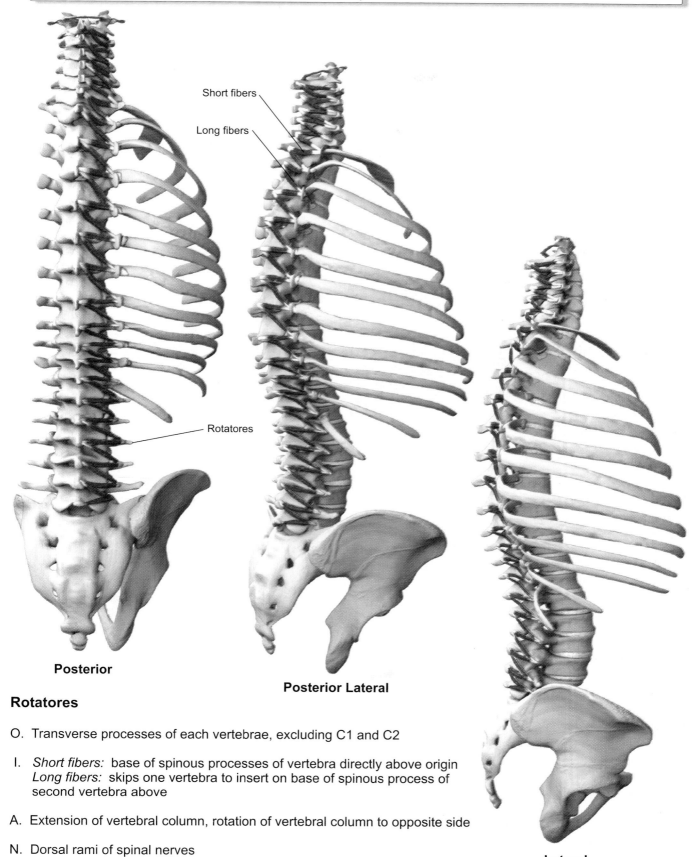

Short fibers

Long fibers

Rotatores

Posterior

Posterior Lateral

Lateral

Rotatores

O. Transverse processes of each vertebrae, excluding C1 and C2

I. *Short fibers:* base of spinous processes of vertebra directly above origin
Long fibers: skips one vertebra to insert on base of spinous process of second vertebra above

A. Extension of vertebral column, rotation of vertebral column to opposite side

N. Dorsal rami of spinal nerves

Unit 3 Muscular System

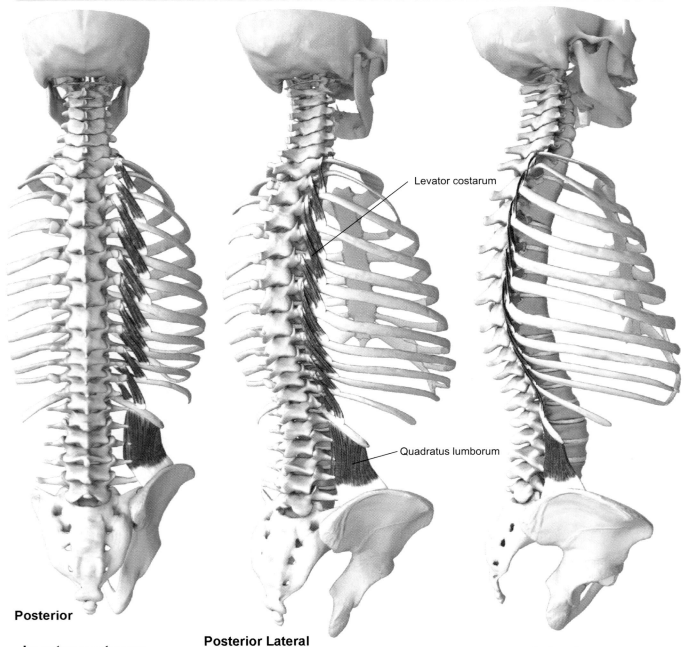

Levator costarum

Quadratus lumborum

Posterior

Posterior Lateral

Lateral

Levator costarum

O. Transverse processes of seventh cervical and first eleven thoracic vertebrae (C7–T11)

I. Costal angle of subadjacent ribs—one through twelve

A. Elevation of ribs, lateral flexion and rotation of vertebral column, assists in respiration

N. Dorsal primary rami of spinal nerves (C8–T11)

Quadratus lumborum

O. Posterior iliac crest and iliolumbar ligament

I. Inferior border of twelfth rib, transverse processes of first through fourth lumbar vertebrae (L1–L4)

A. *Bilaterally:* extension and stabilization of lumbar vertebrae, stabilization of twelfth rib (for inhalation and forced exhalation)
Unilaterally: lateral flexion of lumbar spine
With spine fixed: elevation of hip

N. Lumbar plexus (T12–L3)

Unit 3 Muscular System

Intertransversarii

The intertransversarii are sets of muscles spanning between the vertebrae and are most distinct in the cervical spine. Documentation of placement for these sets is conflicting. Some sources include attachments connecting the transverse vertebrae throughout the entire vertebral column. Other references record connections in the thoracic region, primarily at superior or inferior segments. In addition, there are publications that site a complete absence of these muscles in the thoracic region.

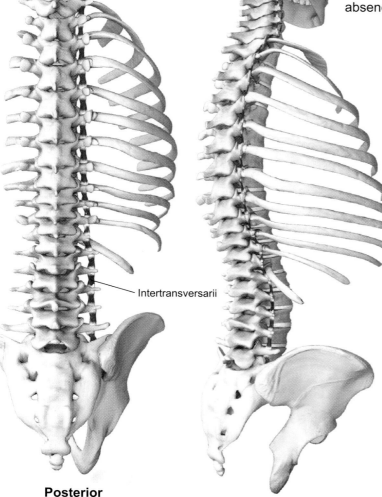

Intertransversarii

Posterior

Posterior Lateral

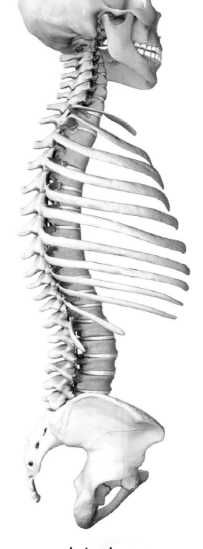

Lateral

Intertransversarii

O. Upper border of transverse processes of all vertebrae

I. Lower border of transverse process of vertebra directly above origin

A. Extension and lateral flexion of vertebral column

N. Ventral and dorsal rami of spinal nerves

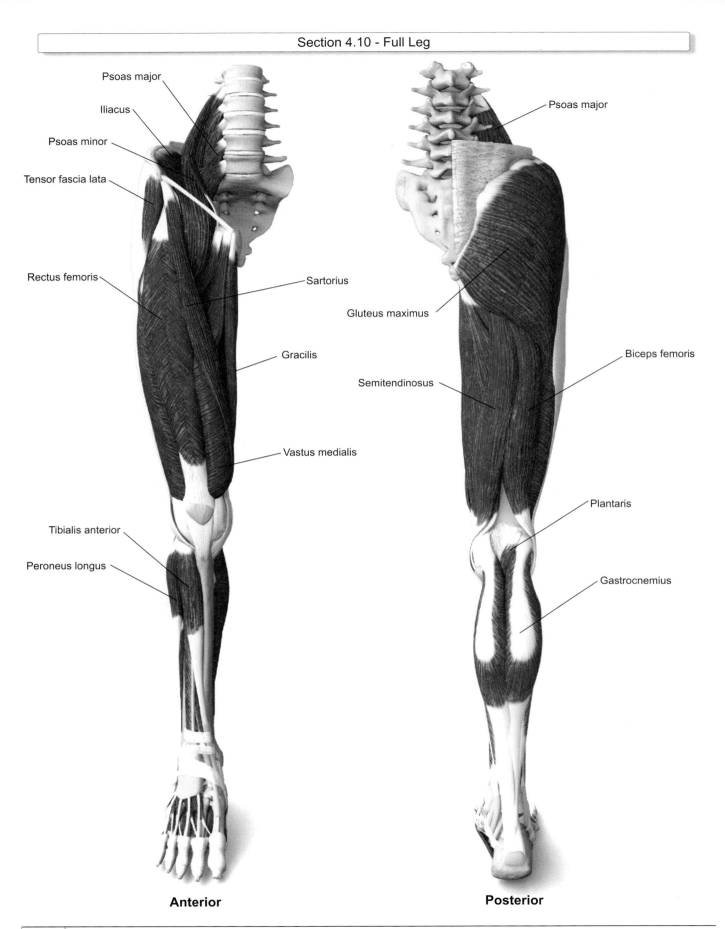

Psoas major

Iliacus

Psoas minor

Tensor fascia lata

Rectus femoris

Psoas major

Sartorius

Gluteus maximus

Gracilis

Biceps femoris

Semitendinosus

Vastus medialis

Plantaris

Tibialis anterior

Peroneus longus

Gastrocnemius

Anterior

Posterior

Unit 3 Muscular System

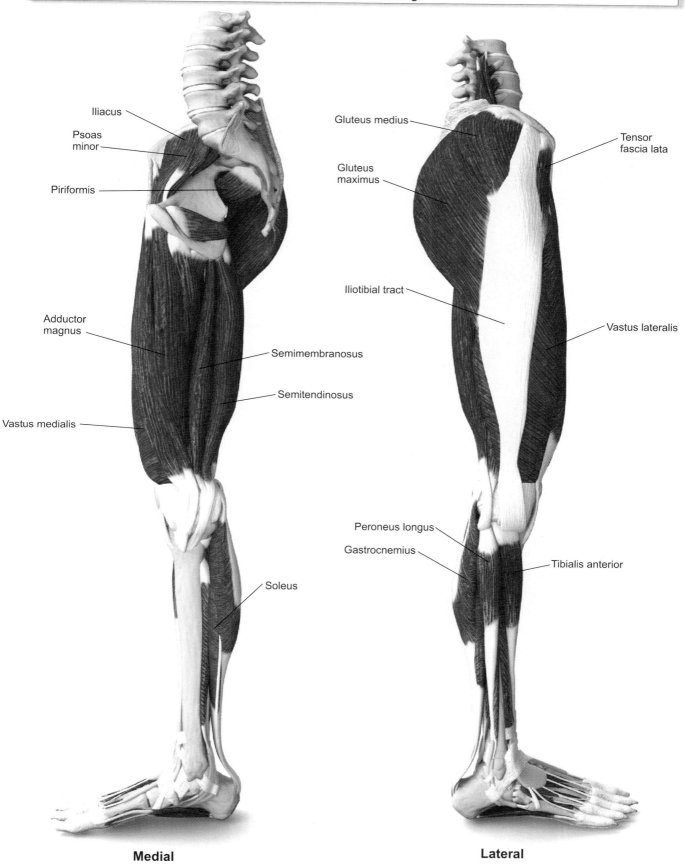

Iliacus

Psoas
minor

Piriformis

Adductor
magnus

Vastus medialis

Semimembranosus

Semitendinosus

Soleus

Gluteus medius

Gluteus
maximus

Tensor
fascia lata

Iliotibial tract

Vastus lateralis

Peroneus longus

Gastrocnemius

Tibialis anterior

Medial

Lateral

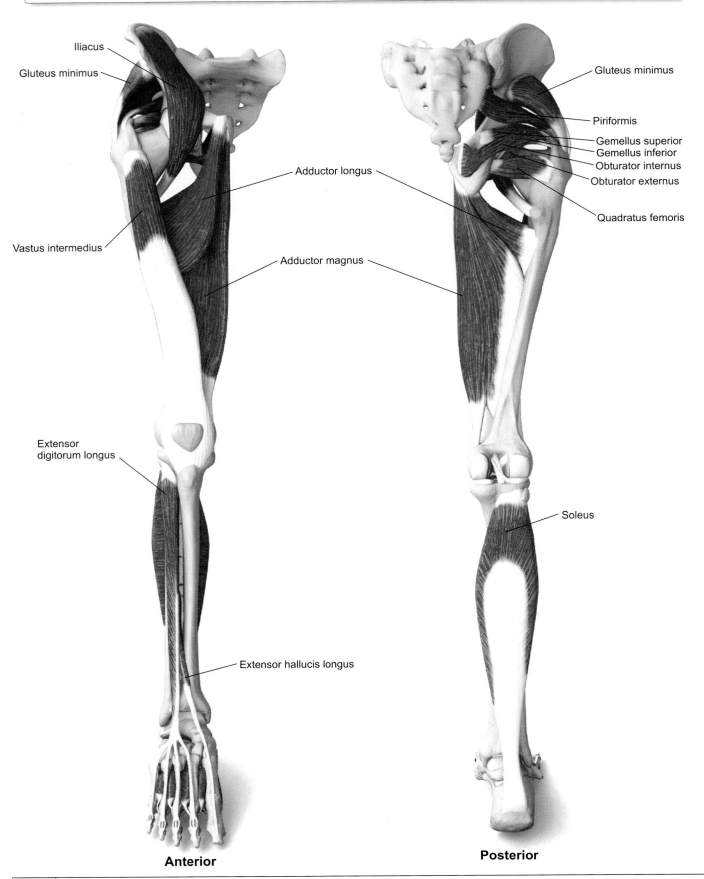

Iliacus

Gluteus minimus

Adductor longus

Vastus intermedius

Adductor magnus

Extensor
digitorum longus

Extensor hallucis longus

Gluteus minimus

Piriformis

Gemellus superior
Gemellus inferior
Obturator internus
Obturator externus

Quadratus femoris

Soleus

Anterior

Posterior

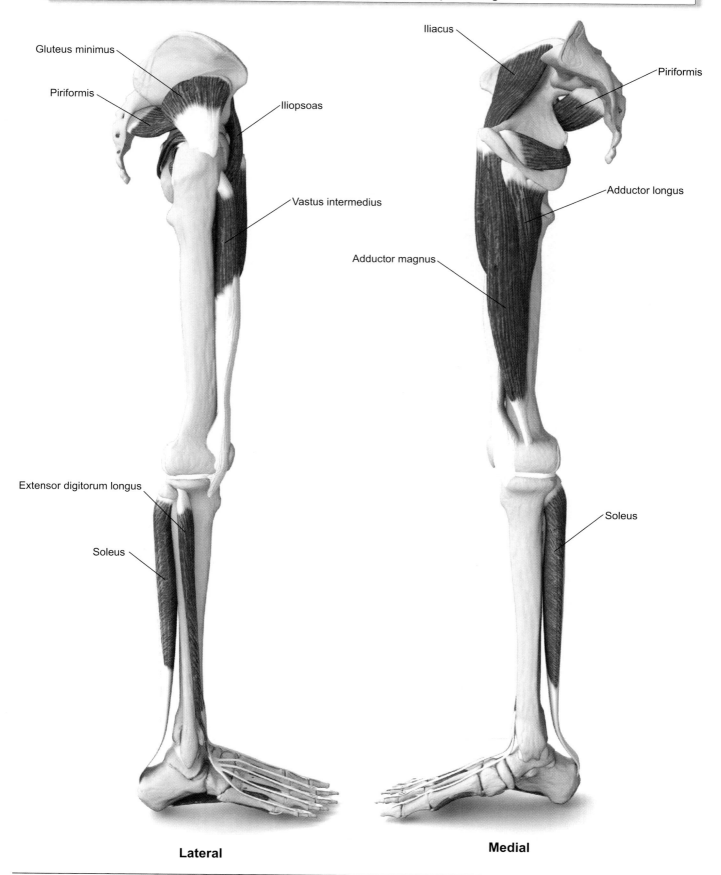

Gluteus minimus

Piriformis

Iliopsoas

Vastus intermedius

Extensor digitorum longus

Soleus

Iliacus

Piriformis

Adductor longus

Adductor magnus

Soleus

Lateral

Medial

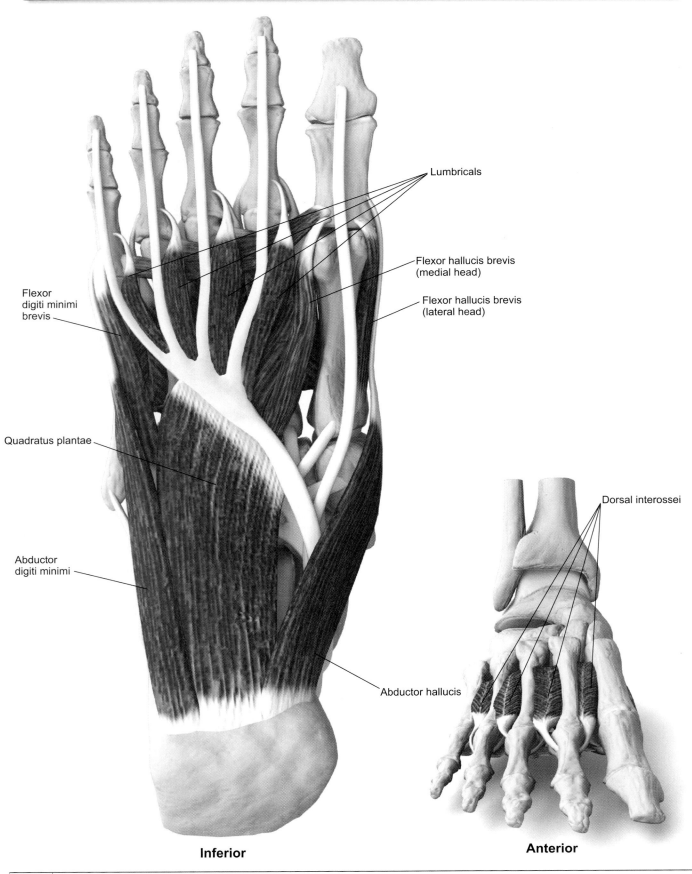

Lumbricals

Flexor hallucis brevis
(medial head)

Flexor hallucis brevis
(lateral head)

Flexor
digiti minimi
brevis

Quadratus plantae

Abductor
digiti minimi

Dorsal interossei

Abductor hallucis

Inferior

Anterior

Unit 3 Muscular System

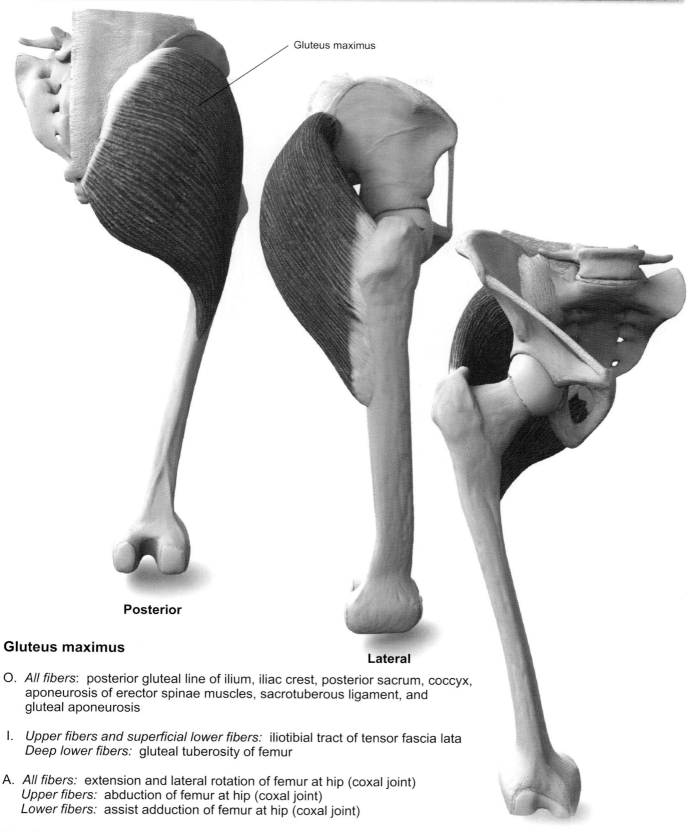

Gluteus maximus

Posterior

Lateral

Anterior

Gluteus maximus

O. *All fibers:* posterior gluteal line of ilium, iliac crest, posterior sacrum, coccyx, aponeurosis of erector spinae muscles, sacrotuberous ligament, and gluteal aponeurosis

I. *Upper fibers and superficial lower fibers:* iliotibial tract of tensor fascia lata
Deep lower fibers: gluteal tuberosity of femur

A. *All fibers:* extension and lateral rotation of femur at hip (coxal joint)
Upper fibers: abduction of femur at hip (coxal joint)
Lower fibers: assist adduction of femur at hip (coxal joint)

N. Inferior gluteal nerve (L5, S1, S2)

Unit 3 Muscular System

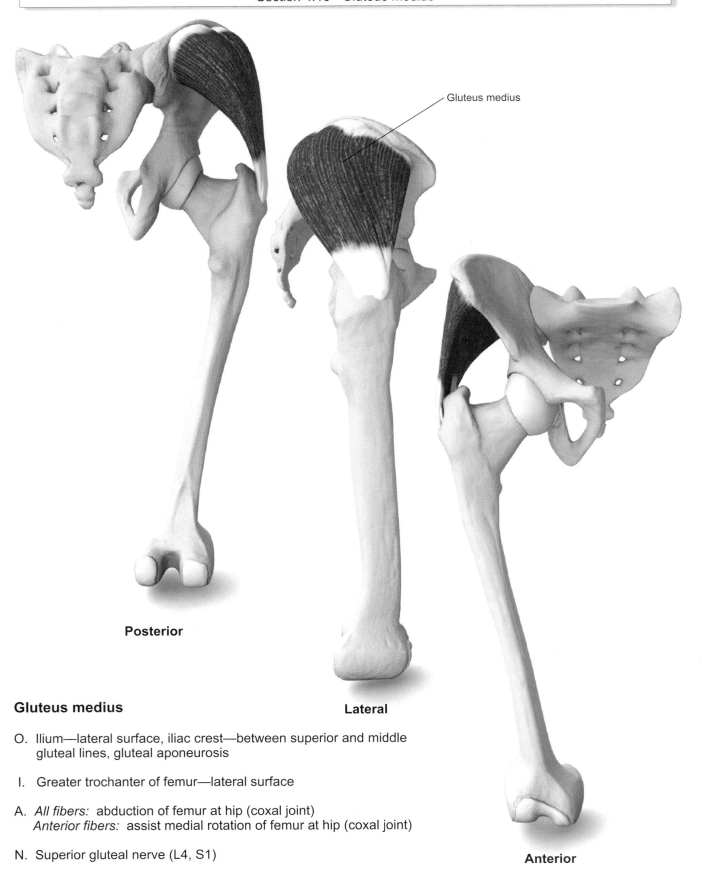

Gluteus medius

Posterior

Lateral

Anterior

Gluteus medius

O. Ilium—lateral surface, iliac crest—between superior and middle gluteal lines, gluteal aponeurosis

I. Greater trochanter of femur—lateral surface

A. *All fibers:* abduction of femur at hip (coxal joint)
    Anterior fibers: assist medial rotation of femur at hip (coxal joint)

N. Superior gluteal nerve (L4, S1)

Unit 3 Muscular System

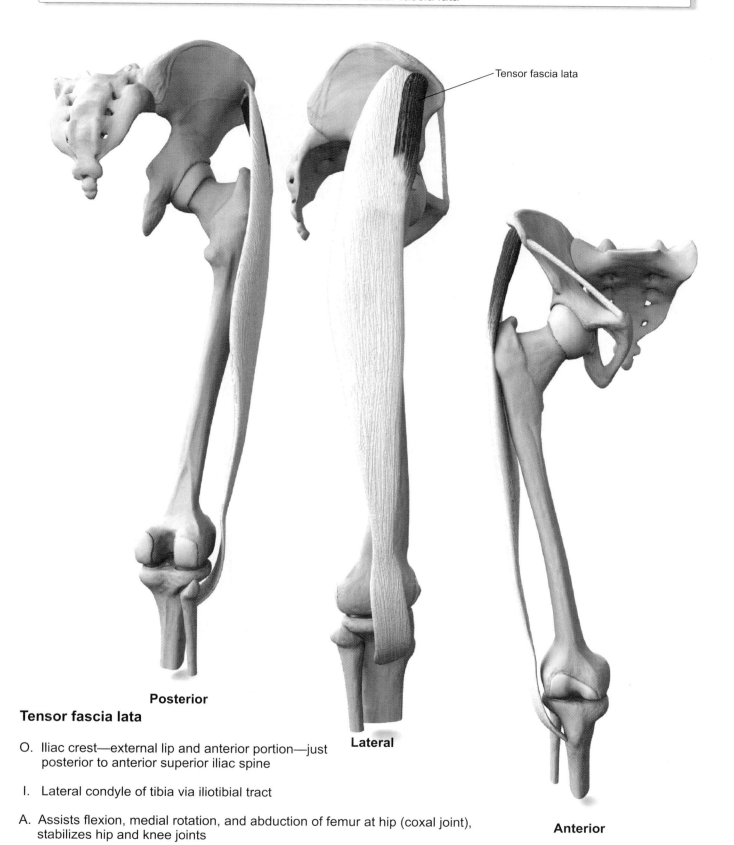

Tensor fascia lata

Posterior

Lateral

Anterior

Tensor fascia lata

O. Iliac crest—external lip and anterior portion—just posterior to anterior superior iliac spine

I. Lateral condyle of tibia via iliotibial tract

A. Assists flexion, medial rotation, and abduction of femur at hip (coxal joint), stabilizes hip and knee joints

N. Superior gluteal nerve (L4, L5, S1)

Unit 3 Muscular System

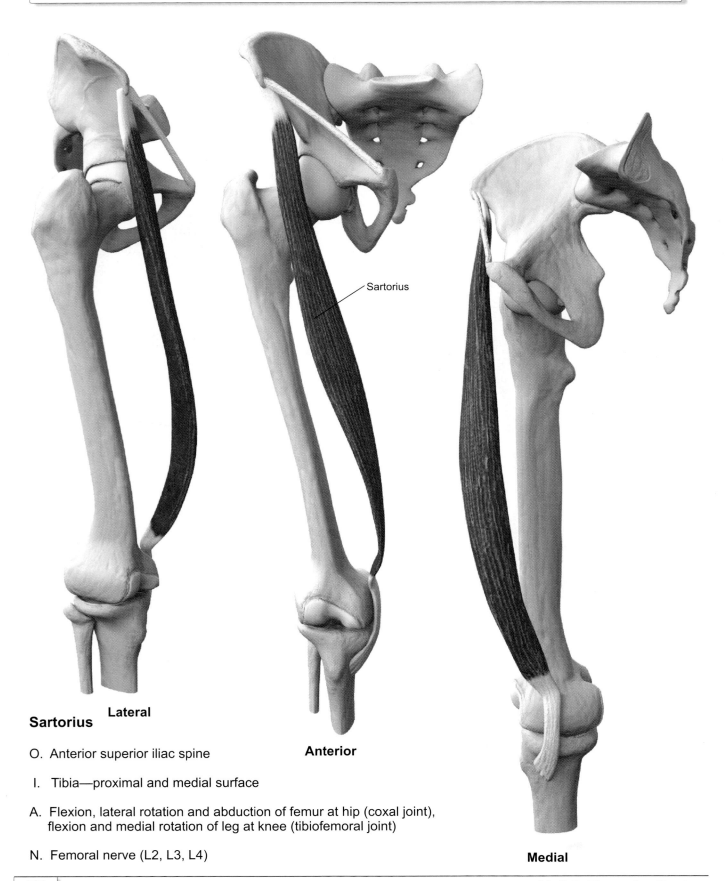

Sartorius

Lateral

Anterior

Medial

Sartorius

O. Anterior superior iliac spine

I. Tibia—proximal and medial surface

A. Flexion, lateral rotation and abduction of femur at hip (coxal joint), flexion and medial rotation of leg at knee (tibiofemoral joint)

N. Femoral nerve (L2, L3, L4)

Unit 3 Muscular System

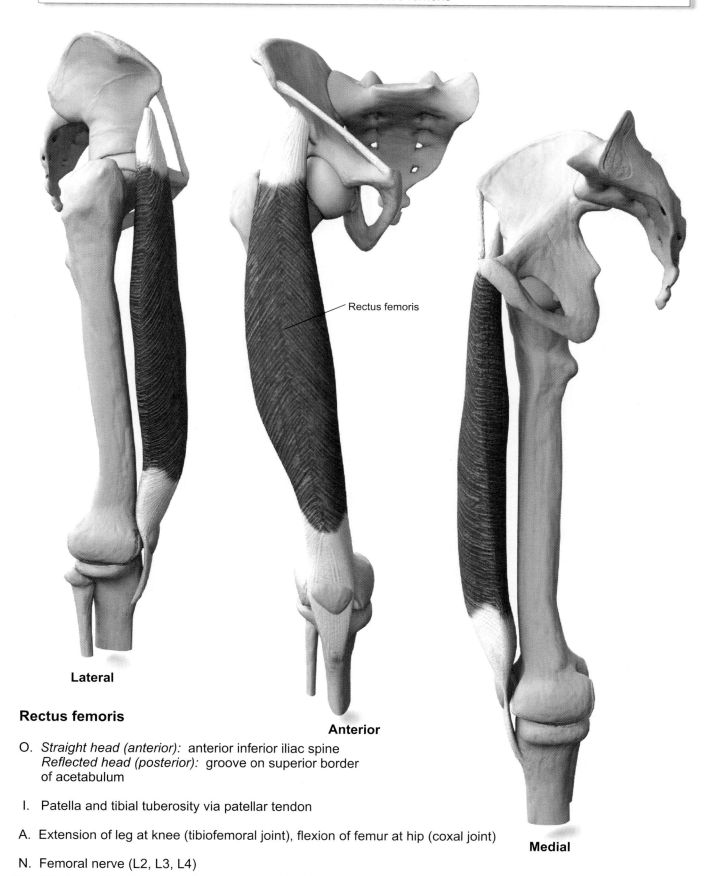

Rectus femoris

Lateral

Anterior

Medial

Rectus femoris

O. *Straight head (anterior):* anterior inferior iliac spine
    Reflected head (posterior): groove on superior border
    of acetabulum

I. Patella and tibial tuberosity via patellar tendon

A. Extension of leg at knee (tibiofemoral joint), flexion of femur at hip (coxal joint)

N. Femoral nerve (L2, L3, L4)

Unit 3 Muscular System

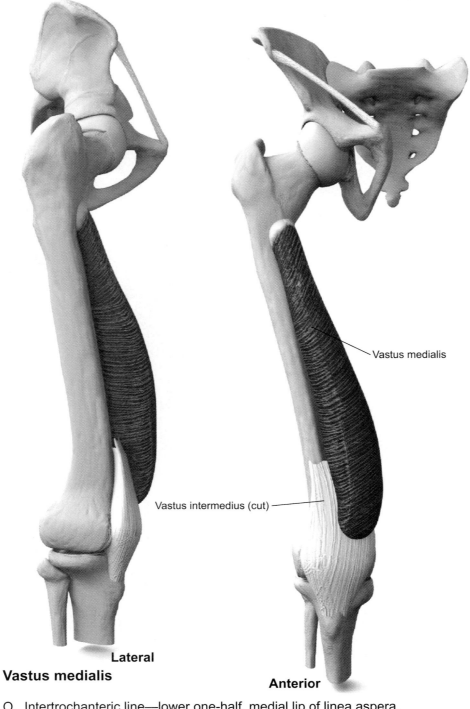

Lateral

Vastus medialis

Vastus intermedius (cut)

Anterior

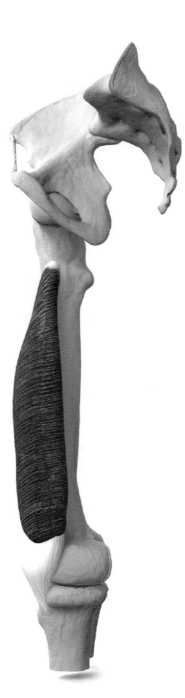

Medial

Vastus medialis

O. Intertrochanteric line—lower one-half, medial lip of linea aspera, medial supracondylar ridge of femur—upper portion, medial intramuscular septum

I. Patella and tibial tuberosity via patellar tendon

A. Extension of leg at knee (tibiofemoral joint), stabilizes patella

N. Femoral nerve (L2, L3, L4)

Unit 3 Muscular System

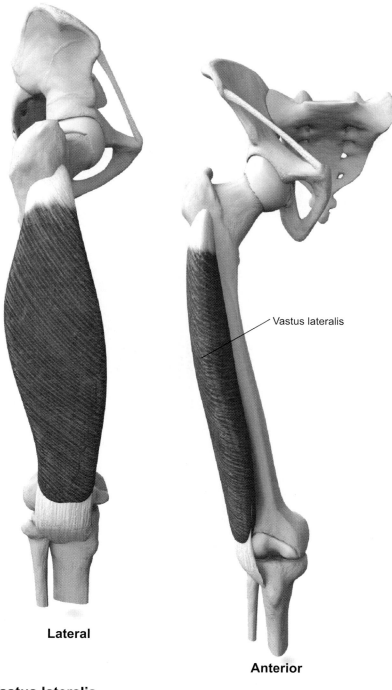

Lateral

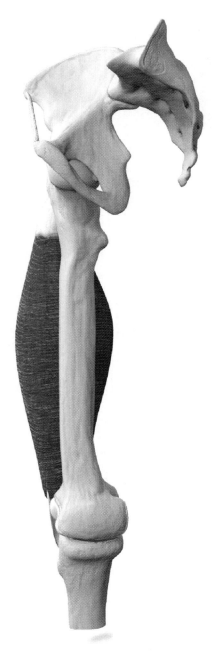

Vastus lateralis

Anterior

Medial

Vastus lateralis

O. Intertrochanteric line—superior portion, greater trochanter, lateral lip of linea aspera and gluteal tuberosity of femur

I. Patella and tibial tuberosity via patellar tendon

A. Extension of leg at knee (tibiofemoral joint), stabilizes patella

N. Femoral nerve (L2, L3, L4)

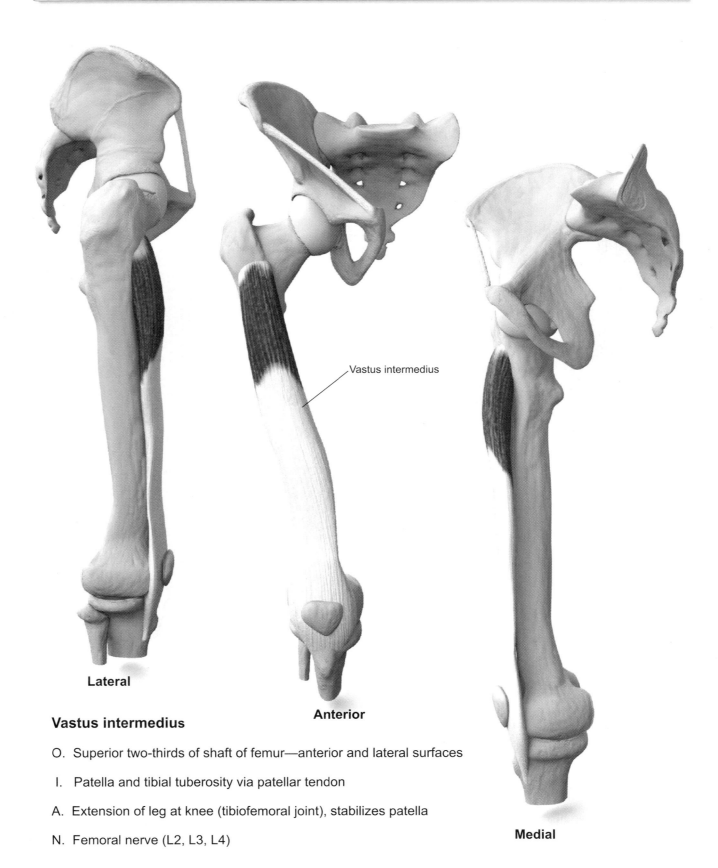

Lateral

Anterior

Vastus intermedius

Medial

Vastus intermedius

O. Superior two-thirds of shaft of femur—anterior and lateral surfaces

I. Patella and tibial tuberosity via patellar tendon

A. Extension of leg at knee (tibiofemoral joint), stabilizes patella

N. Femoral nerve (L2, L3, L4)

Unit 3 Muscular System

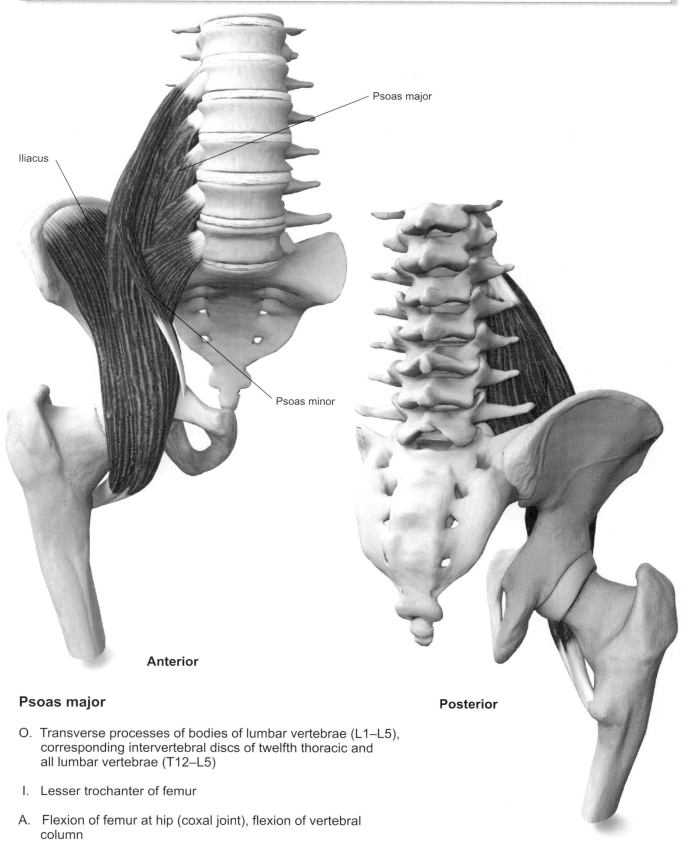

Psoas major

Iliacus

Psoas minor

Anterior

Posterior

Psoas major

O. Transverse processes of bodies of lumbar vertebrae (L1–L5), corresponding intervertebral discs of twelfth thoracic and all lumbar vertebrae (T12–L5)

I. Lesser trochanter of femur

A. Flexion of femur at hip (coxal joint), flexion of vertebral column

N. Ventral rami (L2, L3, L4)

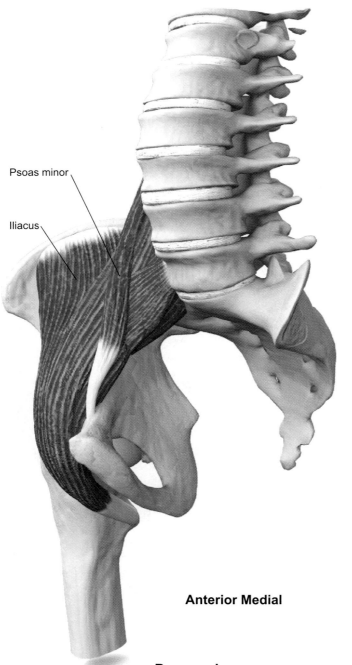

Psoas minor

Iliacus

Anterior Medial

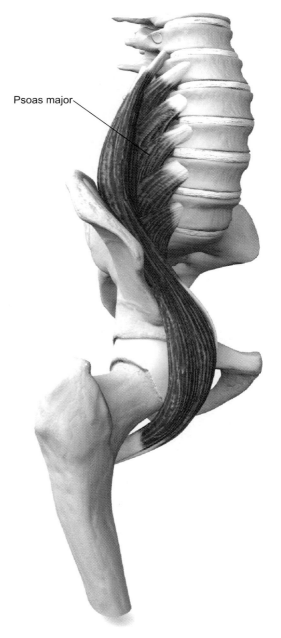

Psoas major

Anterior Lateral

Psoas minor

O. Vertebral body of twelfth thoracic vertebra, first lumbar vertebra and intervertebral disc between the two (T12–L1)

I. Iliopubic eminence, pectineal line of pubis, fascia overlying iliopsoas muscle

A. Flexion of lumbar vertebrae

N. Lumbar plexus (L1, L2)

Unit 3 Muscular System

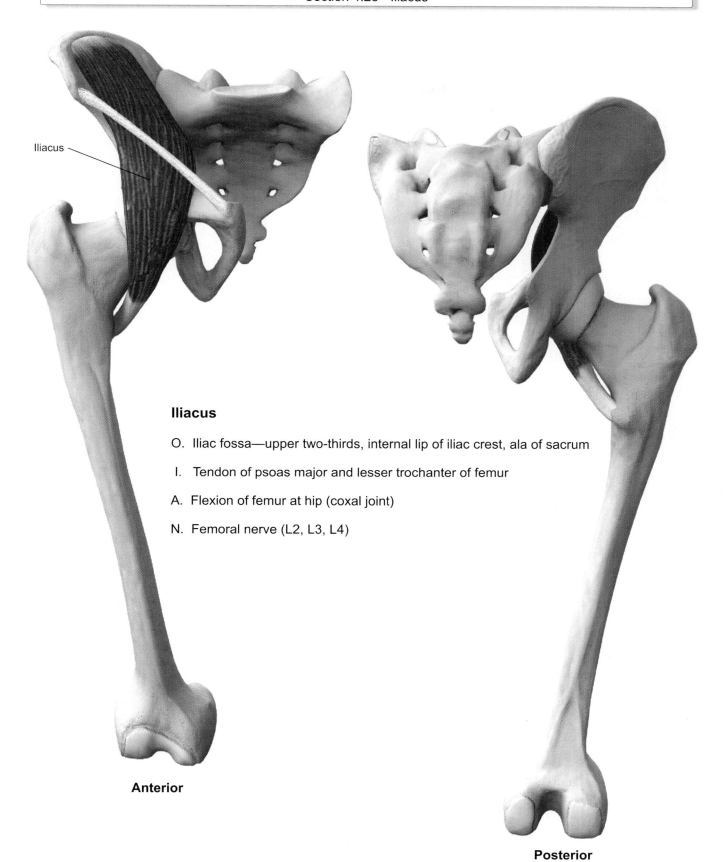

Iliacus

Iliacus

O. Iliac fossa—upper two-thirds, internal lip of iliac crest, ala of sacrum

I. Tendon of psoas major and lesser trochanter of femur

A. Flexion of femur at hip (coxal joint)

N. Femoral nerve (L2, L3, L4)

Anterior

Posterior

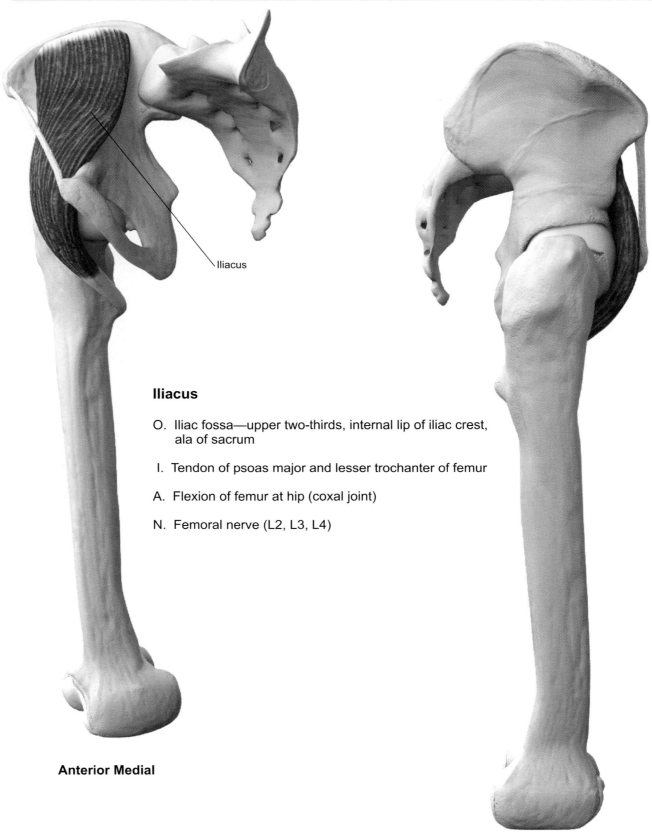

Iliacus

Iliacus

O. Iliac fossa—upper two-thirds, internal lip of iliac crest, ala of sacrum

I. Tendon of psoas major and lesser trochanter of femur

A. Flexion of femur at hip (coxal joint)

N. Femoral nerve (L2, L3, L4)

Anterior Medial

Lateral

Unit 3 Muscular System

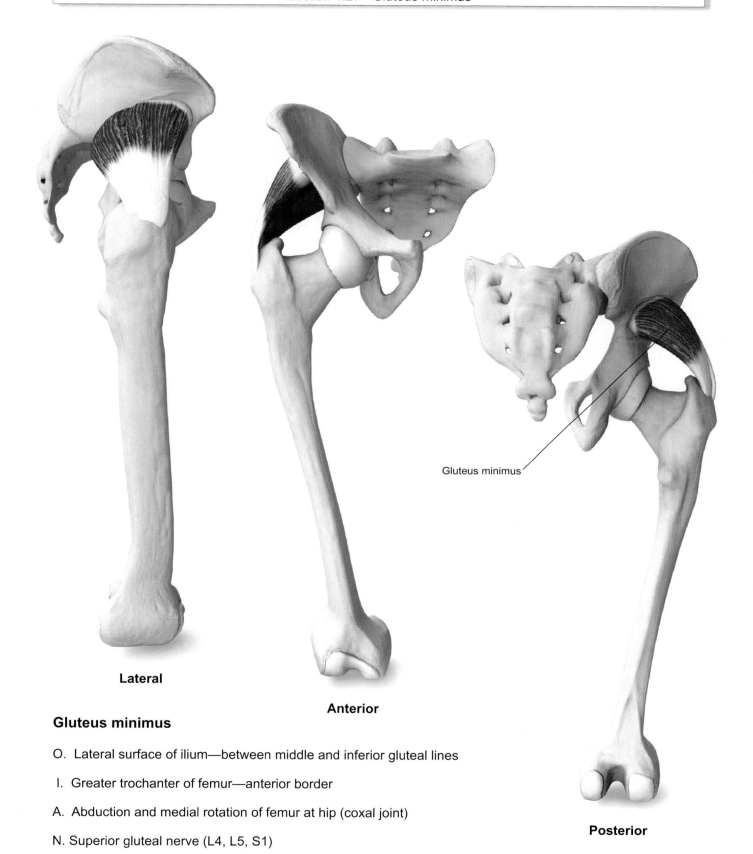

Lateral

Anterior

Gluteus minimus

Posterior

Gluteus minimus

O. Lateral surface of ilium—between middle and inferior gluteal lines

I. Greater trochanter of femur—anterior border

A. Abduction and medial rotation of femur at hip (coxal joint)

N. Superior gluteal nerve (L4, L5, S1)

Unit 3 Muscular System

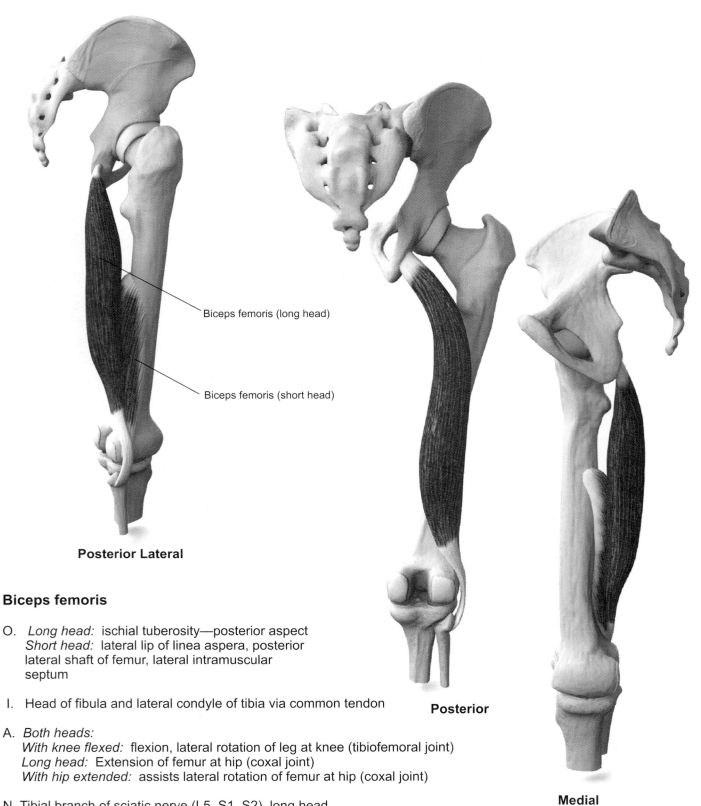

Biceps femoris (long head)

Biceps femoris (short head)

Posterior Lateral

Posterior

Medial

Biceps femoris

O. *Long head:* ischial tuberosity—posterior aspect
Short head: lateral lip of linea aspera, posterior lateral shaft of femur, lateral intramuscular septum

I. Head of fibula and lateral condyle of tibia via common tendon

A. *Both heads:*
With knee flexed: flexion, lateral rotation of leg at knee (tibiofemoral joint)
Long head: Extension of femur at hip (coxal joint)
With hip extended: assists lateral rotation of femur at hip (coxal joint)

N. Tibial branch of sciatic nerve (L5, S1, S2), long head
Peroneal branch of sciatic nerve (L5, S1, S2), short head

Unit 3 Muscular System

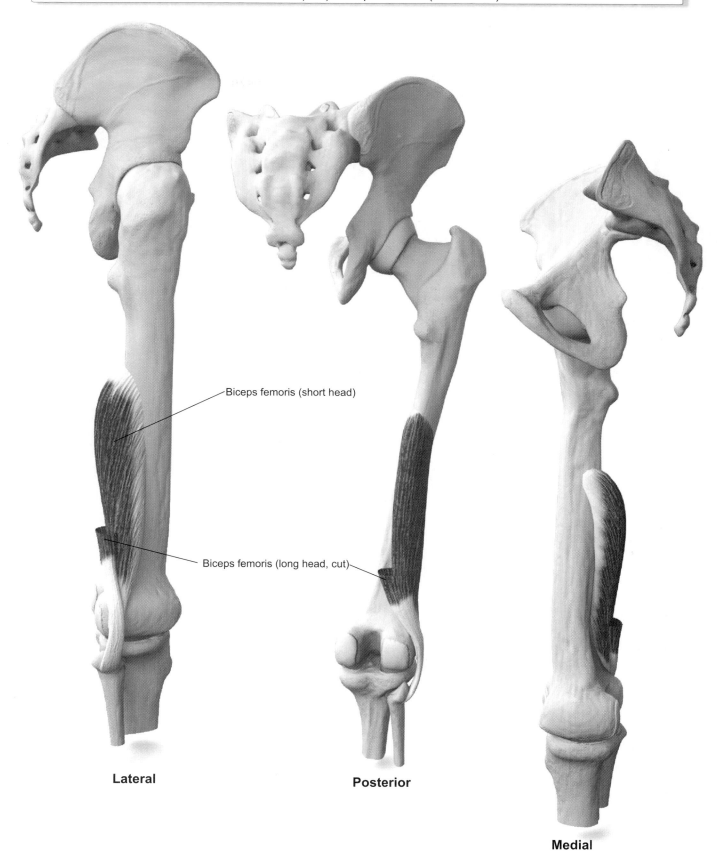

Biceps femoris (short head)

Biceps femoris (long head, cut)

Lateral

Posterior

Medial

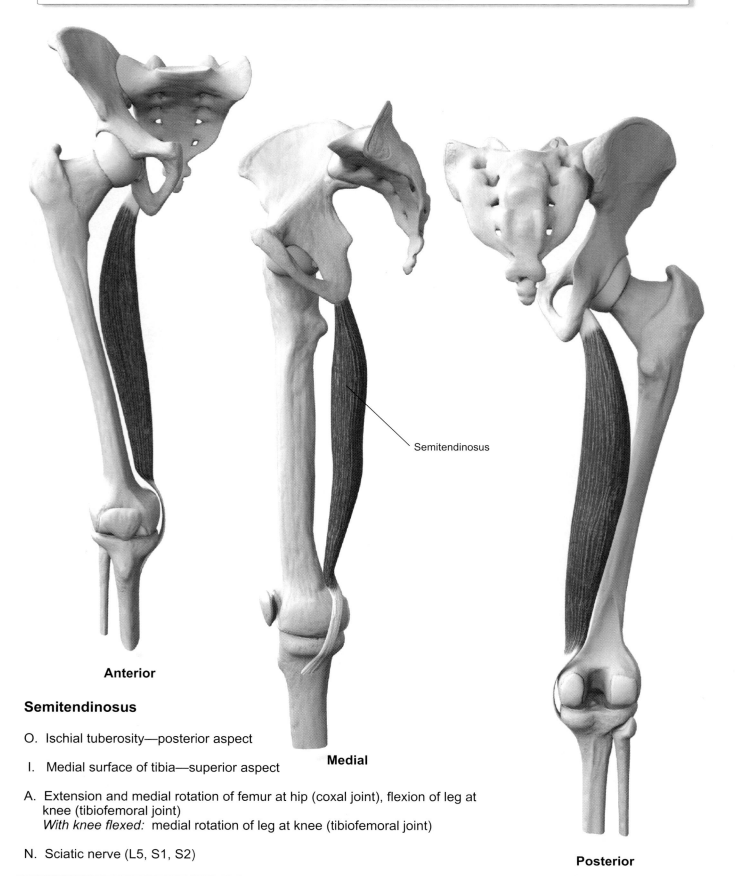

Semitendinosus

Anterior

Medial

Posterior

Semitendinosus

O. Ischial tuberosity—posterior aspect

 I. Medial surface of tibia—superior aspect

A. Extension and medial rotation of femur at hip (coxal joint), flexion of leg at knee (tibiofemoral joint)
With knee flexed: medial rotation of leg at knee (tibiofemoral joint)

N. Sciatic nerve (L5, S1, S2)

Unit 3 Muscular System

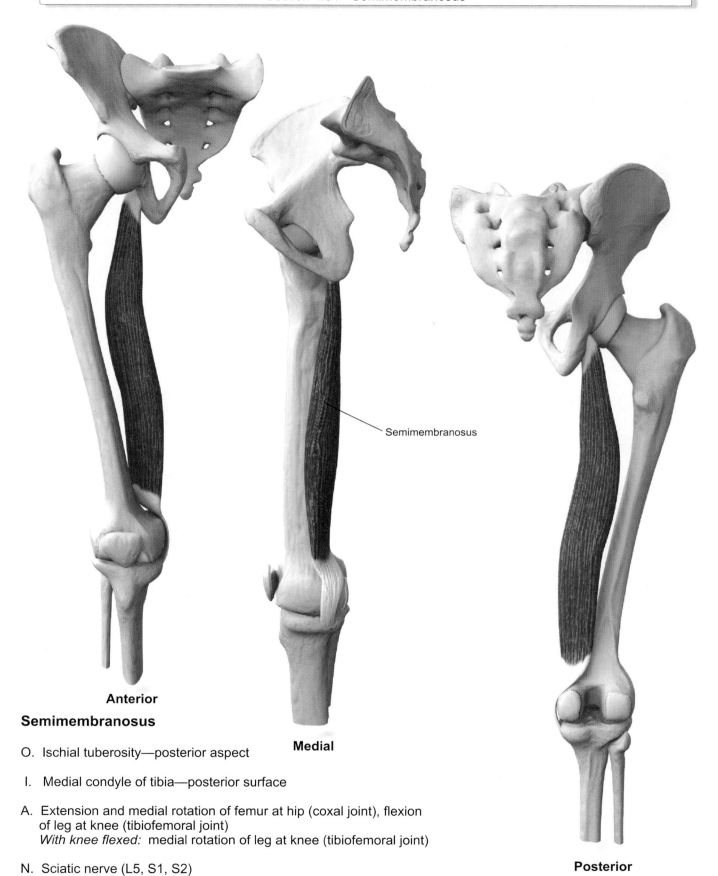

Semimembranosus

Anterior

Medial

Posterior

Semimembranosus

O. Ischial tuberosity—posterior aspect

 I. Medial condyle of tibia—posterior surface

A. Extension and medial rotation of femur at hip (coxal joint), flexion
    of leg at knee (tibiofemoral joint)
    With knee flexed: medial rotation of leg at knee (tibiofemoral joint)

N. Sciatic nerve (L5, S1, S2)

Unit 3 Muscular System

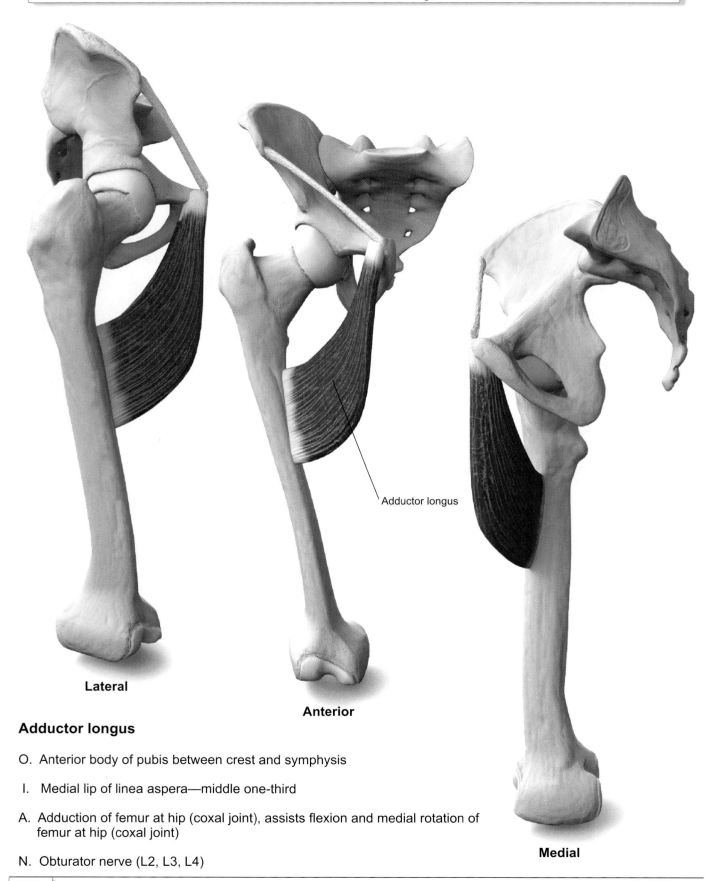

Lateral

Anterior

Adductor longus

Medial

Adductor longus

O. Anterior body of pubis between crest and symphysis

I. Medial lip of linea aspera—middle one-third

A. Adduction of femur at hip (coxal joint), assists flexion and medial rotation of femur at hip (coxal joint)

N. Obturator nerve (L2, L3, L4)

Unit 3 Muscular System

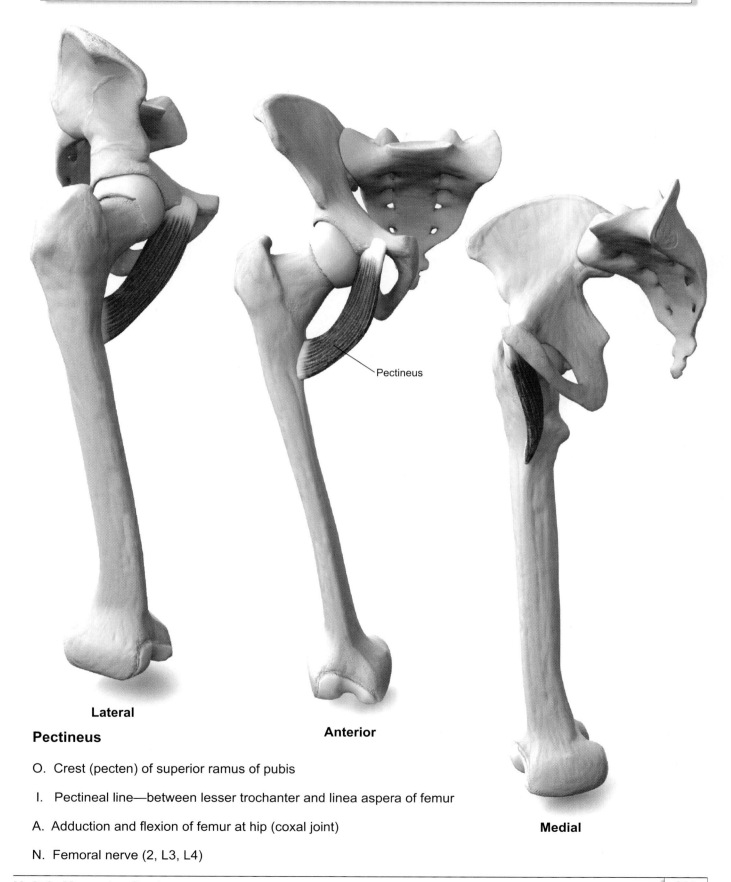

Lateral

Anterior

Pectineus

Medial

Pectineus

O. Crest (pecten) of superior ramus of pubis

I. Pectineal line—between lesser trochanter and linea aspera of femur

A. Adduction and flexion of femur at hip (coxal joint)

N. Femoral nerve (2, L3, L4)

Unit 3 Muscular System

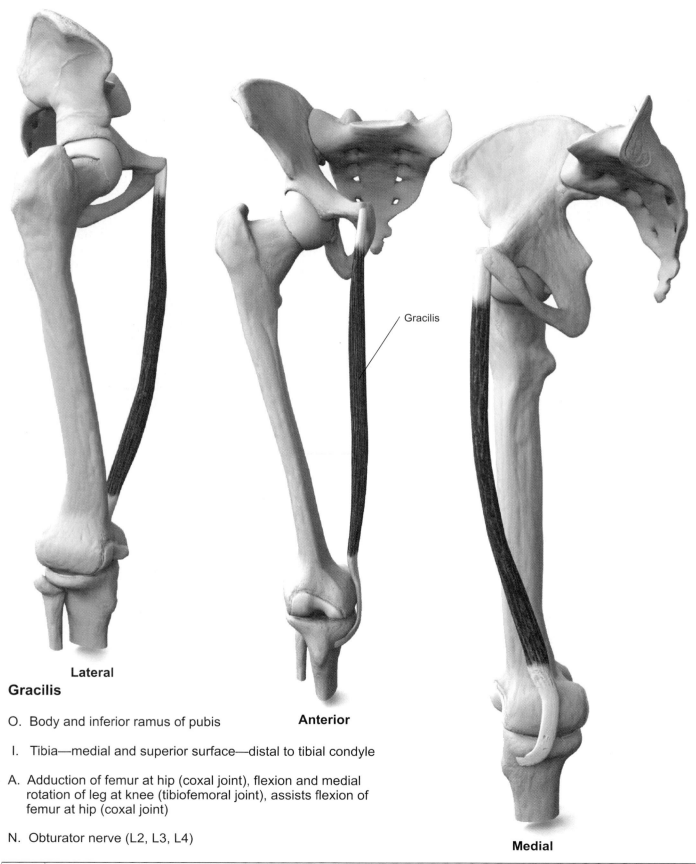

Lateral

Anterior

Gracilis

Medial

Gracilis

O. Body and inferior ramus of pubis

I. Tibia—medial and superior surface—distal to tibial condyle

A. Adduction of femur at hip (coxal joint), flexion and medial rotation of leg at knee (tibiofemoral joint), assists flexion of femur at hip (coxal joint)

N. Obturator nerve (L2, L3, L4)

Unit 3 Muscular System

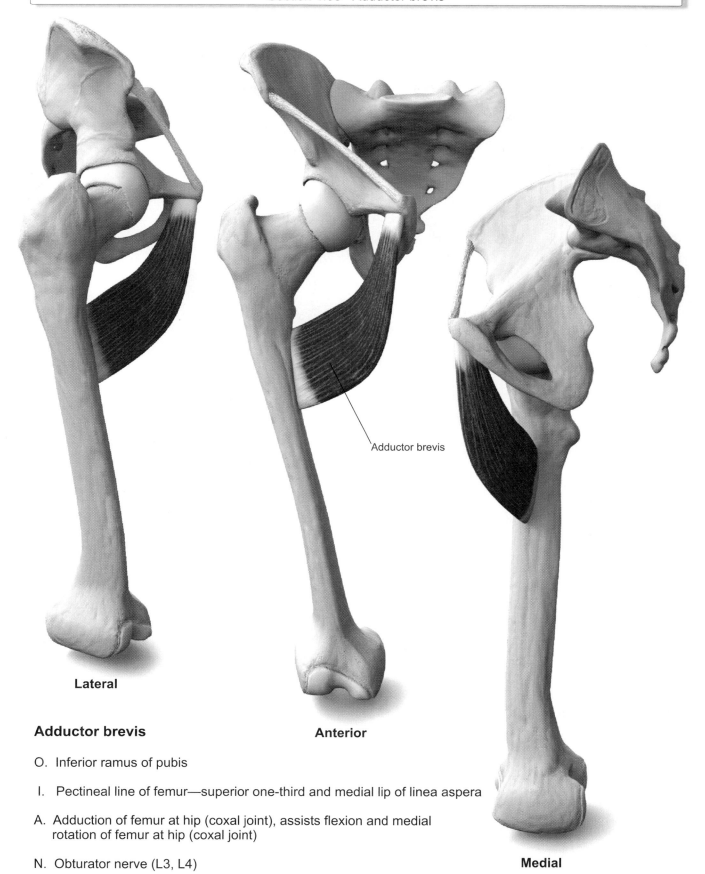

Lateral

Anterior

Adductor brevis

Medial

Adductor brevis

O. Inferior ramus of pubis

I. Pectineal line of femur—superior one-third and medial lip of linea aspera

A. Adduction of femur at hip (coxal joint), assists flexion and medial
    rotation of femur at hip (coxal joint)

N. Obturator nerve (L3, L4)

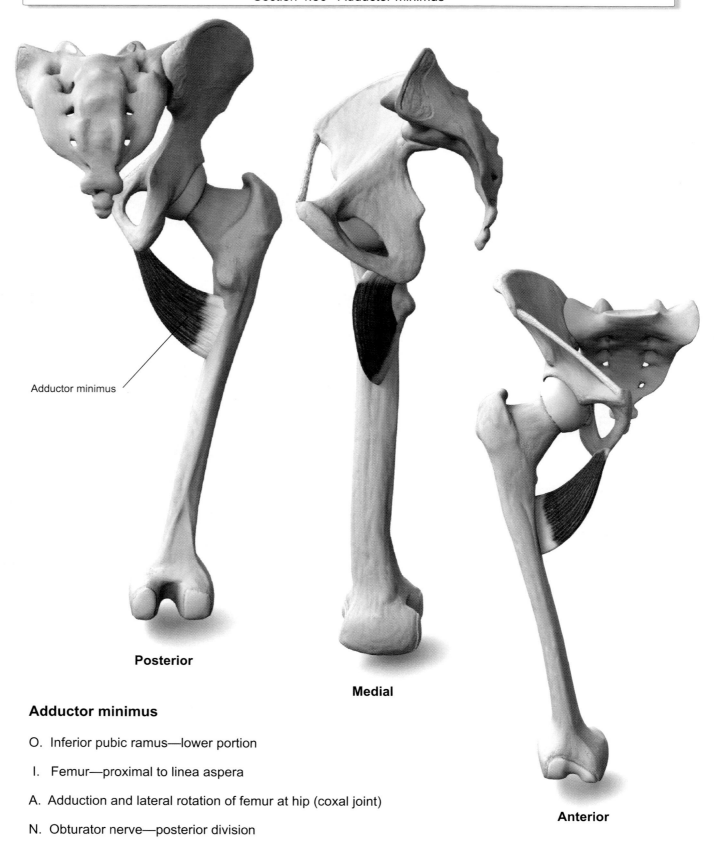

Adductor minimus

Posterior

Medial

Anterior

Adductor minimus

O. Inferior pubic ramus—lower portion

I. Femur—proximal to linea aspera

A. Adduction and lateral rotation of femur at hip (coxal joint)

N. Obturator nerve—posterior division

Unit 3 Muscular System

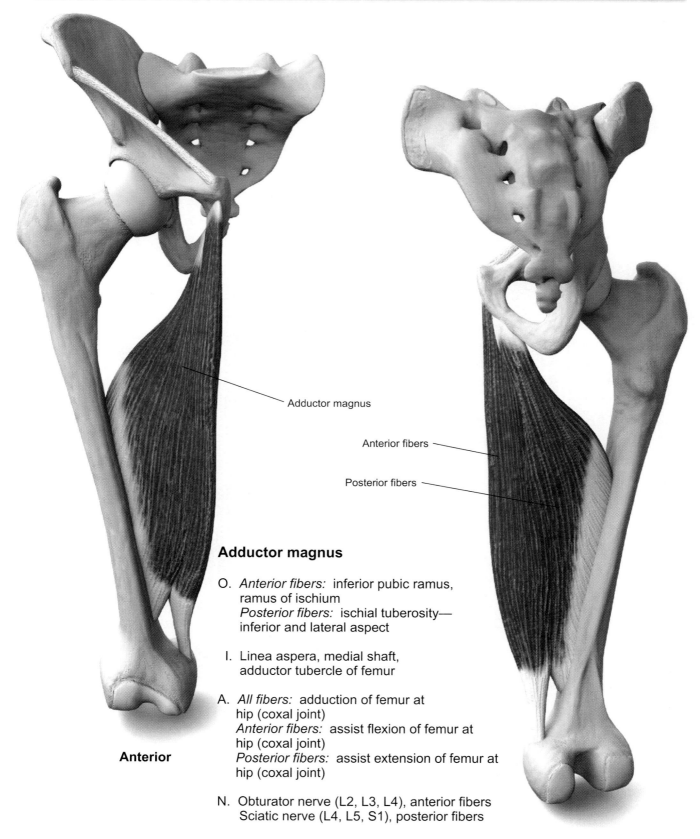

Adductor magnus

Anterior fibers

Posterior fibers

Anterior

Posterior

Adductor magnus

O. *Anterior fibers:* inferior pubic ramus,
   ramus of ischium
   Posterior fibers: ischial tuberosity—
   inferior and lateral aspect

 I. Linea aspera, medial shaft,
    adductor tubercle of femur

A. *All fibers:* adduction of femur at
   hip (coxal joint)
   Anterior fibers: assist flexion of femur at
   hip (coxal joint)
   Posterior fibers: assist extension of femur at
   hip (coxal joint)

N. Obturator nerve (L2, L3, L4), anterior fibers
   Sciatic nerve (L4, L5, S1), posterior fibers

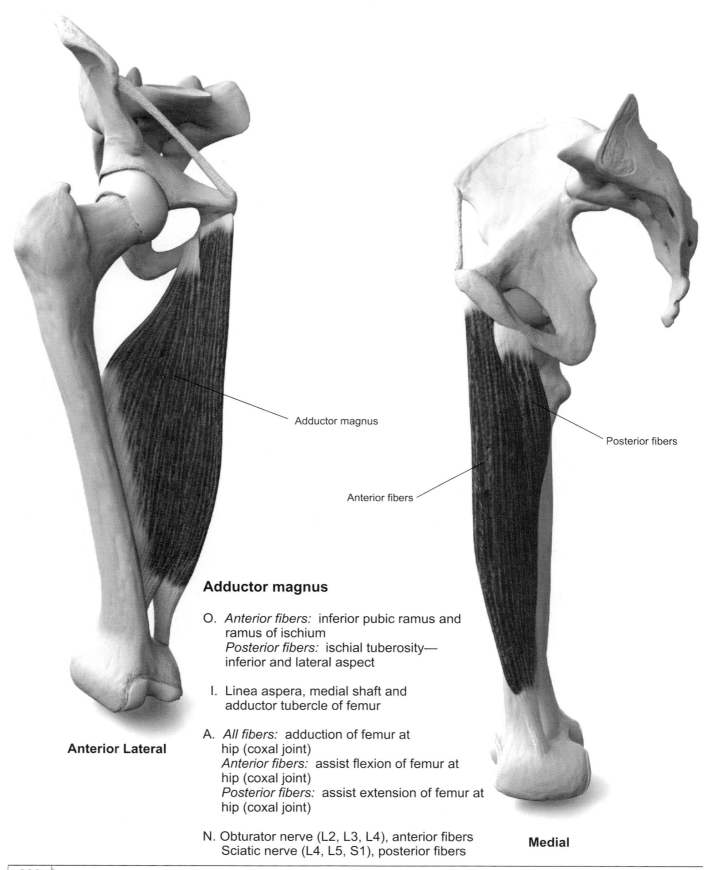

Adductor magnus

Posterior fibers

Anterior fibers

Adductor magnus

O. *Anterior fibers:* inferior pubic ramus and ramus of ischium
Posterior fibers: ischial tuberosity—inferior and lateral aspect

I. Linea aspera, medial shaft and adductor tubercle of femur

A. *All fibers:* adduction of femur at hip (coxal joint)
Anterior fibers: assist flexion of femur at hip (coxal joint)
Posterior fibers: assist extension of femur at hip (coxal joint)

N. Obturator nerve (L2, L3, L4), anterior fibers
Sciatic nerve (L4, L5, S1), posterior fibers

Anterior Lateral

Medial

Unit 3 Muscular System

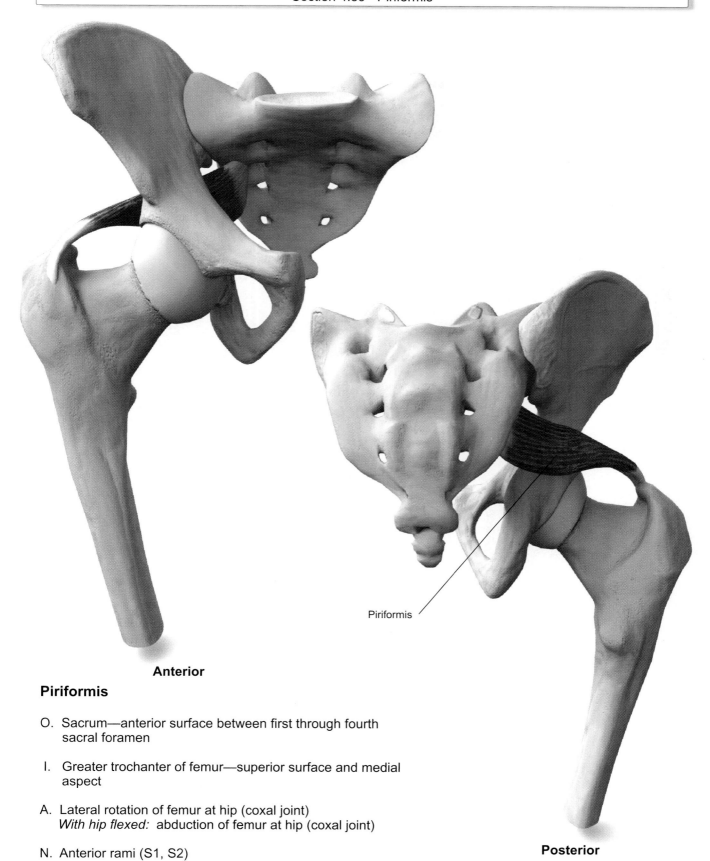

Anterior

Piriformis

Posterior

Piriformis

O. Sacrum—anterior surface between first through fourth sacral foramen

I. Greater trochanter of femur—superior surface and medial aspect

A. Lateral rotation of femur at hip (coxal joint)
With hip flexed: abduction of femur at hip (coxal joint)

N. Anterior rami (S1, S2)

Unit 3 Muscular System

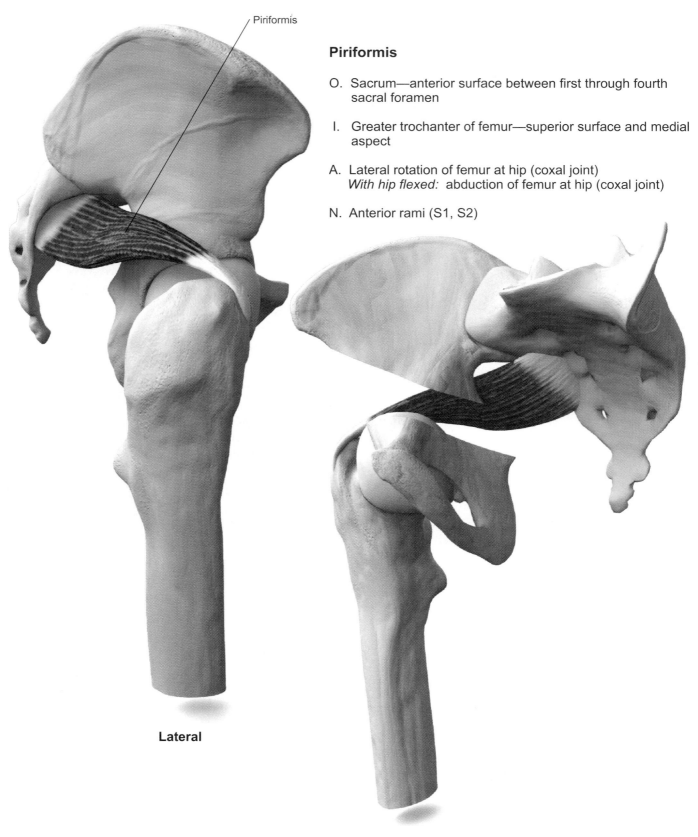

Piriformis

Piriformis

O. Sacrum—anterior surface between first through fourth sacral foramen

I. Greater trochanter of femur—superior surface and medial aspect

A. Lateral rotation of femur at hip (coxal joint)
With hip flexed: abduction of femur at hip (coxal joint)

N. Anterior rami (S1, S2)

Lateral

Anterior Medial

Unit 3 Muscular System

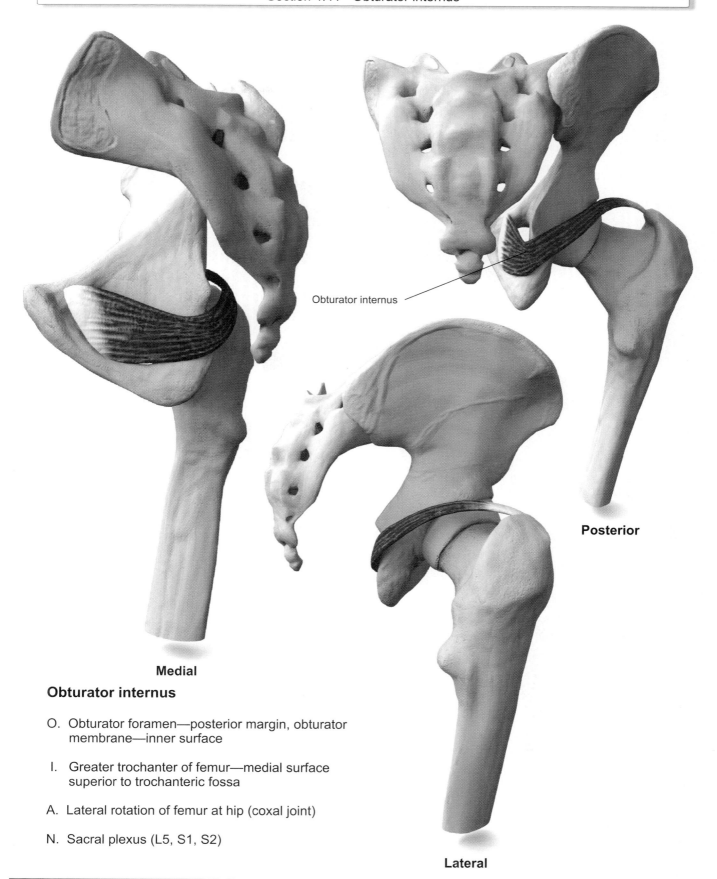

Obturator internus

Medial

Posterior

Lateral

Obturator internus

O. Obturator foramen—posterior margin, obturator membrane—inner surface

I. Greater trochanter of femur—medial surface superior to trochanteric fossa

A. Lateral rotation of femur at hip (coxal joint)

N. Sacral plexus (L5, S1, S2)

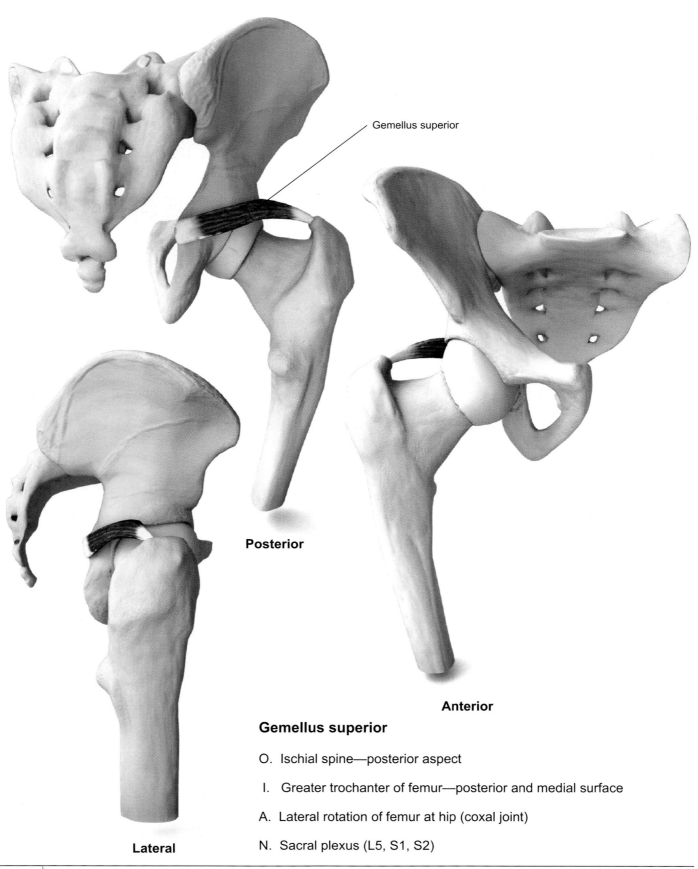

Gemellus superior

Posterior

Anterior

Lateral

Gemellus superior

O. Ischial spine—posterior aspect

I. Greater trochanter of femur—posterior and medial surface

A. Lateral rotation of femur at hip (coxal joint)

N. Sacral plexus (L5, S1, S2)

Unit 3 Muscular System

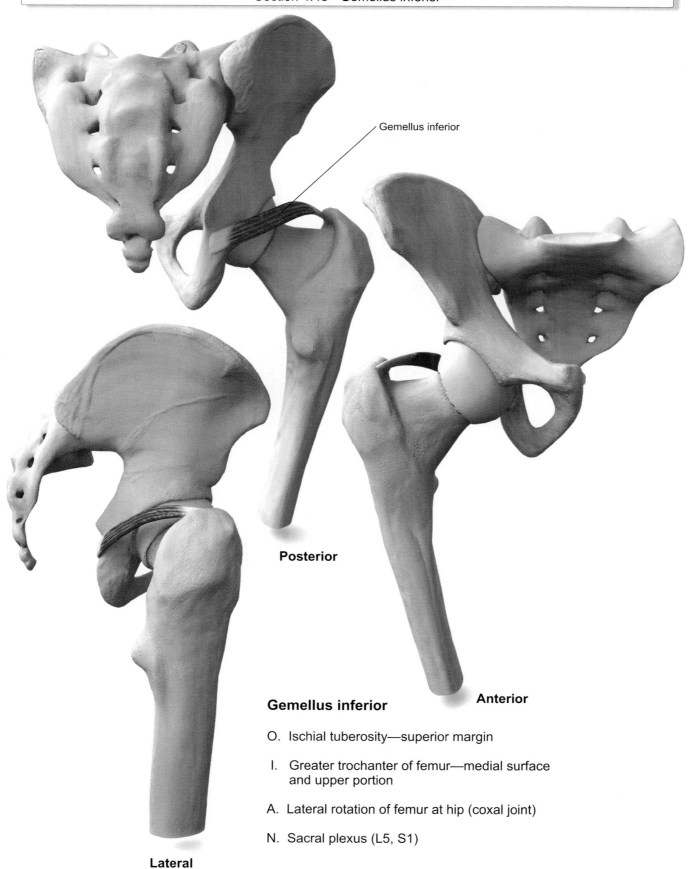

Gemellus inferior

Posterior

Anterior

Lateral

Gemellus inferior

O. Ischial tuberosity—superior margin

I. Greater trochanter of femur—medial surface and upper portion

A. Lateral rotation of femur at hip (coxal joint)

N. Sacral plexus (L5, S1)

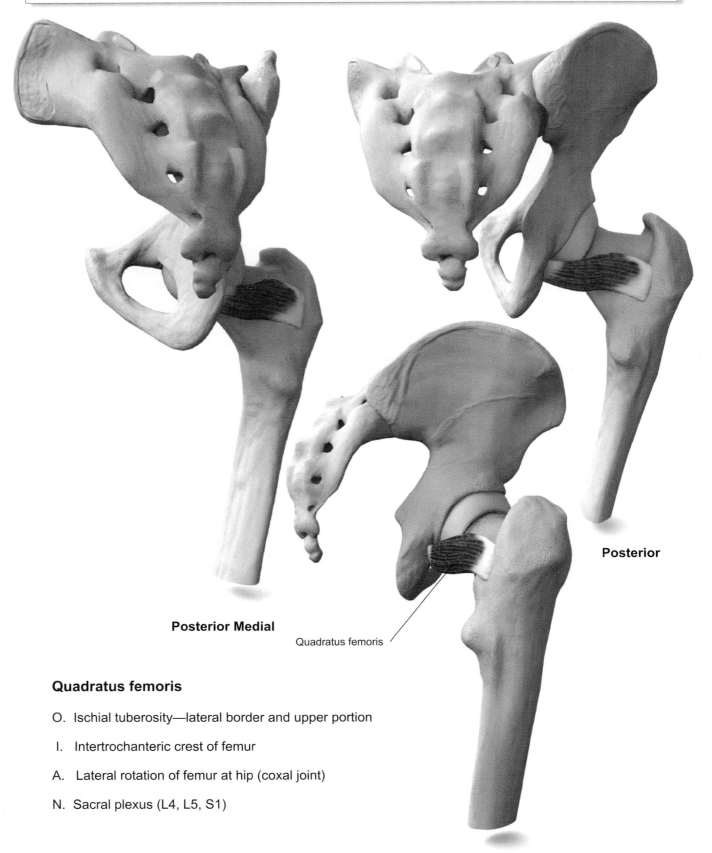

Posterior Medial

Quadratus femoris

Posterior

Posterior Lateral

Quadratus femoris

O. Ischial tuberosity—lateral border and upper portion

I. Intertrochanteric crest of femur

A. Lateral rotation of femur at hip (coxal joint)

N. Sacral plexus (L4, L5, S1)

Unit 3 Muscular System

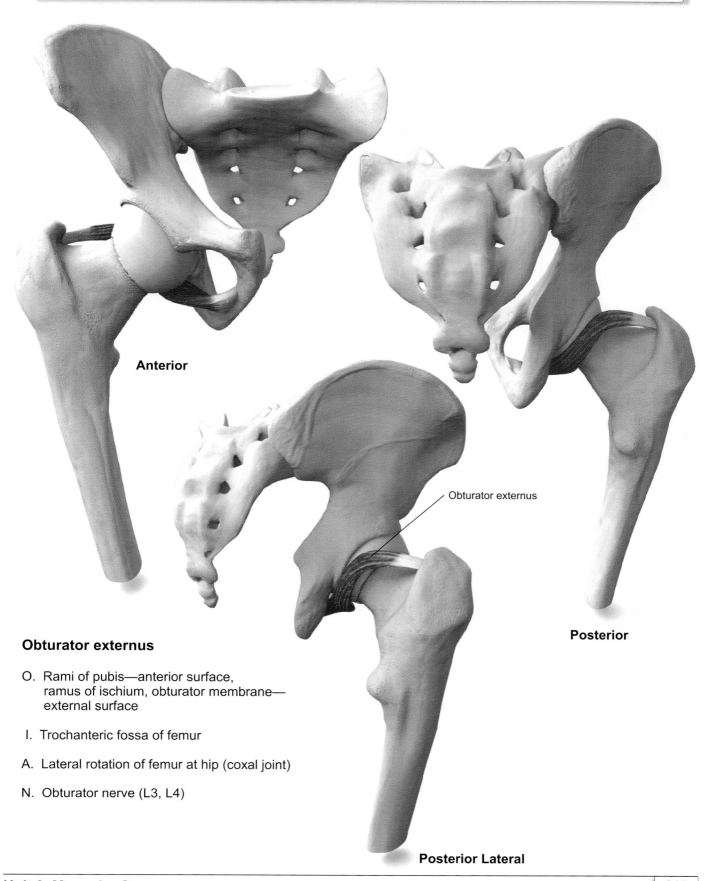

Anterior

Obturator externus

Posterior

Posterior Lateral

Obturator externus

O. Rami of pubis—anterior surface,
ramus of ischium, obturator membrane—
external surface

I. Trochanteric fossa of femur

A. Lateral rotation of femur at hip (coxal joint)

N. Obturator nerve (L3, L4)

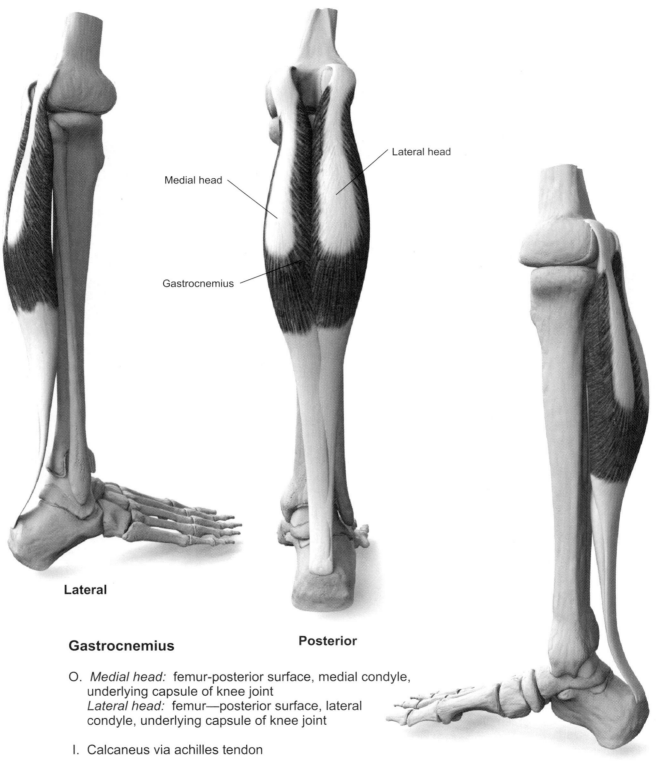

Medial head

Lateral head

Gastrocnemius

Lateral

Posterior

Medial

Gastrocnemius

O. *Medial head:* femur-posterior surface, medial condyle, underlying capsule of knee joint
Lateral head: femur—posterior surface, lateral condyle, underlying capsule of knee joint

I. Calcaneus via achilles tendon

A. Plantarflexion of foot at ankle (talocrural joint), assists in flexion of leg at knee (tibiofemoral joint)

N. Tibial nerve (S1, S2)

Unit 3 Muscular System

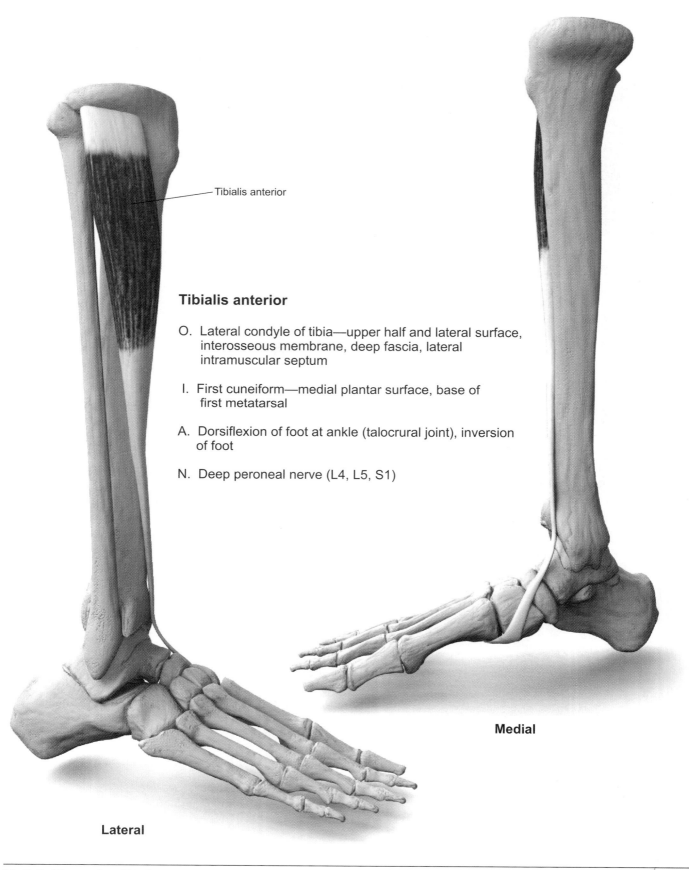

Tibialis anterior

Tibialis anterior

O. Lateral condyle of tibia—upper half and lateral surface, interosseous membrane, deep fascia, lateral intramuscular septum

I. First cuneiform—medial plantar surface, base of first metatarsal

A. Dorsiflexion of foot at ankle (talocrural joint), inversion of foot

N. Deep peroneal nerve (L4, L5, S1)

Medial

Lateral

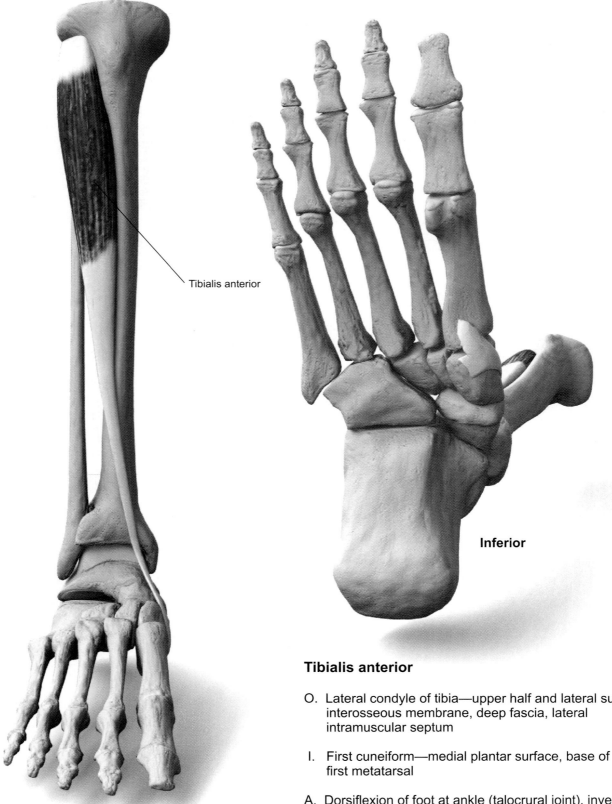

Tibialis anterior

Inferior

Anterior

Tibialis anterior

O. Lateral condyle of tibia—upper half and lateral surface, interosseous membrane, deep fascia, lateral intramuscular septum

 I. First cuneiform—medial plantar surface, base of first metatarsal

A. Dorsiflexion of foot at ankle (talocrural joint), inversion of foot

N. Deep peroneal nerve (L4, L5, S1)

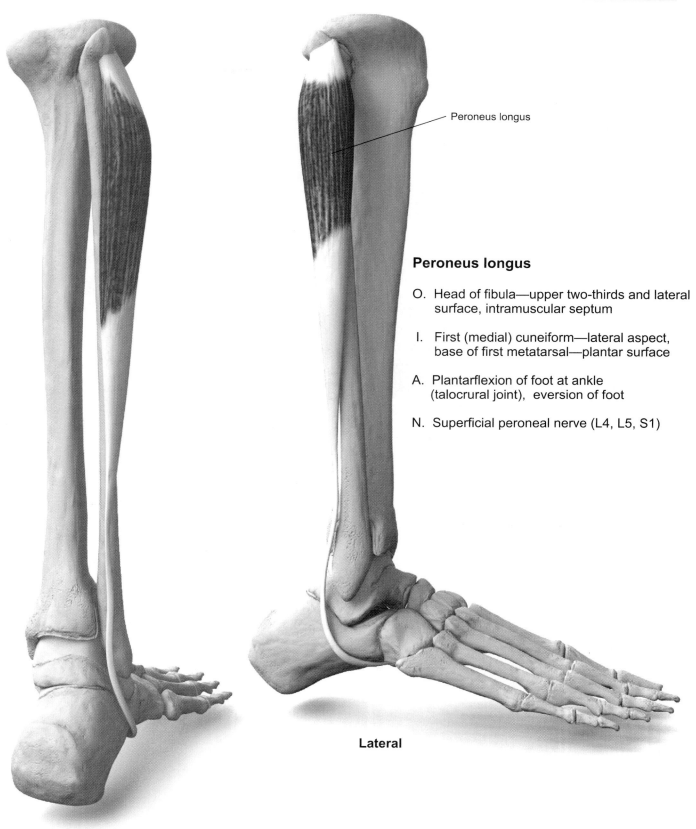

Peroneus longus

Peroneus longus

O. Head of fibula—upper two-thirds and lateral surface, intramuscular septum

I. First (medial) cuneiform—lateral aspect, base of first metatarsal—plantar surface

A. Plantarflexion of foot at ankle (talocrural joint), eversion of foot

N. Superficial peroneal nerve (L4, L5, S1)

Lateral

Posterior

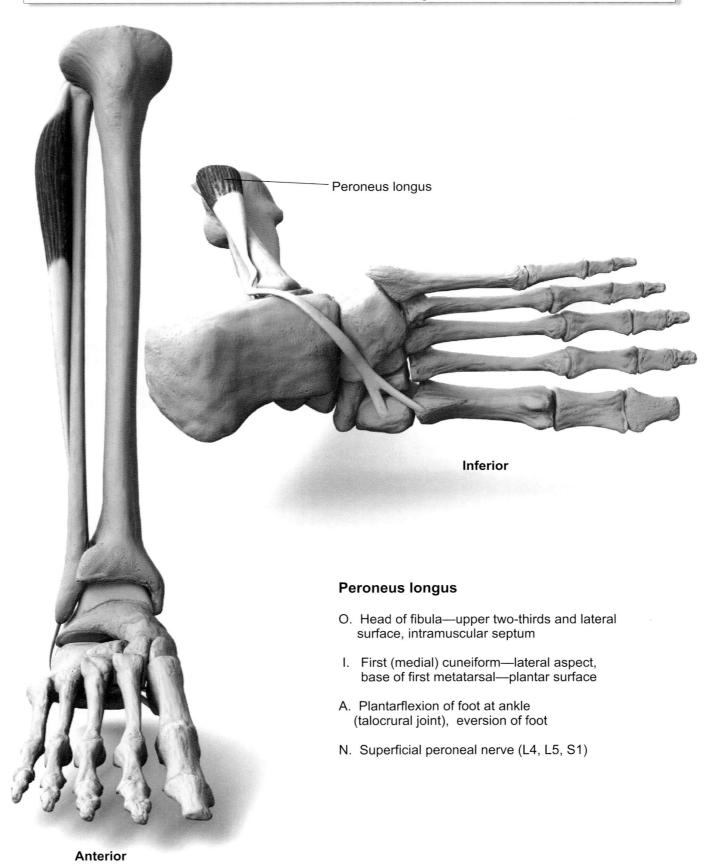

Peroneus longus

Inferior

Anterior

Peroneus longus

O. Head of fibula—upper two-thirds and lateral surface, intramuscular septum

I. First (medial) cuneiform—lateral aspect, base of first metatarsal—plantar surface

A. Plantarflexion of foot at ankle (talocrural joint), eversion of foot

N. Superficial peroneal nerve (L4, L5, S1)

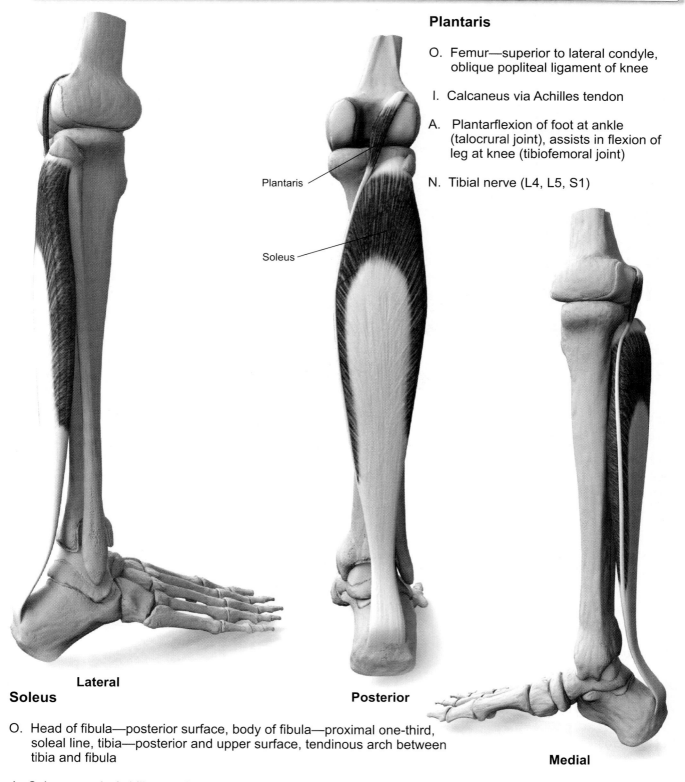

Plantaris

O. Femur—superior to lateral condyle, oblique popliteal ligament of knee

I. Calcaneus via Achilles tendon

A. Plantarflexion of foot at ankle (talocrural joint), assists in flexion of leg at knee (tibiofemoral joint)

N. Tibial nerve (L4, L5, S1)

Plantaris

Soleus

Lateral

Posterior

Medial

Soleus

O. Head of fibula—posterior surface, body of fibula—proximal one-third, soleal line, tibia—posterior and upper surface, tendinous arch between tibia and fibula

I. Calcaneus via Achilles tendon

A. Plantarflexion of foot at ankle (talocrural joint)

N. Tibial nerve (S1, S2)

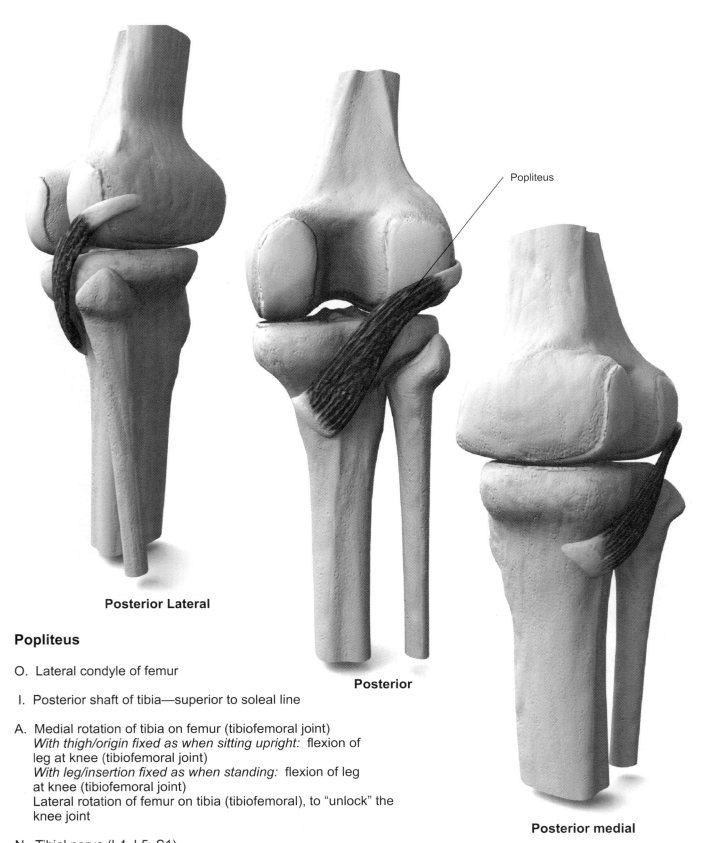

Posterior Lateral

Posterior

Popliteus

Posterior medial

Popliteus

O. Lateral condyle of femur

I. Posterior shaft of tibia—superior to soleal line

A. Medial rotation of tibia on femur (tibiofemoral joint)
    With thigh/origin fixed as when sitting upright: flexion of
    leg at knee (tibiofemoral joint)
    With leg/insertion fixed as when standing: flexion of leg
    at knee (tibiofemoral joint)
    Lateral rotation of femur on tibia (tibiofemoral), to "unlock" the
    knee joint

N. Tibial nerve (L4, L5, S1)

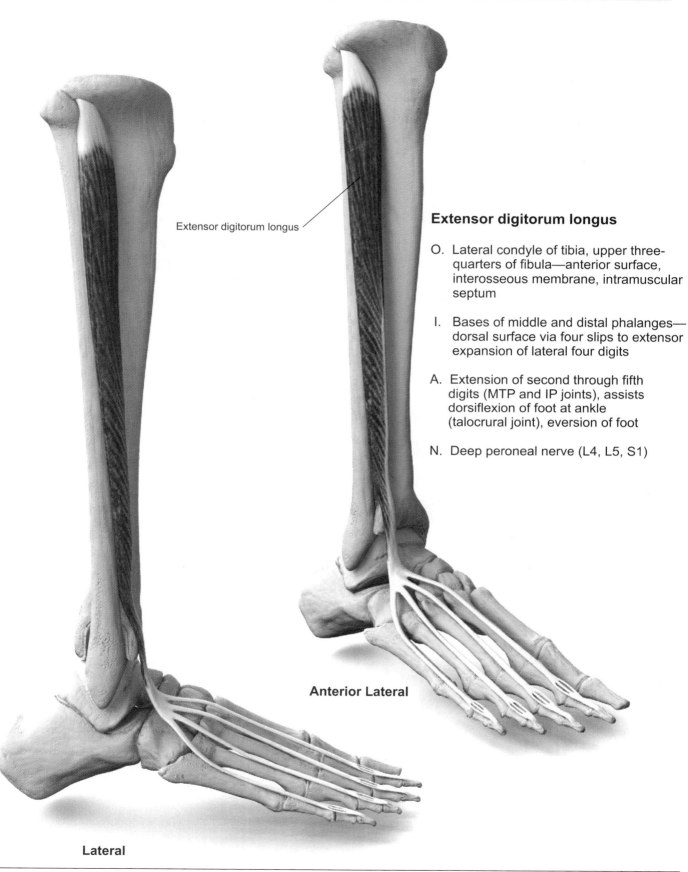

Extensor digitorum longus

Anterior Lateral

Lateral

Extensor digitorum longus

O. Lateral condyle of tibia, upper three-quarters of fibula—anterior surface, interosseous membrane, intramuscular septum

I. Bases of middle and distal phalanges—dorsal surface via four slips to extensor expansion of lateral four digits

A. Extension of second through fifth digits (MTP and IP joints), assists dorsiflexion of foot at ankle (talocrural joint), eversion of foot

N. Deep peroneal nerve (L4, L5, S1)

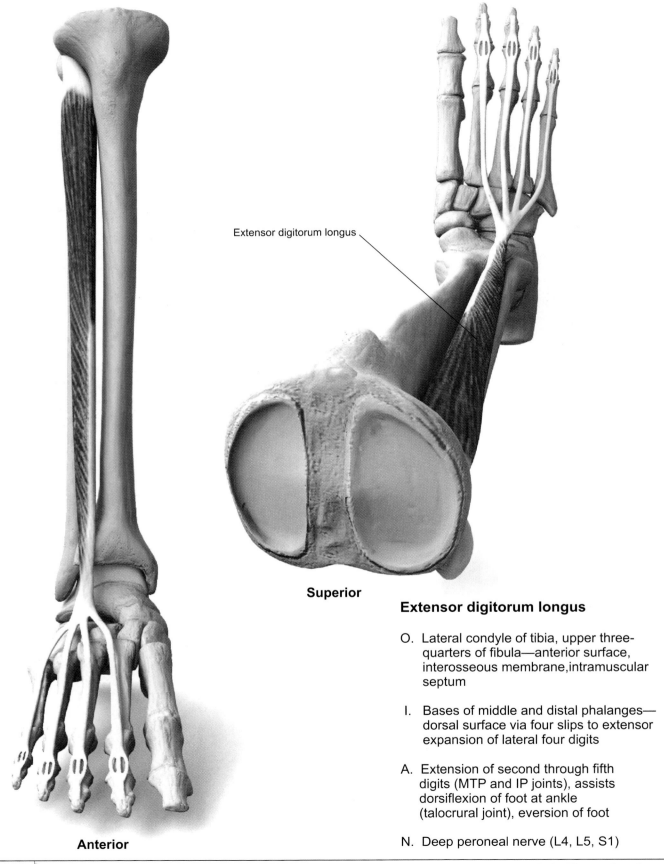

Extensor digitorum longus

Superior

Anterior

Extensor digitorum longus

O. Lateral condyle of tibia, upper three-quarters of fibula—anterior surface, interosseous membrane,intramuscular septum

I. Bases of middle and distal phalanges—dorsal surface via four slips to extensor expansion of lateral four digits

A. Extension of second through fifth digits (MTP and IP joints), assists dorsiflexion of foot at ankle (talocrural joint), eversion of foot

N. Deep peroneal nerve (L4, L5, S1)

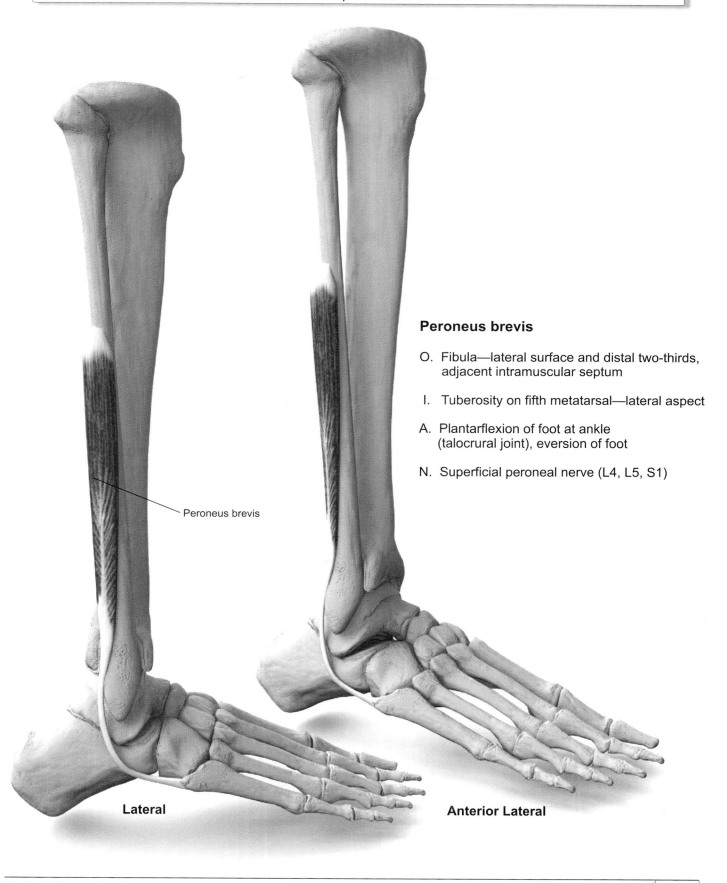

Peroneus brevis

O. Fibula—lateral surface and distal two-thirds, adjacent intramuscular septum

I. Tuberosity on fifth metatarsal—lateral aspect

A. Plantarflexion of foot at ankle (talocrural joint), eversion of foot

N. Superficial peroneal nerve (L4, L5, S1)

Peroneus brevis

Lateral

Anterior Lateral

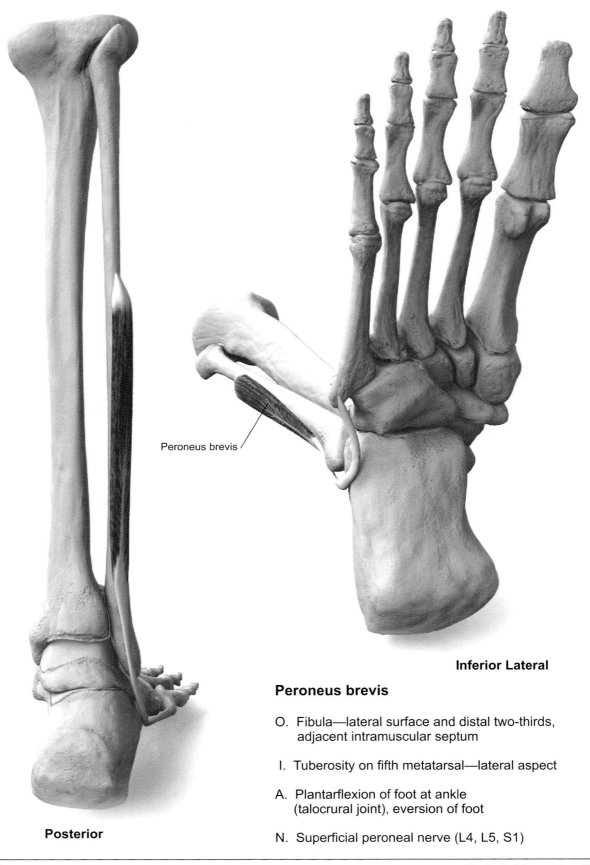

Peroneus brevis

Posterior

Inferior Lateral

Peroneus brevis

O. Fibula—lateral surface and distal two-thirds, adjacent intramuscular septum

I. Tuberosity on fifth metatarsal—lateral aspect

A. Plantarflexion of foot at ankle (talocrural joint), eversion of foot

N. Superficial peroneal nerve (L4, L5, S1)

Unit 3 Muscular System

Peroneus tertius

O. Fibula—anterior margin and distal one-third, interosseous membrane

I. Base of fifth metatarsal—dorsal surface

A. Dorsiflexion of foot at ankle (talocrural joint), eversion of foot

N. Deep peroneal nerve (L5, S1)

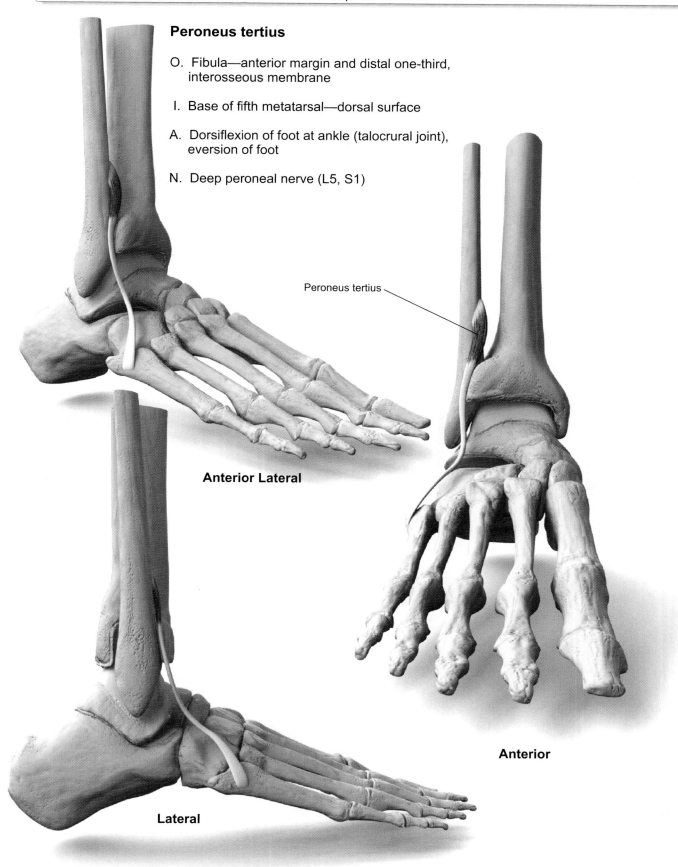

Peroneus tertius

Anterior Lateral

Anterior

Lateral

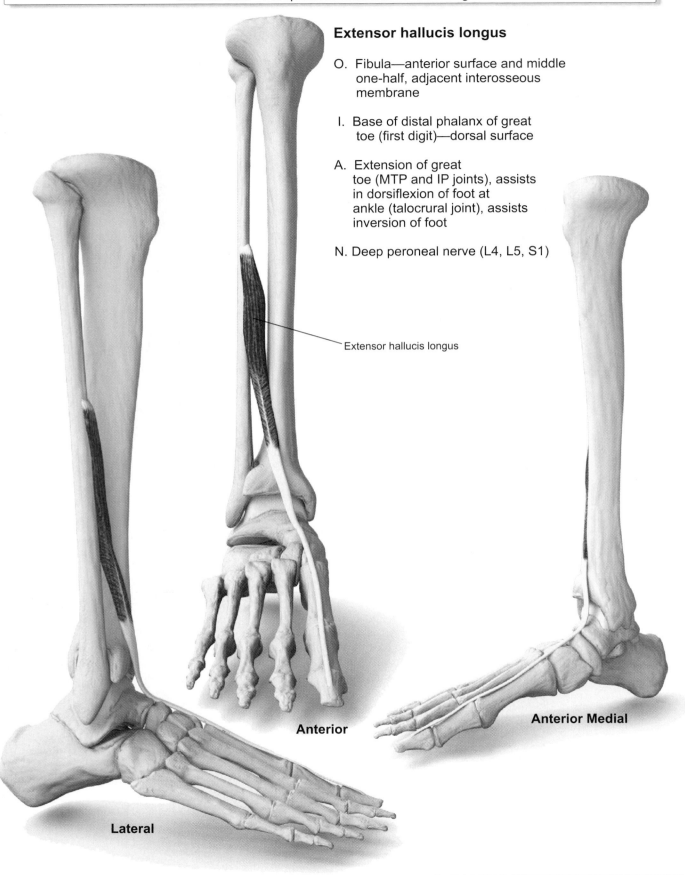

Extensor hallucis longus

O. Fibula—anterior surface and middle one-half, adjacent interosseous membrane

I. Base of distal phalanx of great toe (first digit)—dorsal surface

A. Extension of great toe (MTP and IP joints), assists in dorsiflexion of foot at ankle (talocrural joint), assists inversion of foot

N. Deep peroneal nerve (L4, L5, S1)

Extensor hallucis longus

Anterior

Anterior Medial

Lateral

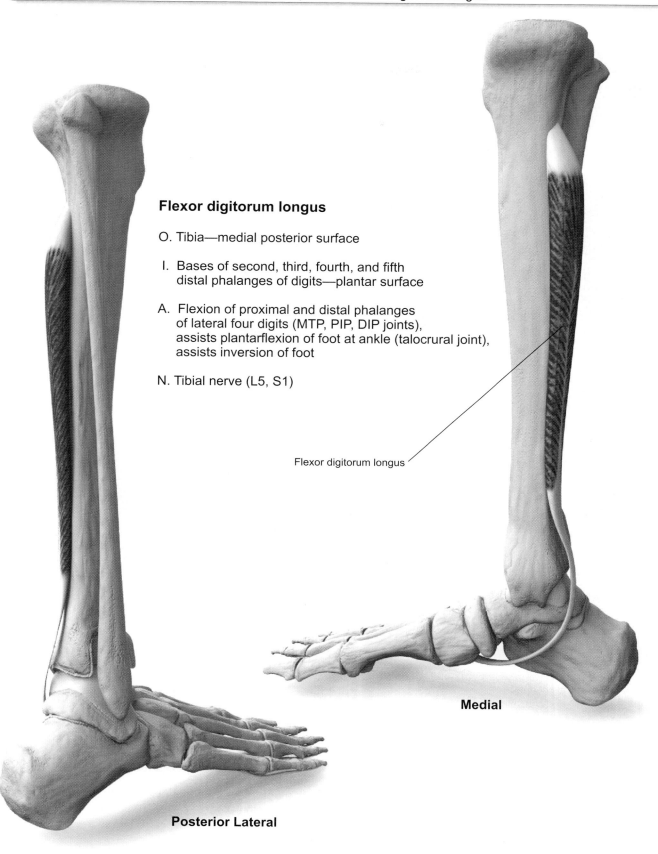

Flexor digitorum longus

O. Tibia—medial posterior surface

I. Bases of second, third, fourth, and fifth
   distal phalanges of digits—plantar surface

A. Flexion of proximal and distal phalanges
   of lateral four digits (MTP, PIP, DIP joints),
   assists plantarflexion of foot at ankle (talocrural joint),
   assists inversion of foot

N. Tibial nerve (L5, S1)

Flexor digitorum longus

Medial

Posterior Lateral

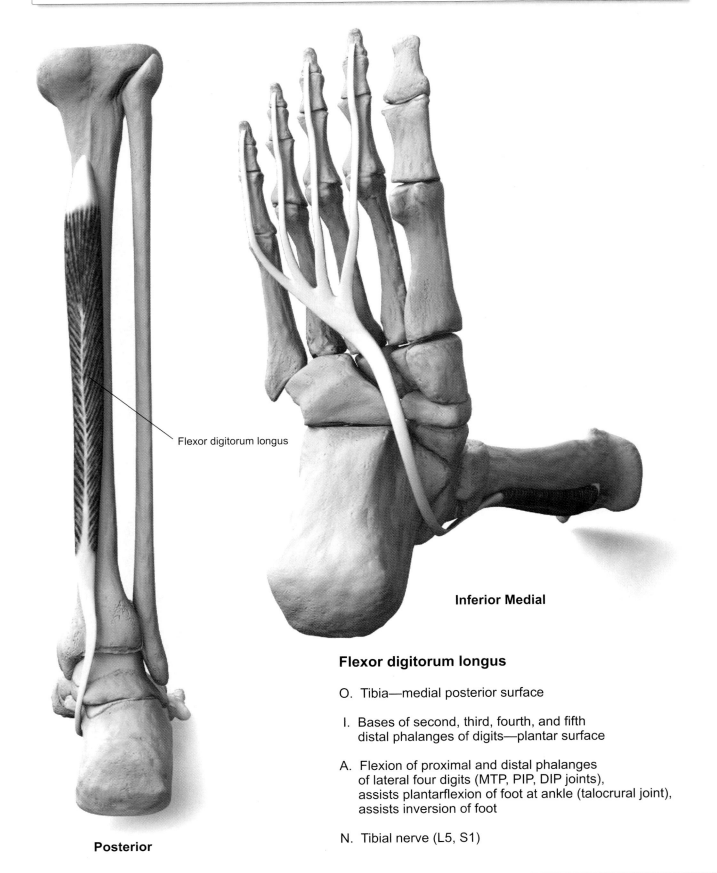

Flexor digitorum longus

Inferior Medial

Flexor digitorum longus

O. Tibia—medial posterior surface

I. Bases of second, third, fourth, and fifth
distal phalanges of digits—plantar surface

A. Flexion of proximal and distal phalanges
of lateral four digits (MTP, PIP, DIP joints),
assists plantarflexion of foot at ankle (talocrural joint),
assists inversion of foot

N. Tibial nerve (L5, S1)

Posterior

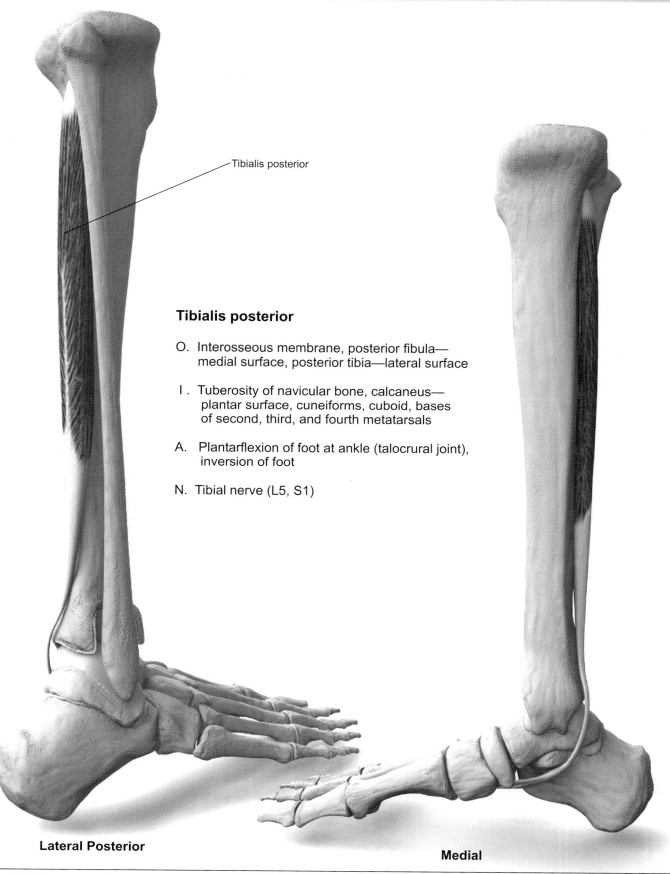

Tibialis posterior

Tibialis posterior

O. Interosseous membrane, posterior fibula—
    medial surface, posterior tibia—lateral surface

I. Tuberosity of navicular bone, calcaneus—
    plantar surface, cuneiforms, cuboid, bases
    of second, third, and fourth metatarsals

A. Plantarflexion of foot at ankle (talocrural joint),
    inversion of foot

N. Tibial nerve (L5, S1)

Lateral Posterior

Medial

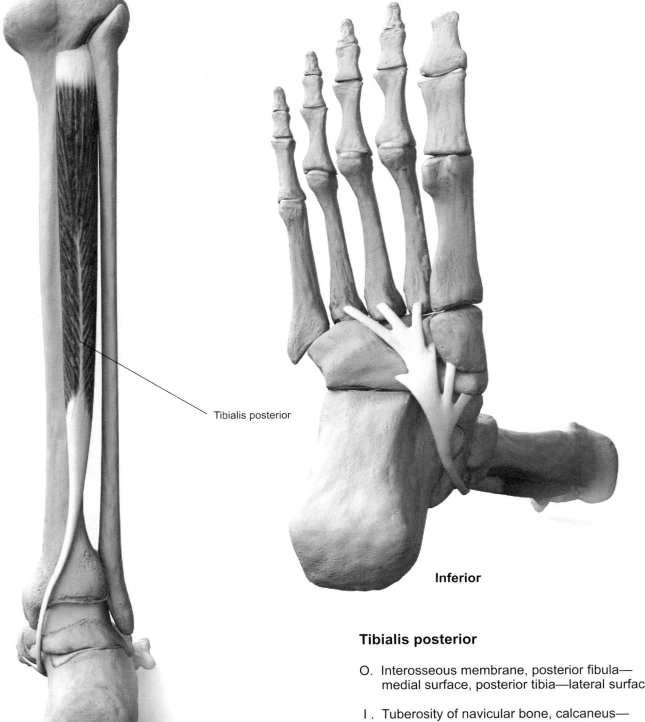

Tibialis posterior

Inferior

Posterior

Tibialis posterior

O. Interosseous membrane, posterior fibula—
medial surface, posterior tibia—lateral surface

I . Tuberosity of navicular bone, calcaneus—
plantar surface, cuneiforms, cuboid, bases
of second, third, and fourth metatarsals

A. Plantarflexion of foot at ankle (talocrural joint),
inversion of foot

N. Tibial nerve (L5, S1)

Unit 3 Muscular System

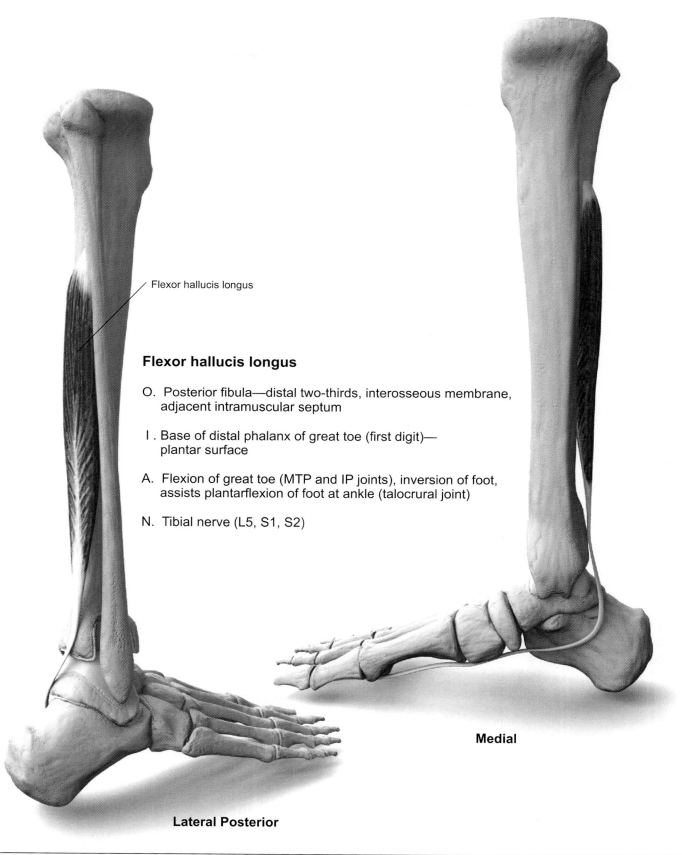

Flexor hallucis longus

Flexor hallucis longus

O. Posterior fibula—distal two-thirds, interosseous membrane, adjacent intramuscular septum

I . Base of distal phalanx of great toe (first digit)— plantar surface

A. Flexion of great toe (MTP and IP joints), inversion of foot, assists plantarflexion of foot at ankle (talocrural joint)

N. Tibial nerve (L5, S1, S2)

Medial

Lateral Posterior

Unit 3 Muscular System

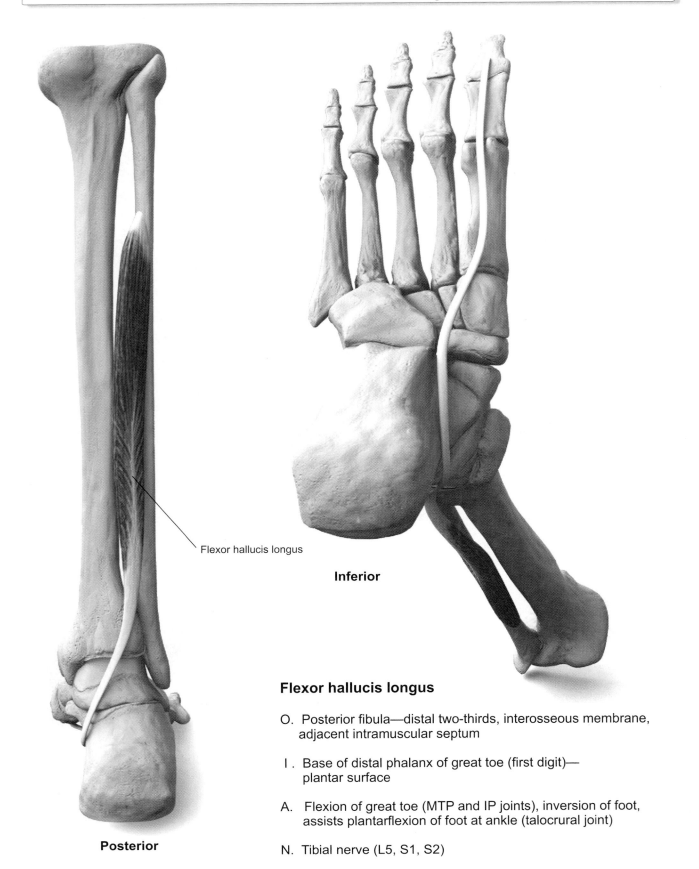

Flexor hallucis longus

Inferior

Posterior

Flexor hallucis longus

O. Posterior fibula—distal two-thirds, interosseous membrane, adjacent intramuscular septum

I. Base of distal phalanx of great toe (first digit)—plantar surface

A. Flexion of great toe (MTP and IP joints), inversion of foot, assists plantarflexion of foot at ankle (talocrural joint)

N. Tibial nerve (L5, S1, S2)

Unit 3 Muscular System

Extensor digitorum brevis

O. Anterior calcaneus—superior lateral surface, lateral talocalcaneal ligament, inferior extensor retinaculum

I. Proximal phalanx of great toe (first digit)—dorsal surface, second, third, and fourth digits via extensor digitorum longus tendons

A. Extension of great toe (MTP joints), extension of second, third, and fourth digits (MTP and IP joints)

N. Deep peroneal nerve (L5, S1)

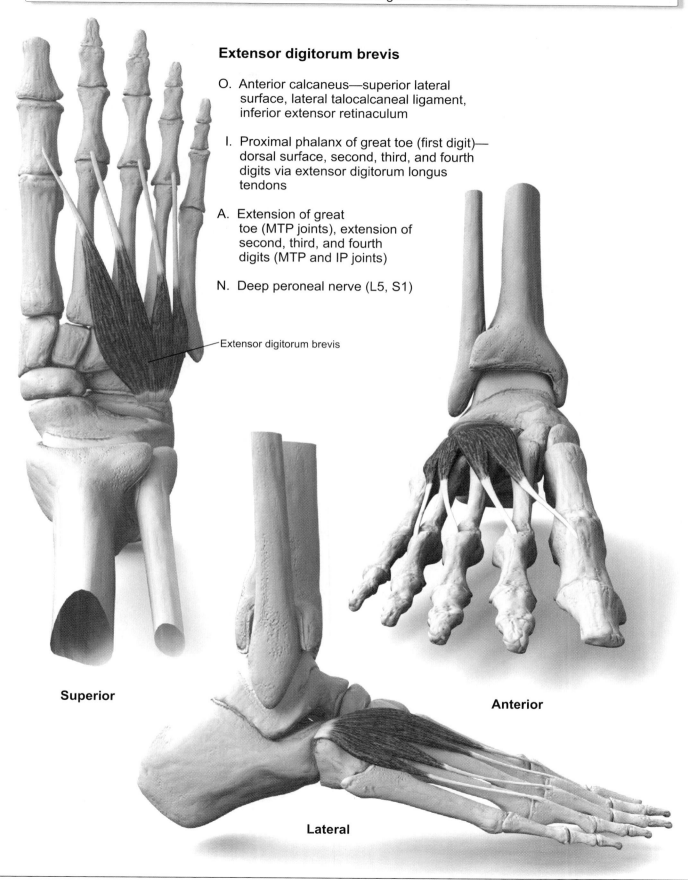

Extensor digitorum brevis

Superior

Lateral

Anterior

Dorsal interossei

O. Adjacent sides of metatarsal bones

I . *First interossei:* base of proximal phalanx of second digit—medial side
Second to fourth interossei: base of proximal phalanx of second to fourth digits—lateral side
All: dorsal extensor expansion of respective digits

A. Abduction of second through fourth digits, assists flexion (MTP joints) and extension (IP joints) of lateral four digits

N. Lateral plantar nerve (S1, S2)

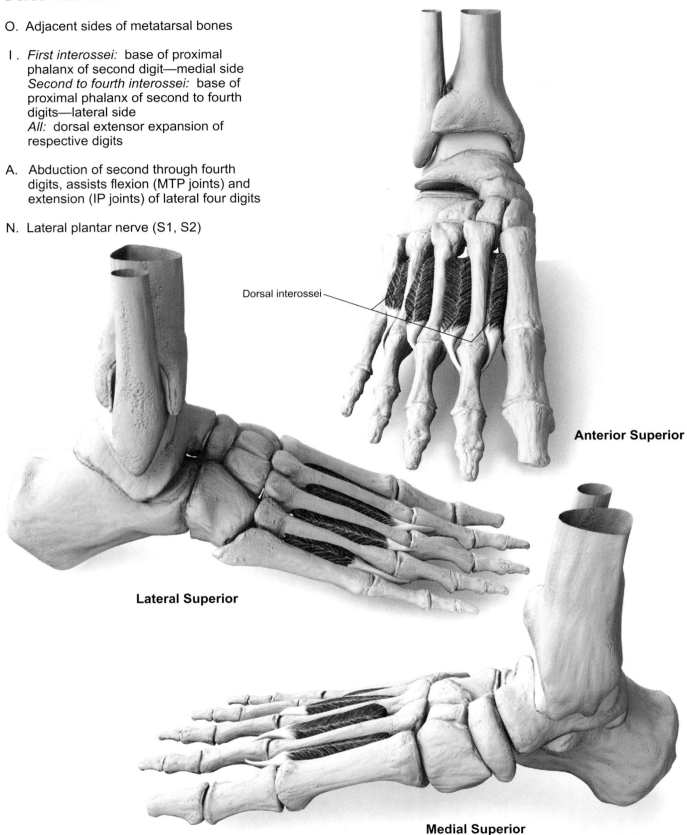

Dorsal interossei

Anterior Superior

Lateral Superior

Medial Superior

Unit 3 Muscular System

Flexor digitorum brevis

O. Tuberosity of calcaneus, plantar aponeurosis

I. Both sides of middle phalanges of second through fifth digits

A. Flexion of lateral four digits (PIP joints)

N. Medial plantar nerve (L4, L5)

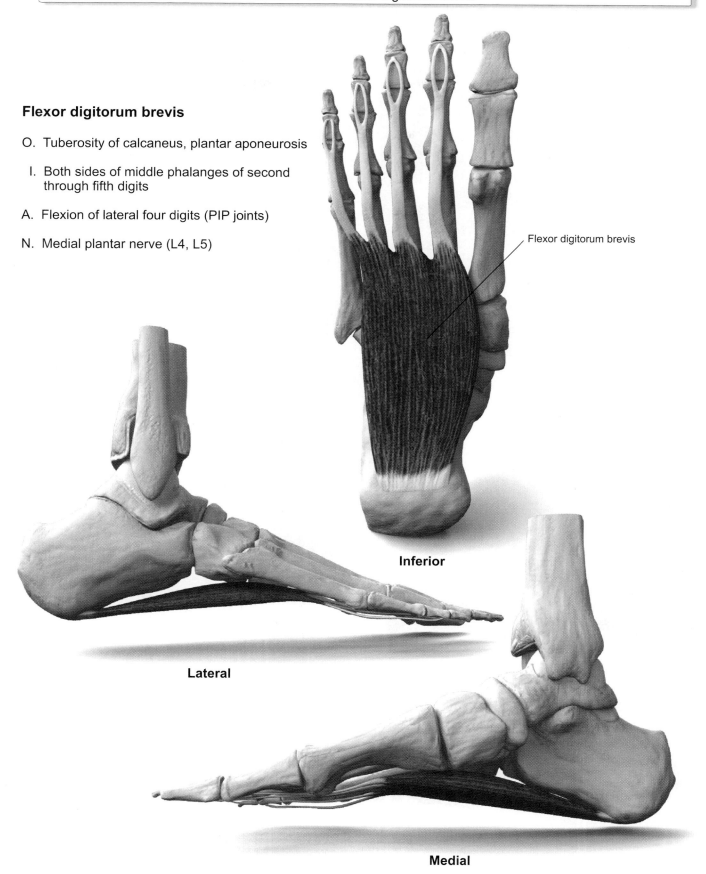

Flexor digitorum brevis

Inferior

Lateral

Medial

Abductor digiti minimi

O. Tuberosity of calcaneus, plantar aponeurosis

I. Proximal phalanx of fifth digit—lateral aspect

A. Abduction of fifth digit (MTP joint), assists flexion of fifth digit (MTP joint)

N. Lateral plantar nerve (S1, S2)

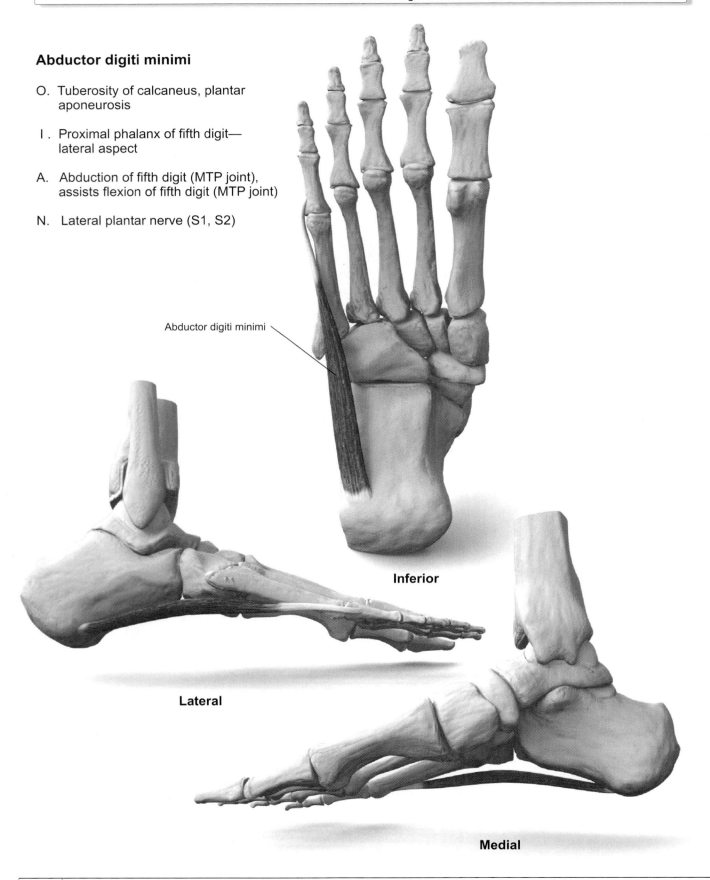

Abductor digiti minimi

Inferior

Lateral

Medial

Unit 3 Muscular System

Abductor hallucis

O. Tuberosity of calcaneus, flexor retinaculum
    of ankle, plantar aponeurosis

I . Base of proximal phalanx of great
    toe (first digit)—medial side, medial
    sesamoid bone of great toe

A. Abduction of great toe (MTP and IP joints),
    assists in flexion of great toe (MTP joint)

N. Medial plantar nerve (L4, L5)

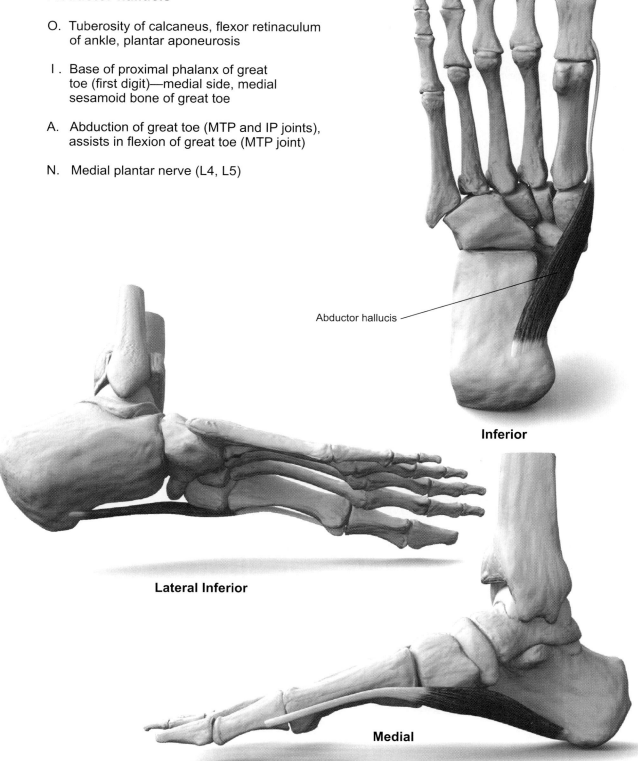

Abductor hallucis

Inferior

Lateral Inferior

Medial

Quadratus plantae

O. *Medial head:* calcaneus—medial side
   Lateral head: calcaneus—lateral side and inferior surface

I. Tendons of flexor digitorum longus

A. Flexion of second through fifth digits (DIP joints)

N. Lateral plantar nerve (S1, S2)

Lumbricals

Quadratus plantae
(lateral head)

Quadratus plantae
(medial head)

Lateral Inferior

Inferior

Lumbricals

O. Tendons of flexor digitorum longus

I. Expansion of tendons to extensor digitorum longus
   on second to fifth digits

A. Flexion of proximal phalanges of second through fifth
   digits (MTP joints), extension of distal phalanges of second
   through fifth digits (DIP joints)

N. Medial plantar nerve (L4, L5), first lumbrical
   Lateral plantar nerve (S1, S2), second third and fourth lumbricals

Medial Inferior

Flexor digiti brevis

O. Base of fifth metatarsal, adjacent tendinous sheath of peroneus longus

I . Base of proximal phalanx of fifth digit—lateral aspect

A. Flexion of proximal phalanx of fifth digit (MP joint)

N. Lateral plantar nerve (S1, S2)

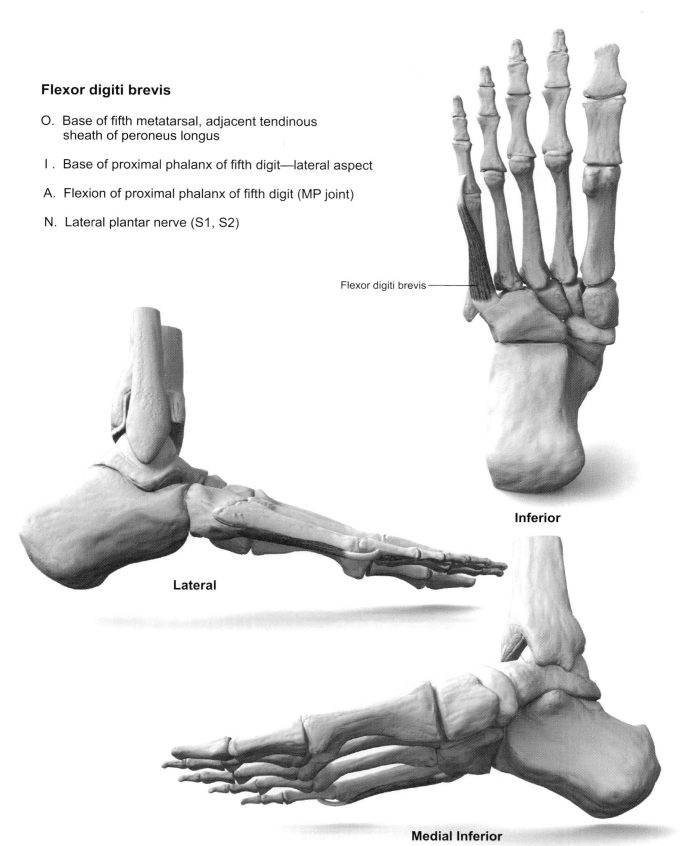

Flexor digiti brevis

Inferior

Lateral

Medial Inferior

Flexor hallucis brevis

O. Cuboid—plantar surface, lateral cuneiforms, and prolongation of tibialis posterior tendon

I. Base of proximal phalanx of great toe (first digit)—medial and lateral aspects

A. Flexion of great toe (MTP joint)

N. Medial plantar nerve (L4, L5, S1)

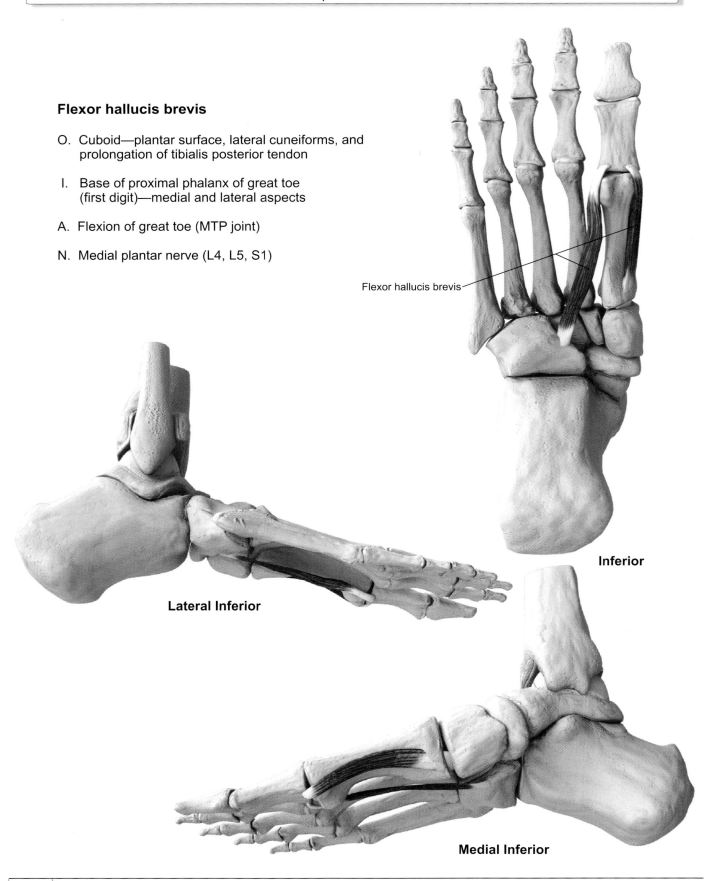

Flexor hallucis brevis

Inferior

Lateral Inferior

Medial Inferior

Unit 3 Muscular System

Adductor hallucis

O. *Oblique head:* Bases of second, third, and fourth metatarsal bones, tendinous sheath of peroneus longus
Transverse head: Plantar metatarsophalangeal ligaments and transverse metatarsal ligaments of third, fourth, and fifth digits

I. Base of phalanx of great toe (first digit)—lateral aspect

A. Adduction of great toe, assists flexion of great toe

N. Lateral plantar nerve (S1, S2)

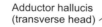

Adductor hallucis
(transverse head)

Adductor hallucis
(oblique head)

Inferior

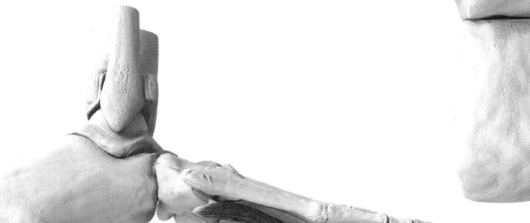

Inferior Lateral

Inferior Medial

Plantar interossei

O. Third, fourth, and fifth metatarsals—inferior and medial sides

I. Base of proximal phalanx of corresponding digit—medial side

A. Adduction of third, fourth, and fifth digits toward second digit, flexion of third, fourth, and fifth digits (MTP joints)

N. Lateral plantar nerve (S1, S2)

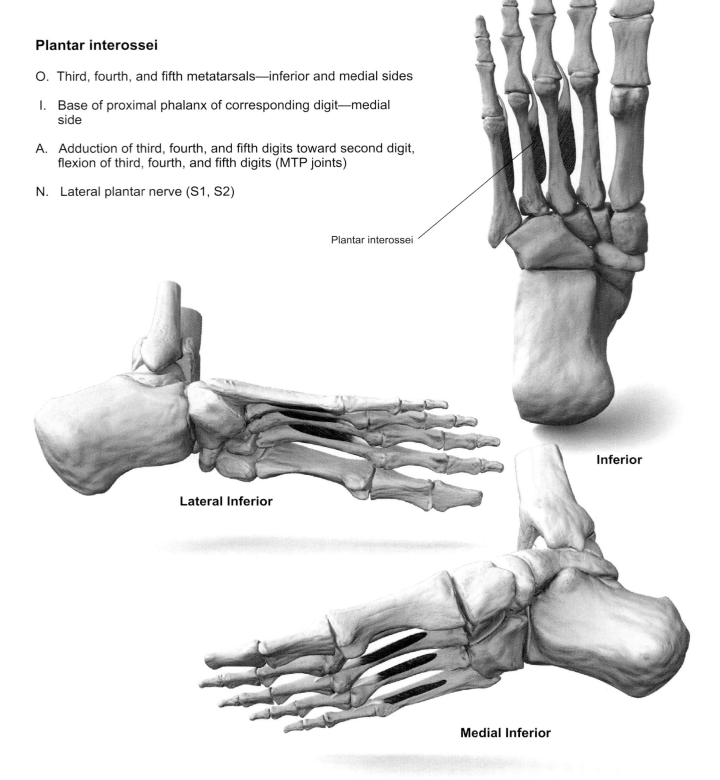

Plantar interossei

Inferior

Lateral Inferior

Medial Inferior

Unit 3 Muscular System

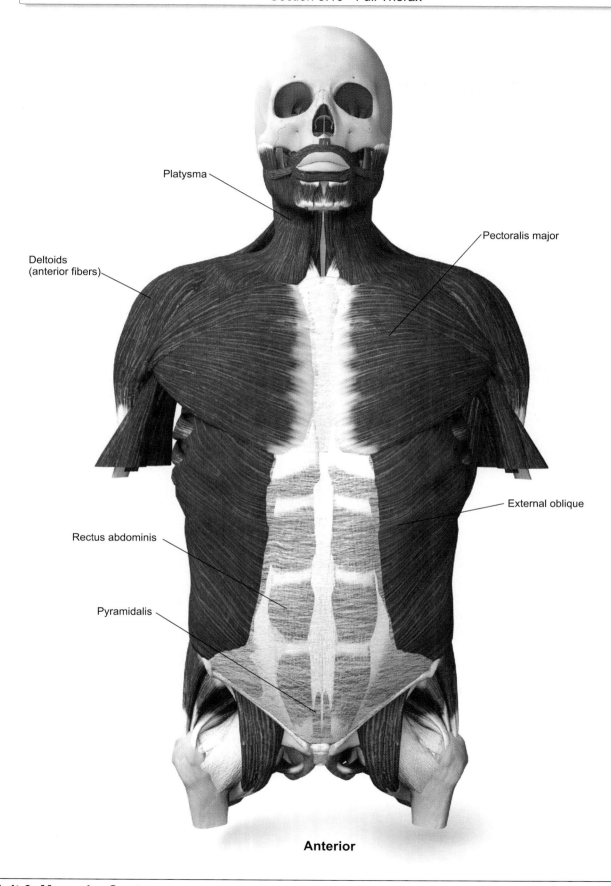

Platysma

Pectoralis major

Deltoids
(anterior fibers)

External oblique

Rectus abdominis

Pyramidalis

Anterior

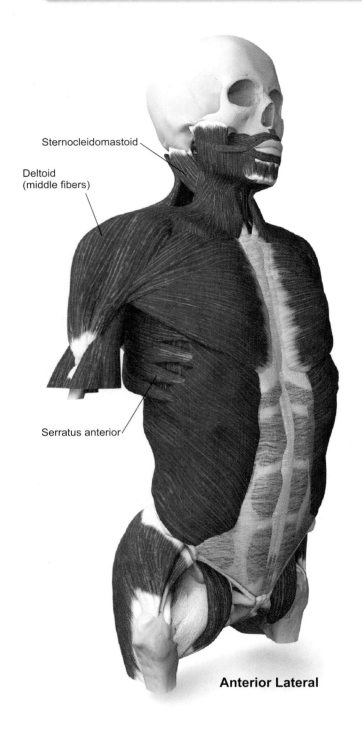

Sternocleidomastoid

Deltoid
(middle fibers)

Serratus anterior

Anterior Lateral

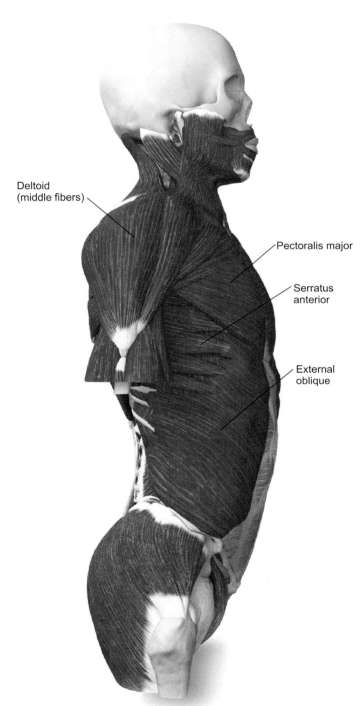

Deltoid
(middle fibers)

Pectoralis major

Serratus
anterior

External
oblique

Lateral

Unit 3 Muscular System

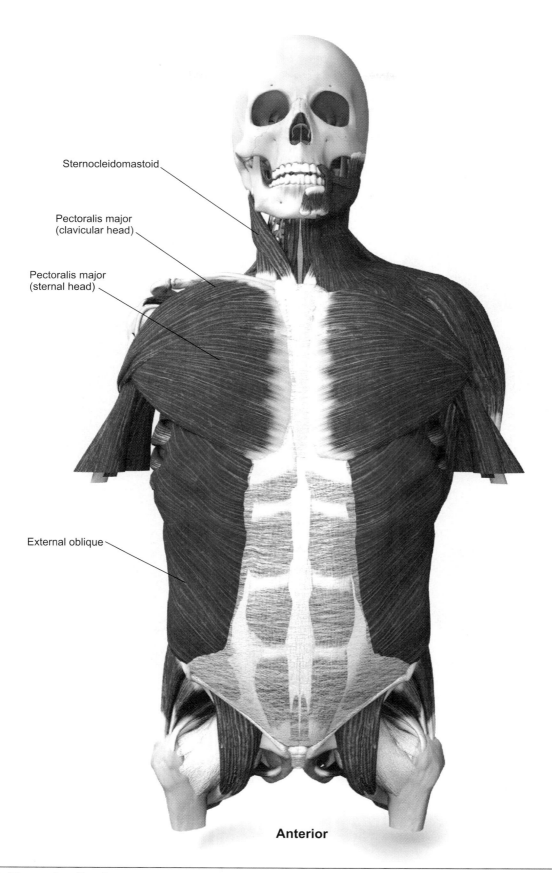

Sternocleidomastoid

Pectoralis major
(clavicular head)

Pectoralis major
(sternal head)

External oblique

Anterior

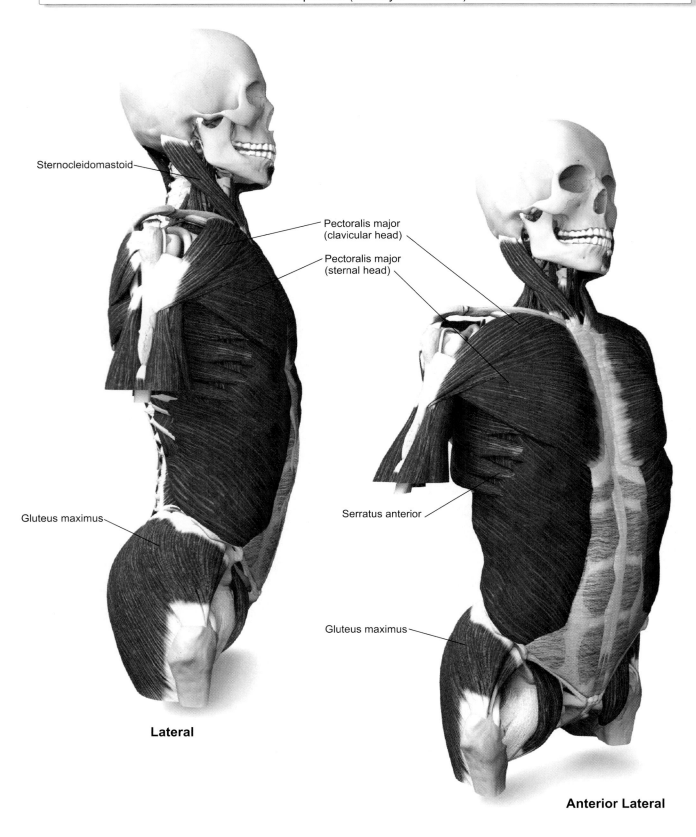

Sternocleidomastoid

Pectoralis major
(clavicular head)

Pectoralis major
(sternal head)

Gluteus maximus

Serratus anterior

Gluteus maximus

Lateral

Anterior Lateral

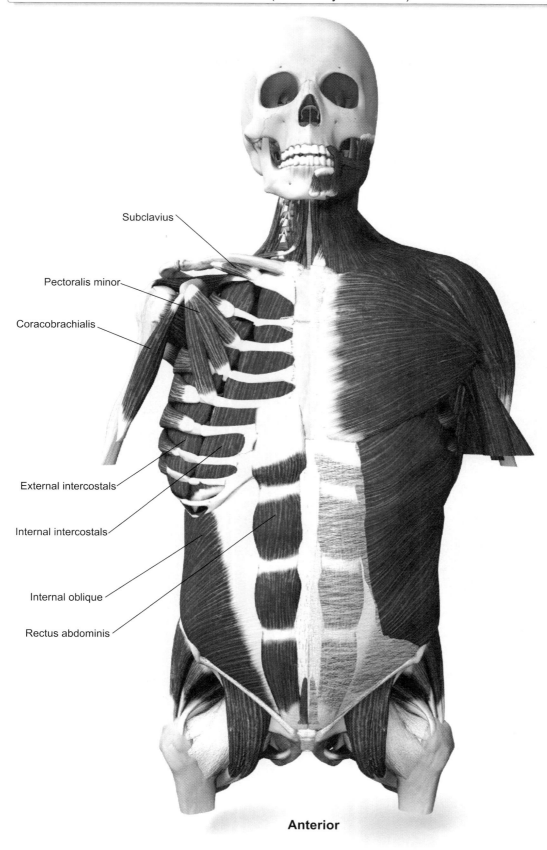

Subclavius

Pectoralis minor

Coracobrachialis

External intercostals

Internal intercostals

Internal oblique

Rectus abdominis

Anterior

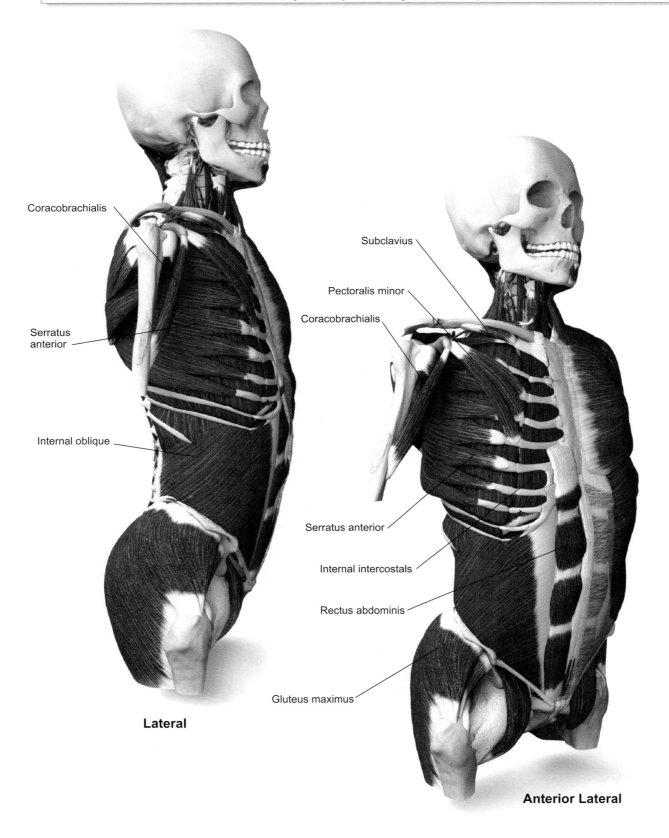

Coracobrachialis

Serratus
anterior

Internal oblique

Subclavius

Pectoralis minor

Coracobrachialis

Serratus anterior

Internal intercostals

Rectus abdominis

Gluteus maximus

Lateral

Anterior Lateral

Unit 3 Muscular System

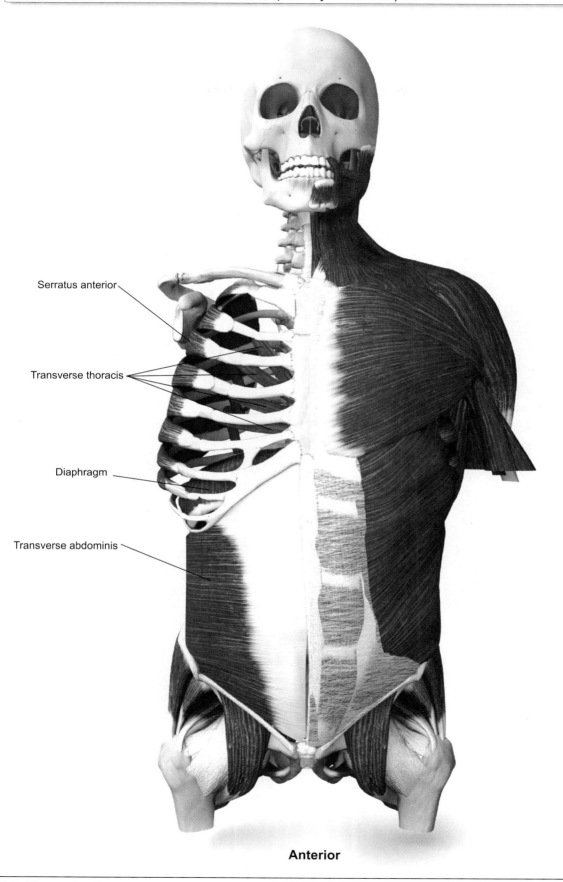

Serratus anterior

Transverse thoracis

Diaphragm

Transverse abdominis

Anterior

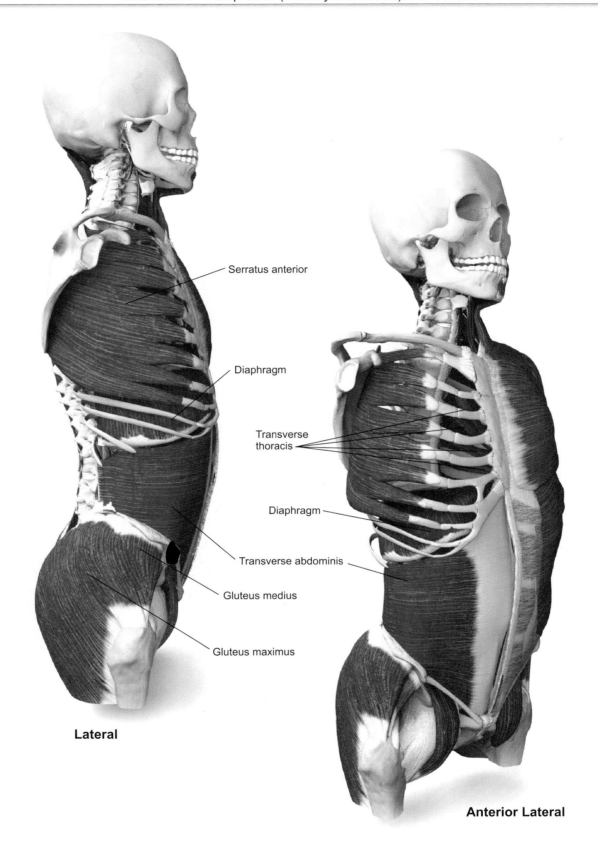

Serratus anterior

Diaphragm

Transverse
thoracis

Diaphragm

Transverse abdominis

Gluteus medius

Gluteus maximus

Lateral

Anterior Lateral

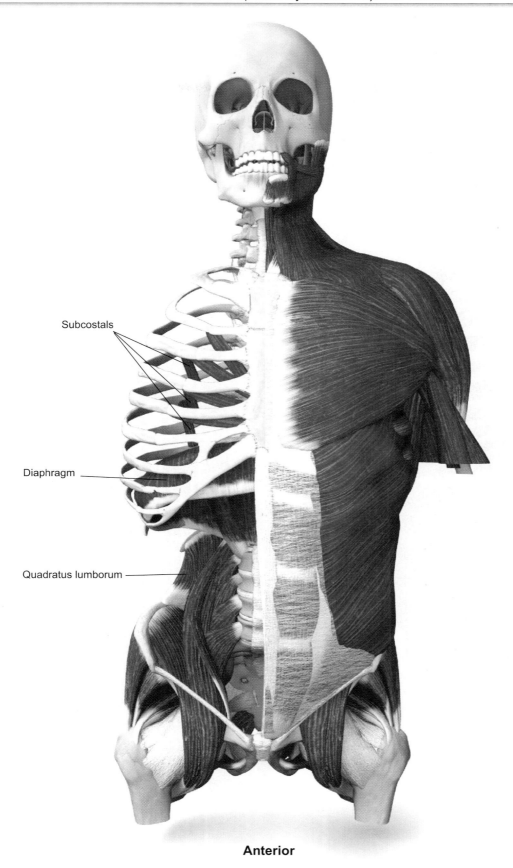

Subcostals

Diaphragm

Quadratus lumborum

Anterior

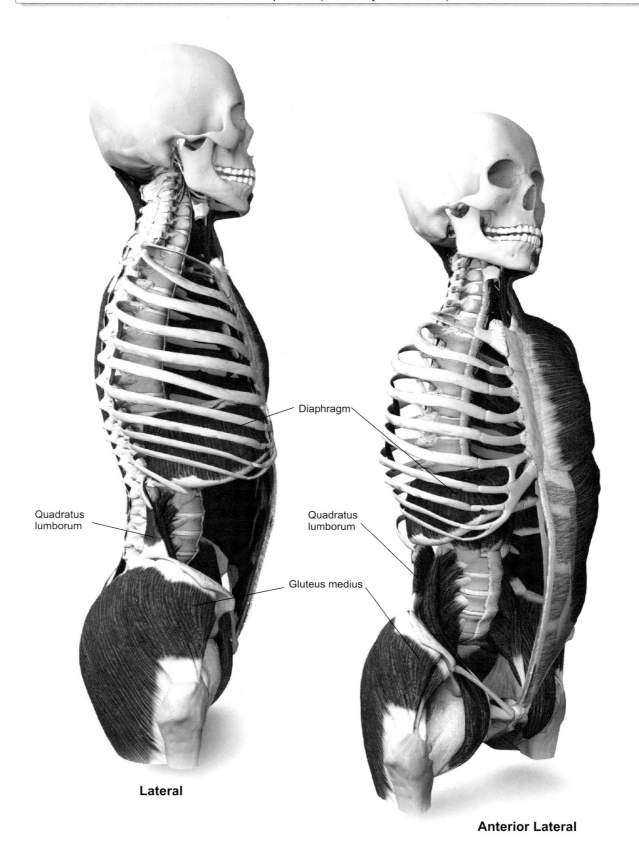

Diaphragm

Quadratus
lumborum

Quadratus
lumborum

Gluteus medius

Lateral

Anterior Lateral

Unit 3 Muscular System

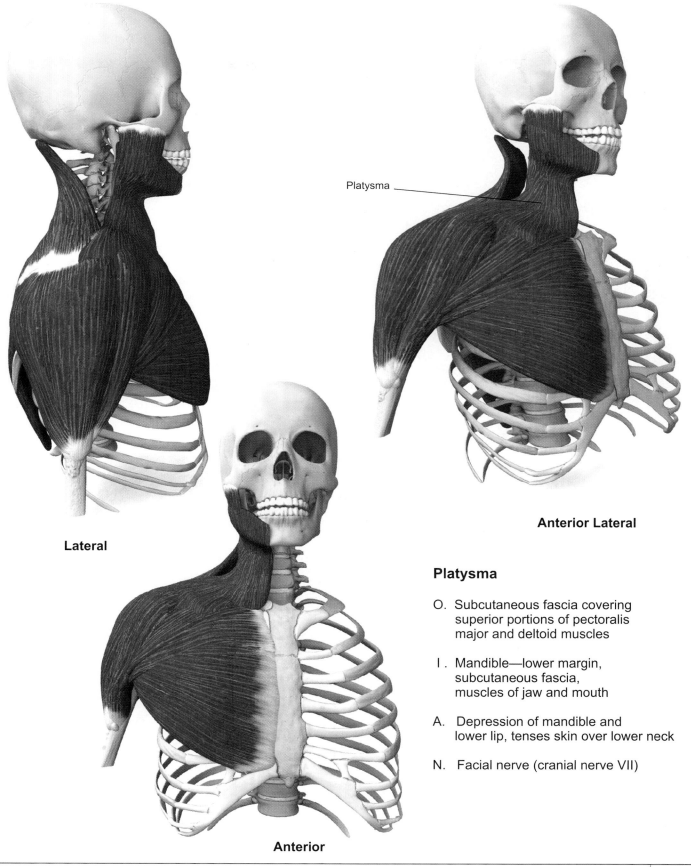

Lateral

Platysma

Anterior Lateral

Anterior

Platysma

O. Subcutaneous fascia covering superior portions of pectoralis major and deltoid muscles

I . Mandible—lower margin, subcutaneous fascia, muscles of jaw and mouth

A. Depression of mandible and lower lip, tenses skin over lower neck

N. Facial nerve (cranial nerve VII)

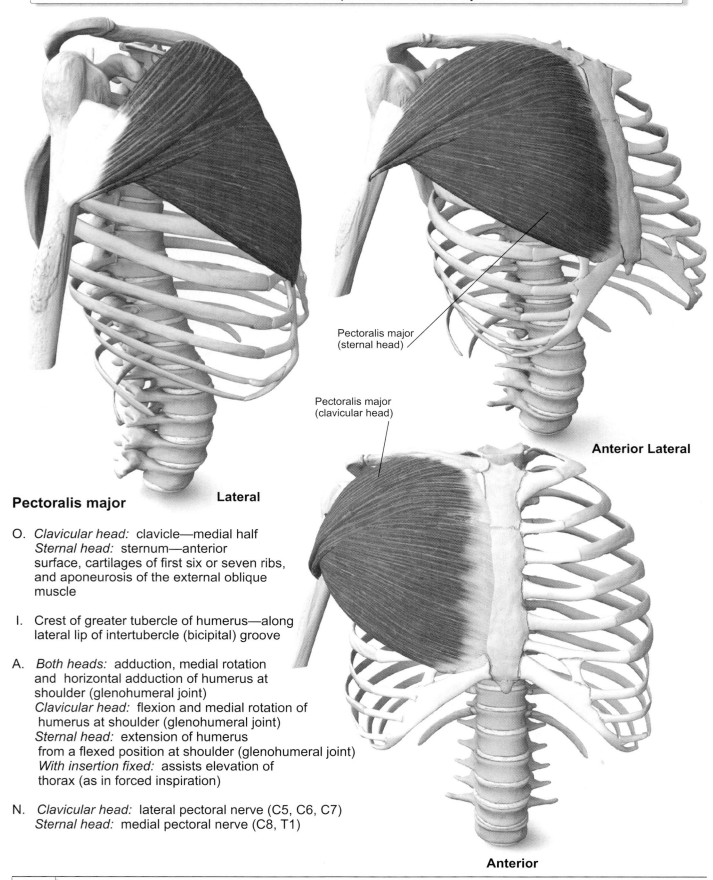

Pectoralis major
(sternal head)

Pectoralis major
(clavicular head)

Anterior Lateral

Lateral

Anterior

Pectoralis major

O. *Clavicular head:* clavicle—medial half
Sternal head: sternum—anterior
surface, cartilages of first six or seven ribs,
and aponeurosis of the external oblique
muscle

I. Crest of greater tubercle of humerus—along
lateral lip of intertubercle (bicipital) groove

A. *Both heads:* adduction, medial rotation
and horizontal adduction of humerus at
shoulder (glenohumeral joint)
Clavicular head: flexion and medial rotation of
humerus at shoulder (glenohumeral joint)
Sternal head: extension of humerus
from a flexed position at shoulder (glenohumeral joint)
With insertion fixed: assists elevation of
thorax (as in forced inspiration)

N. *Clavicular head:* lateral pectoral nerve (C5, C6, C7)
Sternal head: medial pectoral nerve (C8, T1)

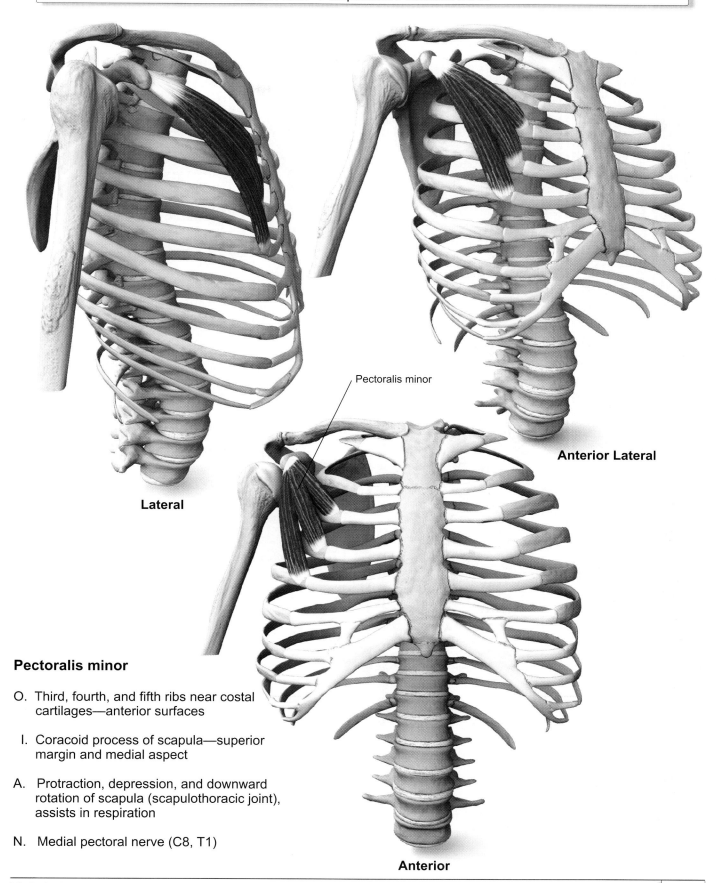

Pectoralis minor

Anterior Lateral

Lateral

Pectoralis minor

O. Third, fourth, and fifth ribs near costal cartilages—anterior surfaces

I. Coracoid process of scapula—superior margin and medial aspect

A. Protraction, depression, and downward rotation of scapula (scapulothoracic joint), assists in respiration

N. Medial pectoral nerve (C8, T1)

Anterior

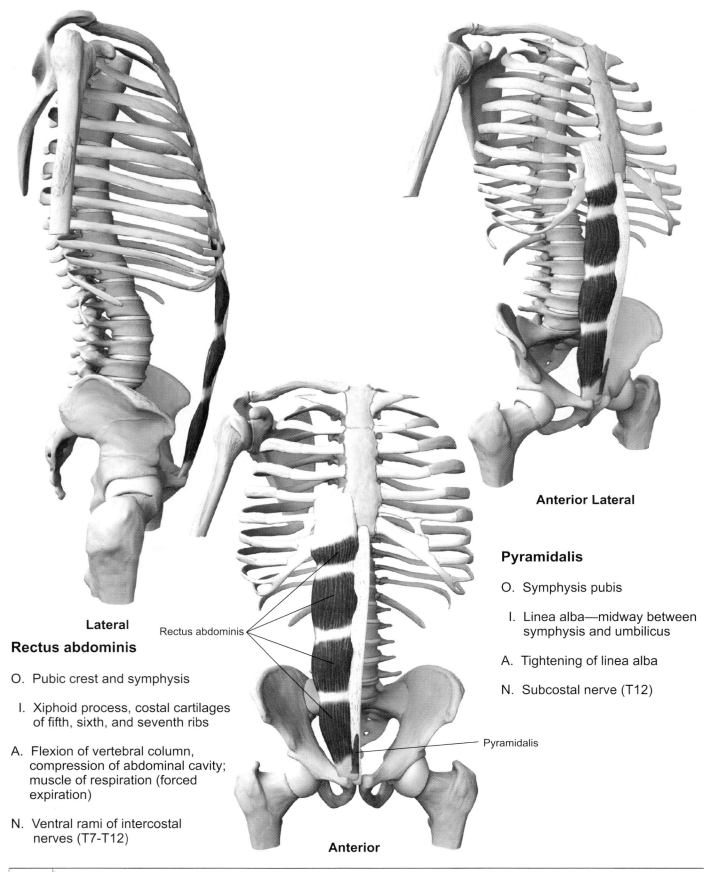

Lateral

Rectus abdominis

O. Pubic crest and symphysis

I. Xiphoid process, costal cartilages of fifth, sixth, and seventh ribs

A. Flexion of vertebral column, compression of abdominal cavity; muscle of respiration (forced expiration)

N. Ventral rami of intercostal nerves (T7-T12)

Rectus abdominis

Anterior

Anterior Lateral

Pyramidalis

O. Symphysis pubis

I. Linea alba—midway between symphysis and umbilicus

A. Tightening of linea alba

N. Subcostal nerve (T12)

Pyramidalis

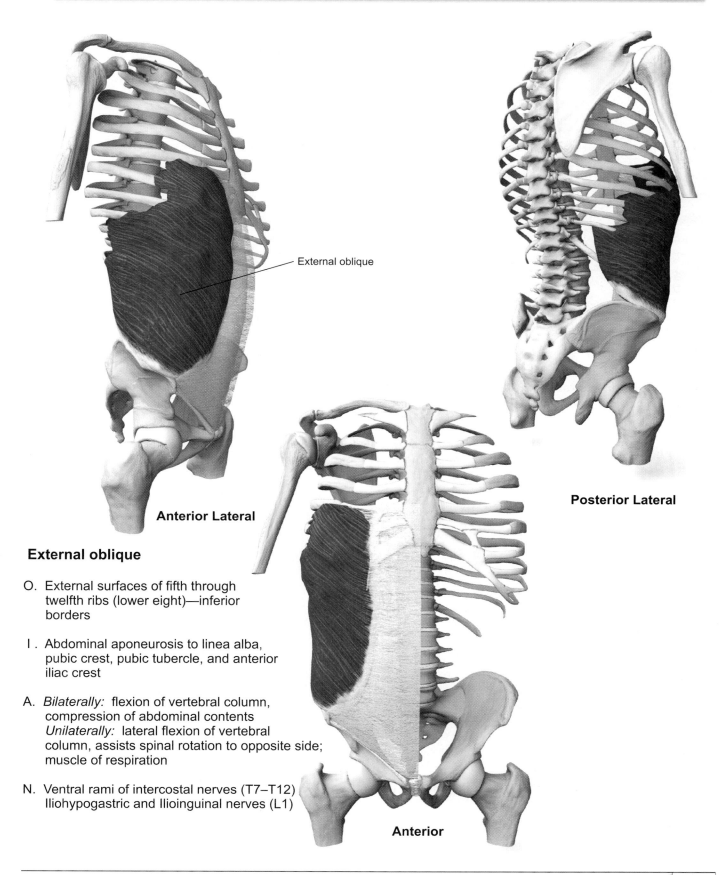

External oblique

Anterior Lateral

Posterior Lateral

Anterior

External oblique

O. External surfaces of fifth through twelfth ribs (lower eight)—inferior borders

I. Abdominal aponeurosis to linea alba, pubic crest, pubic tubercle, and anterior iliac crest

A. *Bilaterally:* flexion of vertebral column, compression of abdominal contents
Unilaterally: lateral flexion of vertebral column, assists spinal rotation to opposite side; muscle of respiration

N. Ventral rami of intercostal nerves (T7–T12) Iliohypogastric and Ilioinguinal nerves (L1)

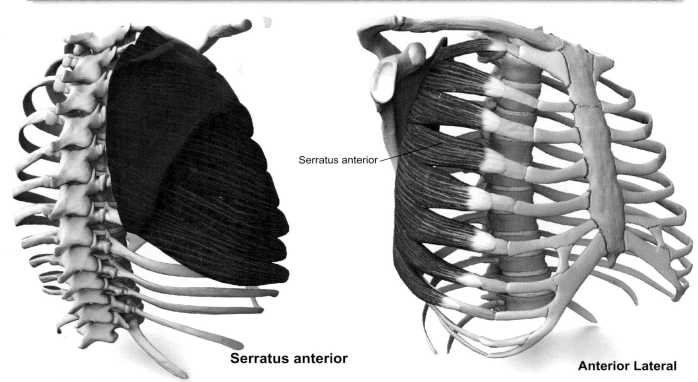

Serratus anterior

Posterior Lateral

Anterior Lateral

Serratus anterior

O. Upper eight or nine ribs—lateral surfaces and superior borders

I. Vertebral border of scapula—anterior surface

A. Protraction and upward rotation of scapula (scapulothoracic joint), secures medial border of scapula firmly against rib cage, assists in respiration

N. Long thoracic nerve (C5, C6, C7)

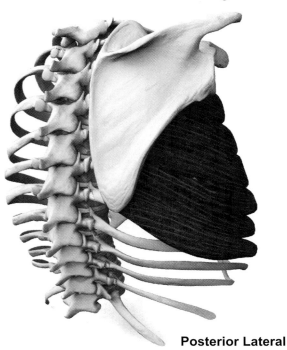

Posterior Lateral

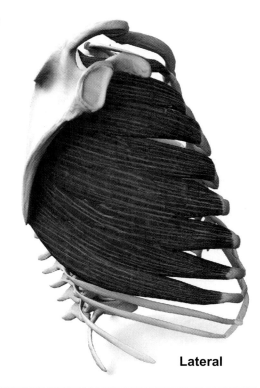

Lateral

Unit 3 Muscular System

Internal oblique

O. Thoracolumbar fascia, inguinal ligament—anterior one-half, iliac crest—anterior two thirds

I . Tenth, eleventh, and twelfth ribs—anterior borders, linea alba, and crest of pubis via conjoint tendon

A. *Bilaterally:* flexion of vertebral column, compression of abdomen
Unilaterally: lateral flexion of vertebral column, rotation to same side; muscle of respiration

N. Ventral rami of intercostal nerves (T7–T12) Iliohypogastric and Ilioinguinal nerves (L1)

Internal oblique

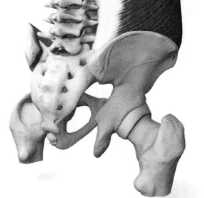

Lateral

Posterior Lateral

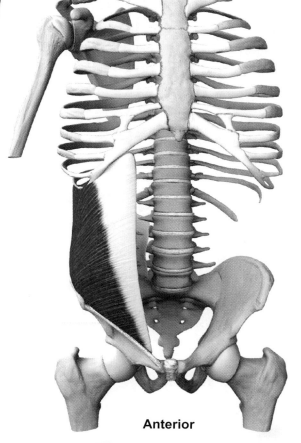

Anterior

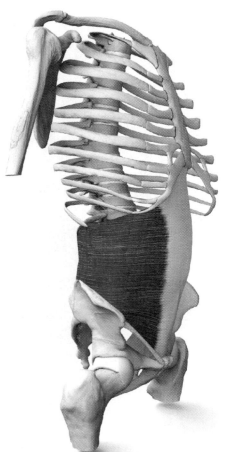

Transverse abdominis

O. Inguinal ligament—lateral one-third, iliac crest, thoracolumbar fascia, internal surfaces of costal cartilages of seventh through twelfth ribs (lower six)

I. Linea alba, pubic crest, and pecten of pubis via conjoint tendon

A. Compression of abdomen; muscle of respiration

N. Ventral rami of intercostal nerves (T7–T12) Iliohypogastric and Ilioinguinal nerves (L1)

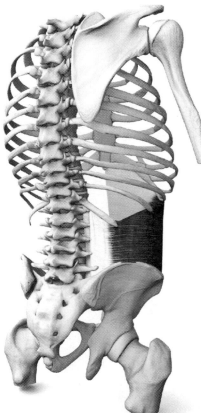

Anterior Lateral

Posterior Lateral

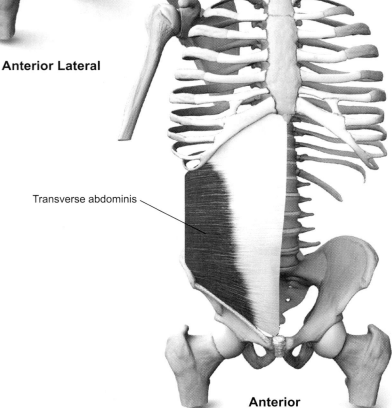

Transverse abdominis

Anterior

Unit 3 Muscular System

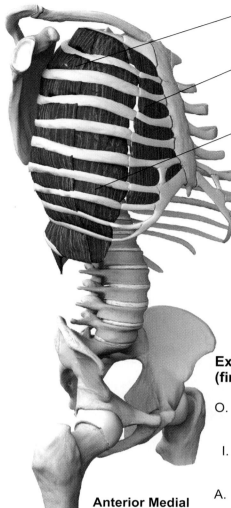

External intercostals

Internal intercostals

Innermost intercostals

Anterior Medial

Posterior Lateral

External intercostals
(first layer—most superficial) 11 pairs

O. Inferior border of rib directly
   above—within an intercostal space

I. Superior border of rib directly
   below—within an intercostal space

A. Stabilization and maintenance of
   integrity of rib cage, assists in
   forced inspiration by elevation of ribs

N. Intercostal nerves

Internal intercostals
(second layer—middle) 11 pairs

O. Inferior border of rib directly above,
   inner surface of rib and costal
   cartilages—within an intercostal space

I. Superior border of rib directly
   below—within an intercostal space

A. Depression and approximation of ribs

N. Intercostal nerves

Innermost intercostals
(third layer—deepest) part of innermost layer

O. Internal and inferior surface of rib directly
   above—within an intercostal space

I. Internal and superior surface of rib
   directly below—within an intercostal space

A. Fixation of ribs during respiration

N. Intercostal nerves

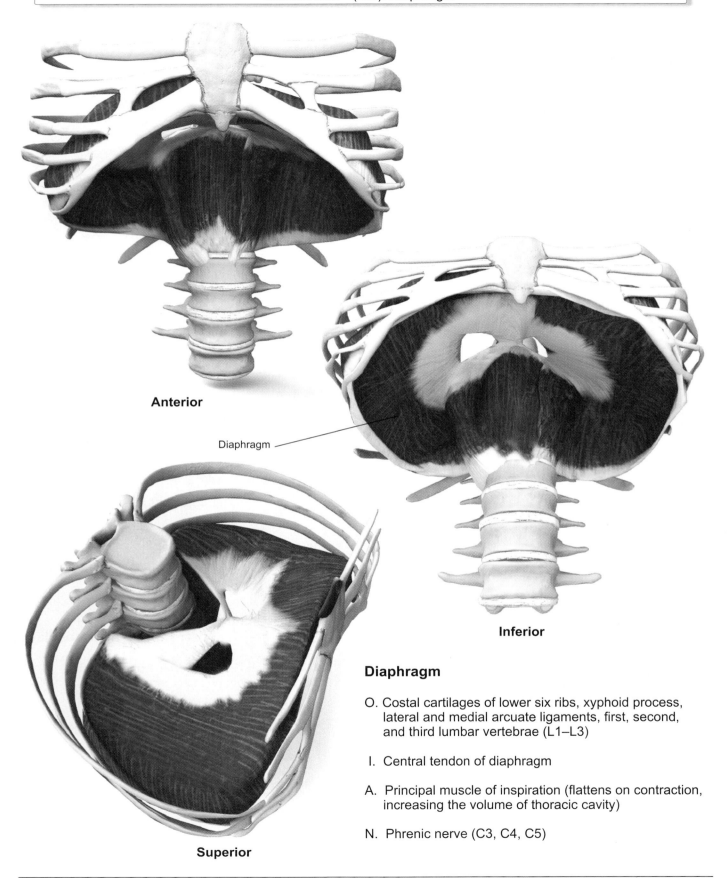

Anterior

Diaphragm

Inferior

Superior

Diaphragm

O. Costal cartilages of lower six ribs, xyphoid process, lateral and medial arcuate ligaments, first, second, and third lumbar vertebrae (L1–L3)

I. Central tendon of diaphragm

A. Principal muscle of inspiration (flattens on contraction, increasing the volume of thoracic cavity)

N. Phrenic nerve (C3, C4, C5)

Unit 3 Muscular System

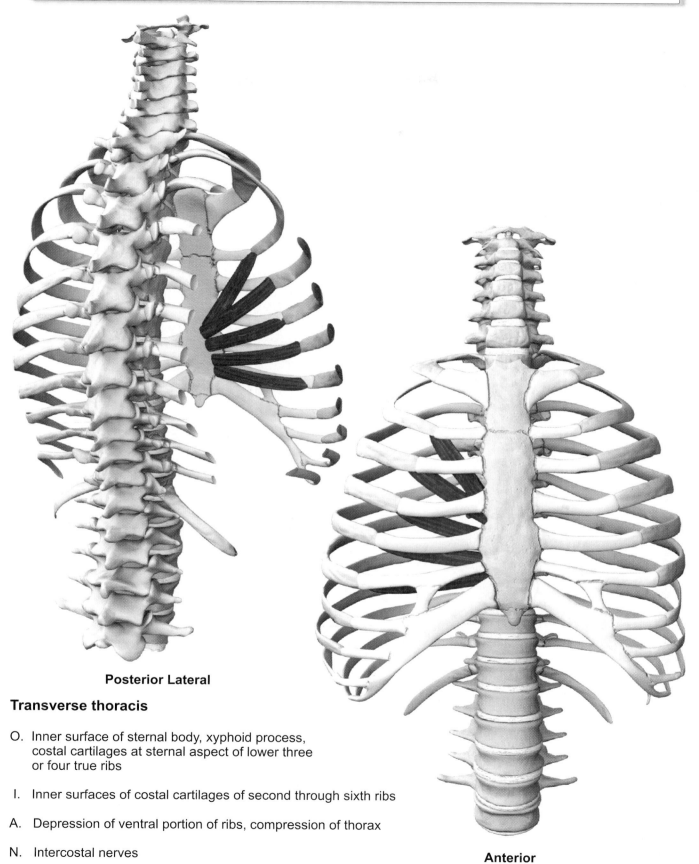

Posterior Lateral

Transverse thoracis

O. Inner surface of sternal body, xyphoid process, costal cartilages at sternal aspect of lower three or four true ribs

I. Inner surfaces of costal cartilages of second through sixth ribs

A. Depression of ventral portion of ribs, compression of thorax

N. Intercostal nerves

Anterior

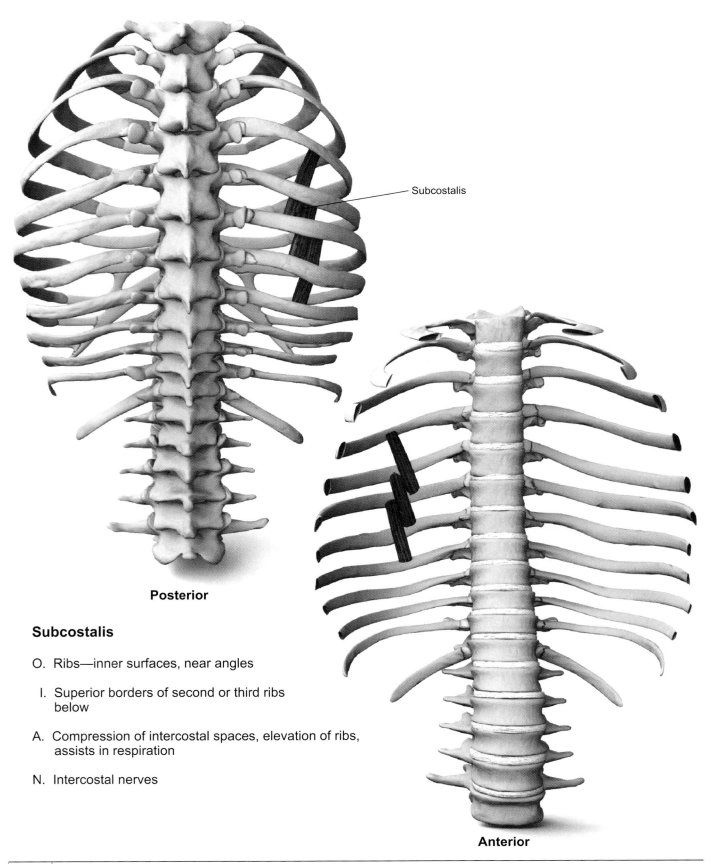

Subcostalis

Posterior

Anterior

Subcostalis

O. Ribs—inner surfaces, near angles

I. Superior borders of second or third ribs below

A. Compression of intercostal spaces, elevation of ribs, assists in respiration

N. Intercostal nerves

Unit 3 Muscular System

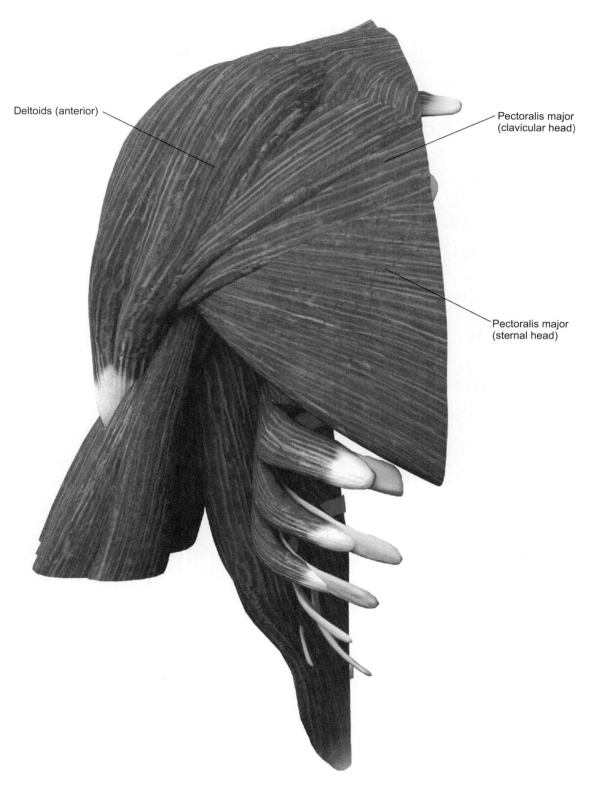

Deltoids (anterior)

Pectoralis major
(clavicular head)

Pectoralis major
(sternal head)

Anterior

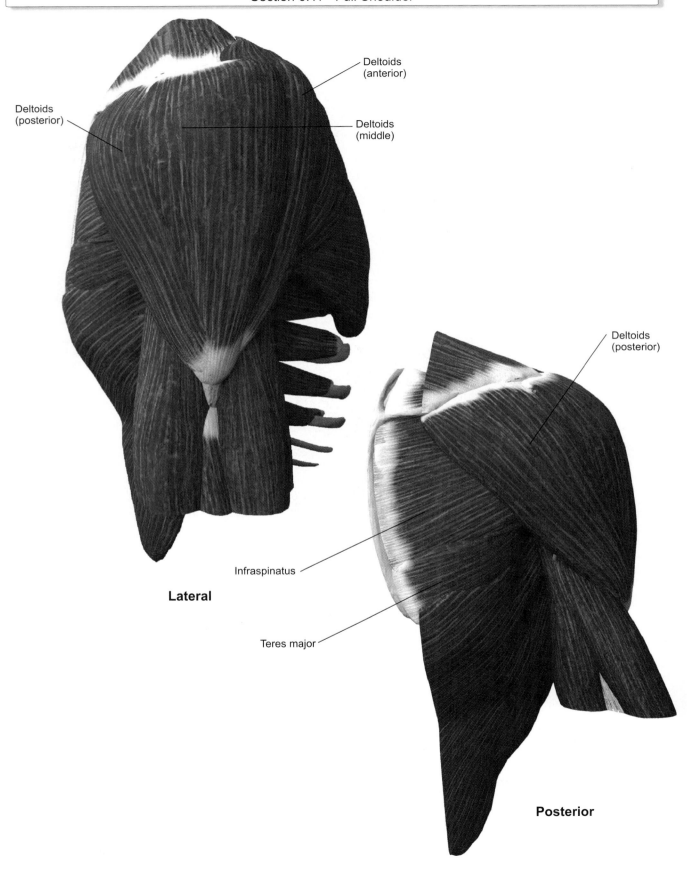

Deltoids
(anterior)

Deltoids
(posterior)

Deltoids
(middle)

Deltoids
(posterior)

Lateral

Infraspinatus

Teres major

Posterior

Unit 3 Muscular System

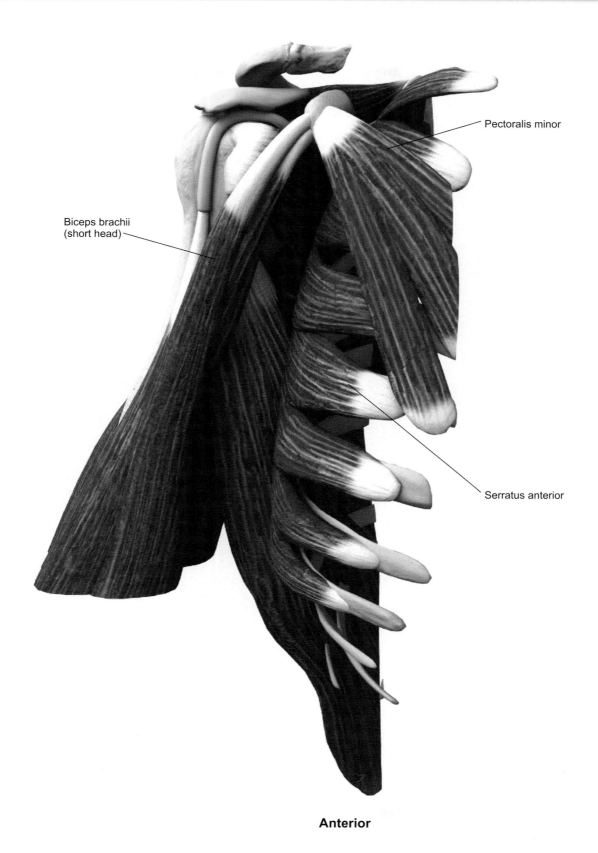

Pectoralis minor

Biceps brachii
(short head)

Serratus anterior

Anterior

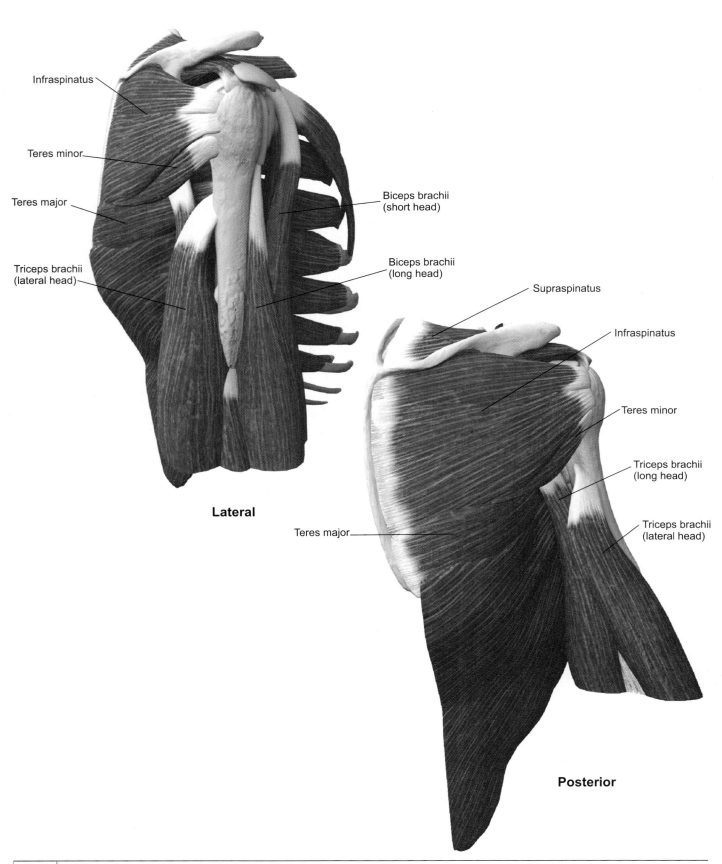

Infraspinatus

Teres minor

Teres major

Triceps brachii
(lateral head)

Biceps brachii
(short head)

Biceps brachii
(long head)

Lateral

Supraspinatus

Infraspinatus

Teres minor

Triceps brachii
(long head)

Teres major

Triceps brachii
(lateral head)

Posterior

Unit 3 Muscular System

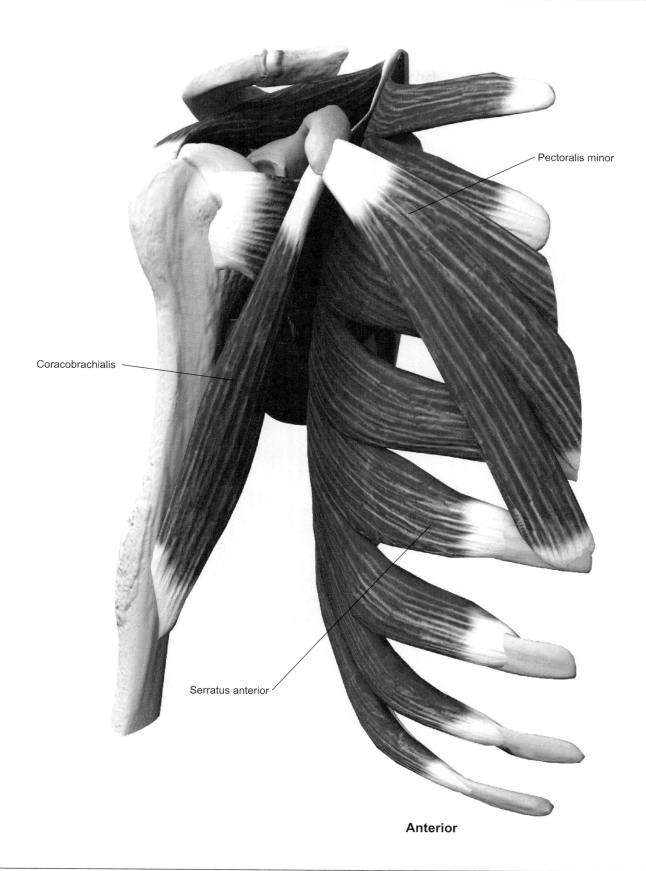

Pectoralis minor

Coracobrachialis

Serratus anterior

Anterior

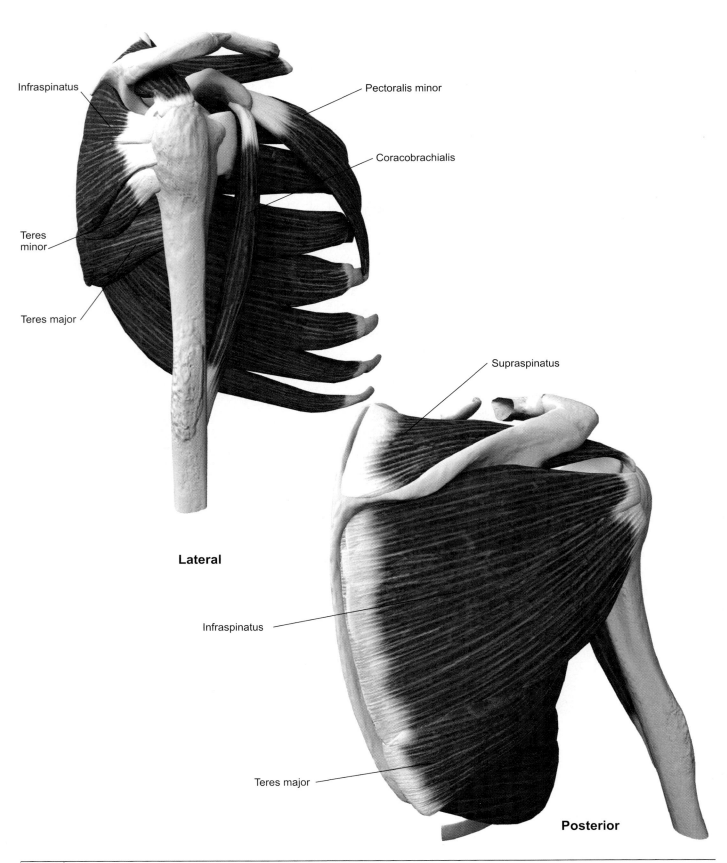

Infraspinatus

Pectoralis minor

Coracobrachialis

Teres
minor

Teres major

Supraspinatus

Lateral

Infraspinatus

Teres major

Posterior

Unit 3 Muscular System

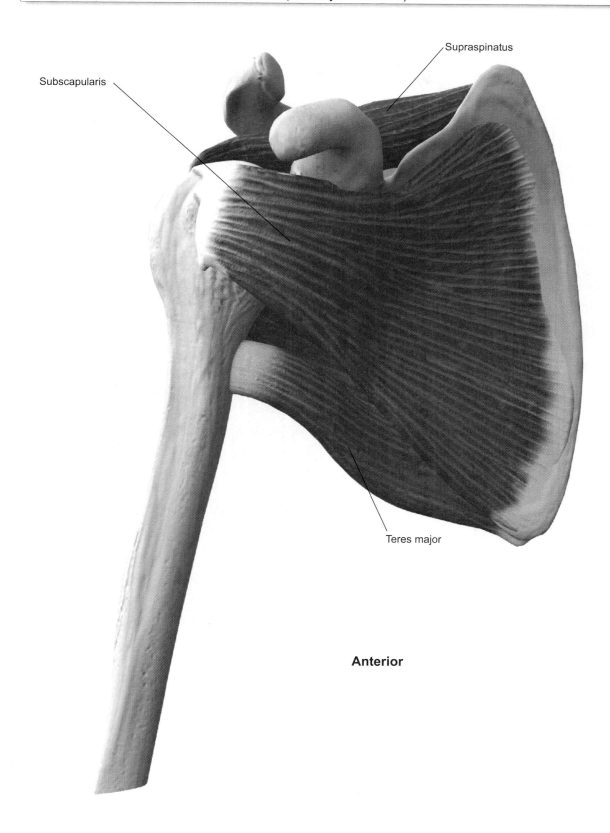

Supraspinatus

Subscapularis

Teres major

Anterior

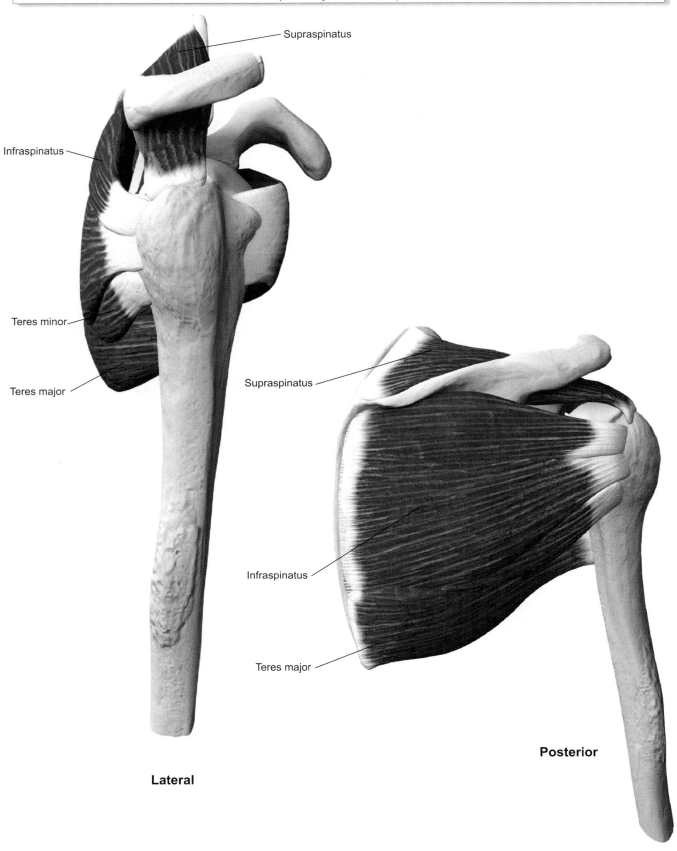

Supraspinatus

Infraspinatus

Teres minor

Teres major

Supraspinatus

Infraspinatus

Teres major

Posterior

Lateral

Unit 3 Muscular System

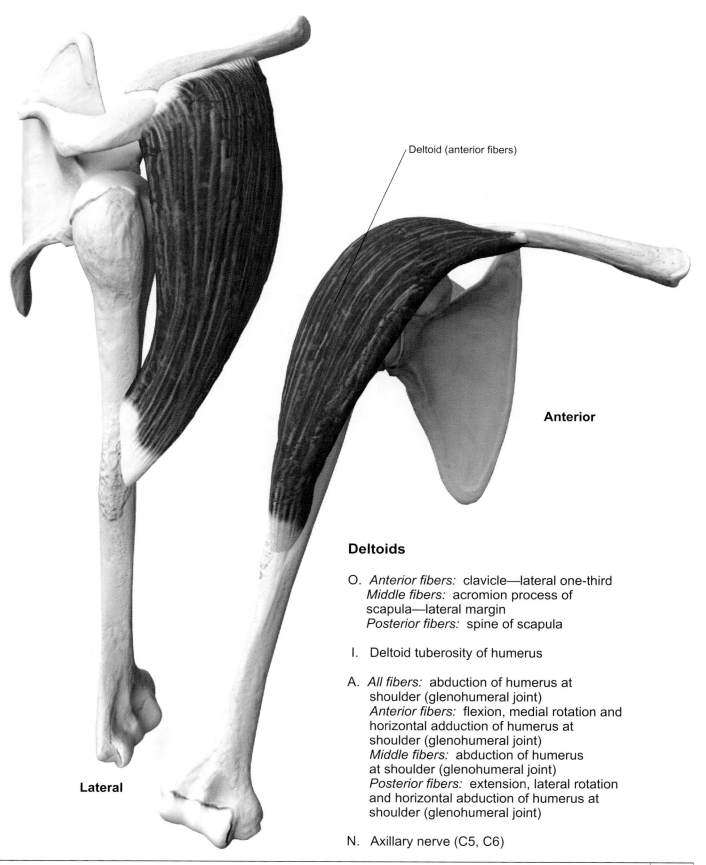

Deltoid (anterior fibers)

Anterior

Lateral

Deltoids

O. *Anterior fibers:* clavicle—lateral one-third
Middle fibers: acromion process of
scapula—lateral margin
Posterior fibers: spine of scapula

I. Deltoid tuberosity of humerus

A. *All fibers:* abduction of humerus at
shoulder (glenohumeral joint)
Anterior fibers: flexion, medial rotation and
horizontal adduction of humerus at
shoulder (glenohumeral joint)
Middle fibers: abduction of humerus
at shoulder (glenohumeral joint)
Posterior fibers: extension, lateral rotation
and horizontal abduction of humerus at
shoulder (glenohumeral joint)

N. Axillary nerve (C5, C6)

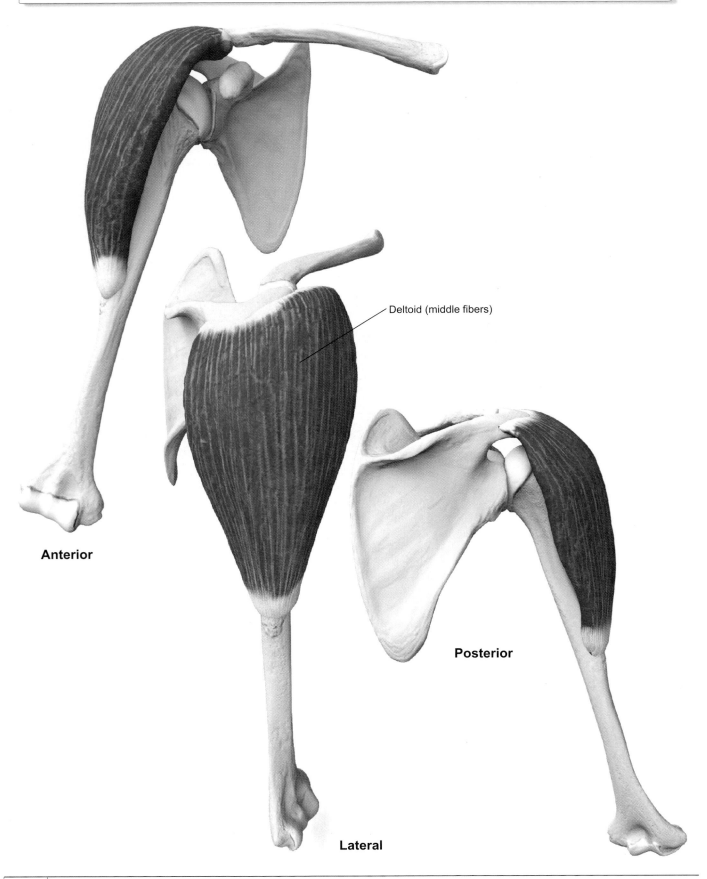

Deltoid (middle fibers)

Anterior

Lateral

Posterior

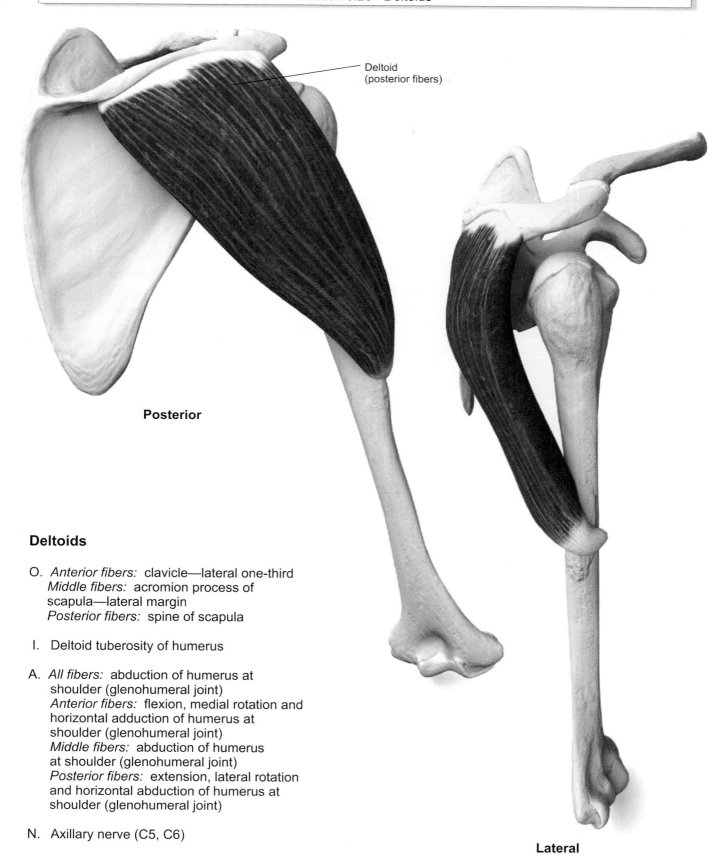

Deltoid
(posterior fibers)

Posterior

Lateral

Deltoids

O. *Anterior fibers:* clavicle—lateral one-third
   Middle fibers: acromion process of
   scapula—lateral margin
   Posterior fibers: spine of scapula

I. Deltoid tuberosity of humerus

A. *All fibers:* abduction of humerus at
   shoulder (glenohumeral joint)
   Anterior fibers: flexion, medial rotation and
   horizontal adduction of humerus at
   shoulder (glenohumeral joint)
   Middle fibers: abduction of humerus
   at shoulder (glenohumeral joint)
   Posterior fibers: extension, lateral rotation
   and horizontal abduction of humerus at
   shoulder (glenohumeral joint)

N. Axillary nerve (C5, C6)

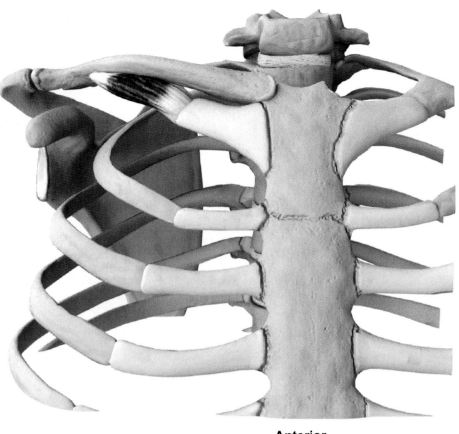

Anterior

Subclavius

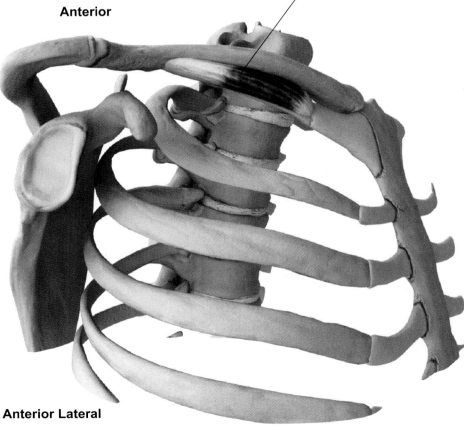

Subclavius

O. Junction of first rib with adjacent costal cartilage

I. Clavicle—inferior lateral aspect

A. Stabilization of clavicle and depression of clavicle

N. Spinal nerves (C5, C6)

Anterior Lateral

Unit 3 Muscular System

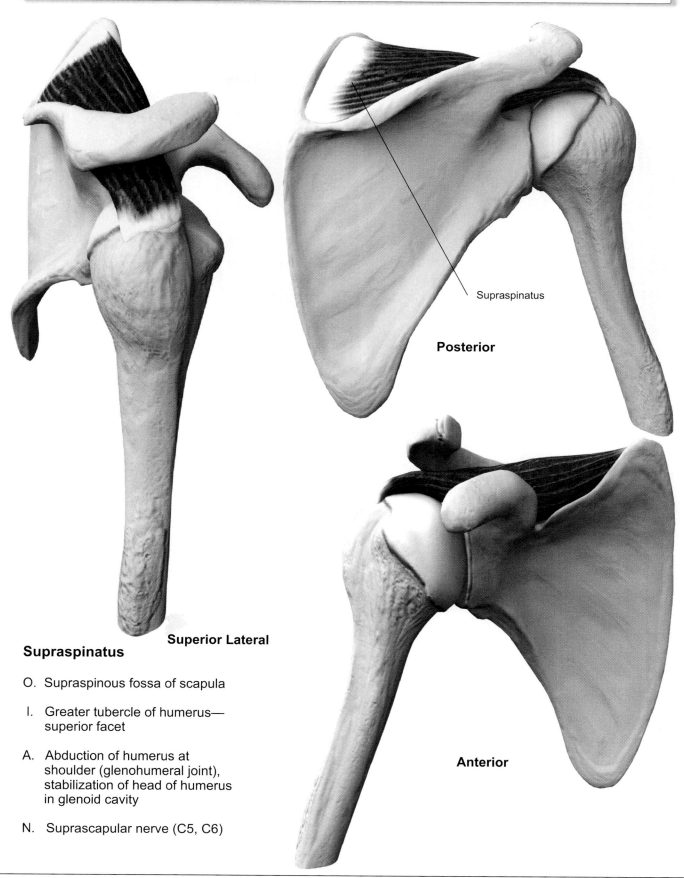

Supraspinatus

Posterior

Superior Lateral

Anterior

Supraspinatus

O. Supraspinous fossa of scapula

I. Greater tubercle of humerus—
   superior facet

A. Abduction of humerus at
   shoulder (glenohumeral joint),
   stabilization of head of humerus
   in glenoid cavity

N. Suprascapular nerve (C5, C6)

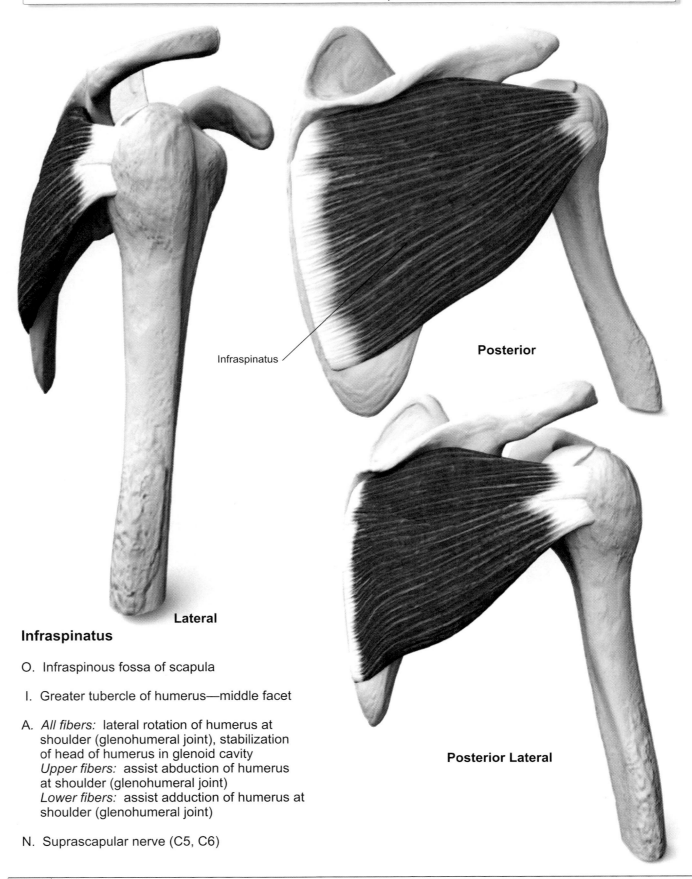

Infraspinatus

Lateral

Posterior

Posterior Lateral

Infraspinatus

O. Infraspinous fossa of scapula

I. Greater tubercle of humerus—middle facet

A. *All fibers:* lateral rotation of humerus at
shoulder (glenohumeral joint), stabilization
of head of humerus in glenoid cavity
Upper fibers: assist abduction of humerus
at shoulder (glenohumeral joint)
Lower fibers: assist adduction of humerus at
shoulder (glenohumeral joint)

N. Suprascapular nerve (C5, C6)

Unit 3 Muscular System

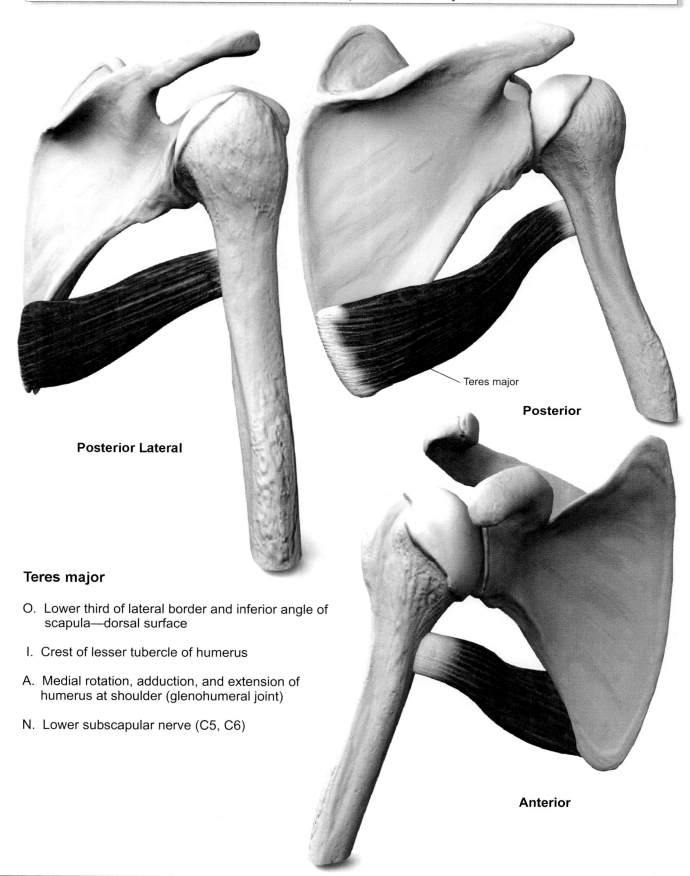

Posterior Lateral

Teres major

Posterior

Anterior

Teres major

O. Lower third of lateral border and inferior angle of scapula—dorsal surface

I. Crest of lesser tubercle of humerus

A. Medial rotation, adduction, and extension of humerus at shoulder (glenohumeral joint)

N. Lower subscapular nerve (C5, C6)

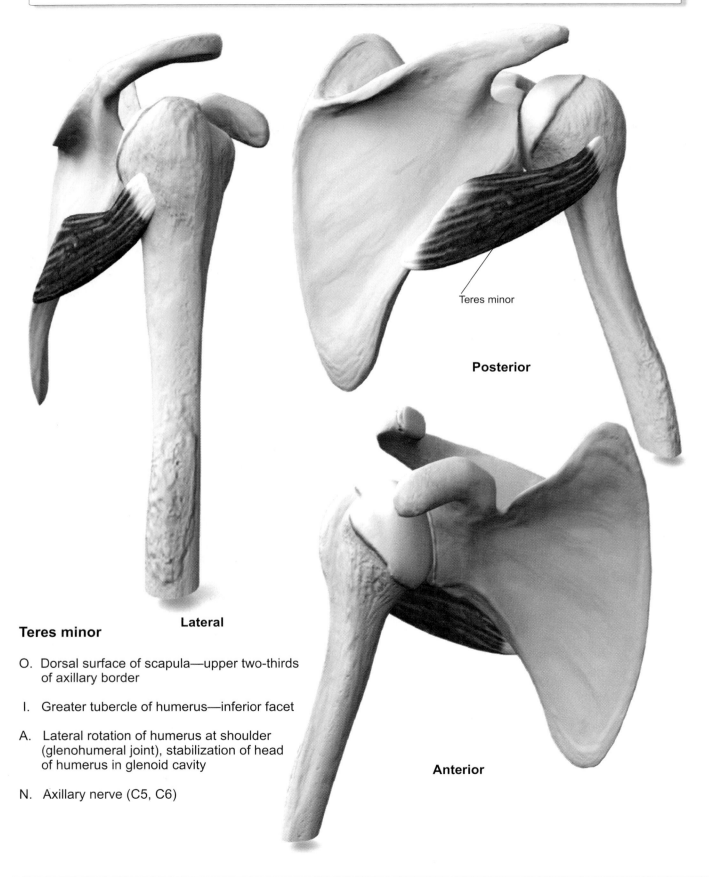

Teres minor

Posterior

Lateral

Anterior

Teres minor

O. Dorsal surface of scapula—upper two-thirds of axillary border

I.   Greater tubercle of humerus—inferior facet

A. Lateral rotation of humerus at shoulder (glenohumeral joint), stabilization of head of humerus in glenoid cavity

N. Axillary nerve (C5, C6)

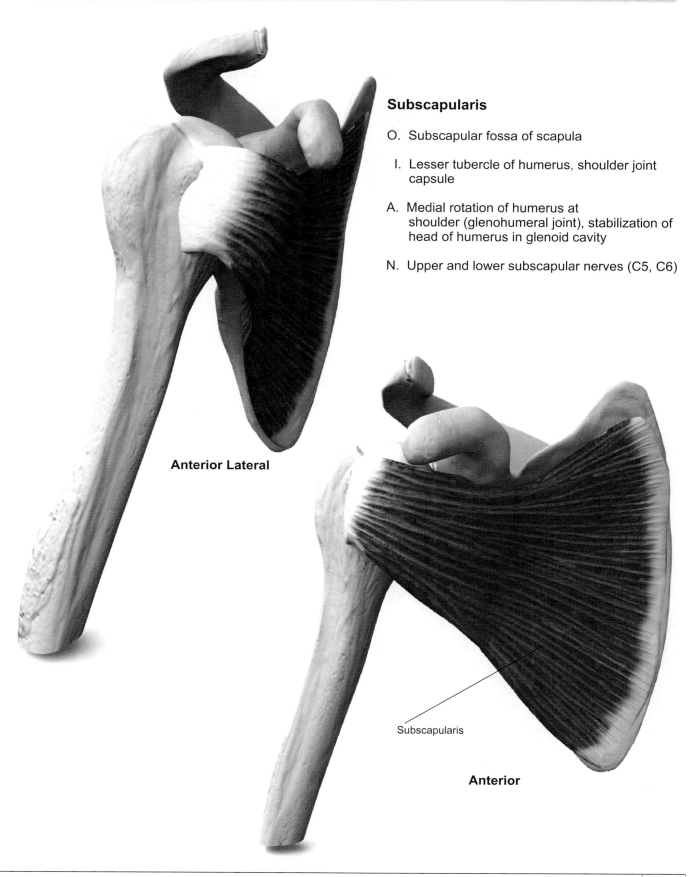

Subscapularis

O. Subscapular fossa of scapula

I. Lesser tubercle of humerus, shoulder joint capsule

A. Medial rotation of humerus at shoulder (glenohumeral joint), stabilization of head of humerus in glenoid cavity

N. Upper and lower subscapular nerves (C5, C6)

Anterior Lateral

Subscapularis

Anterior

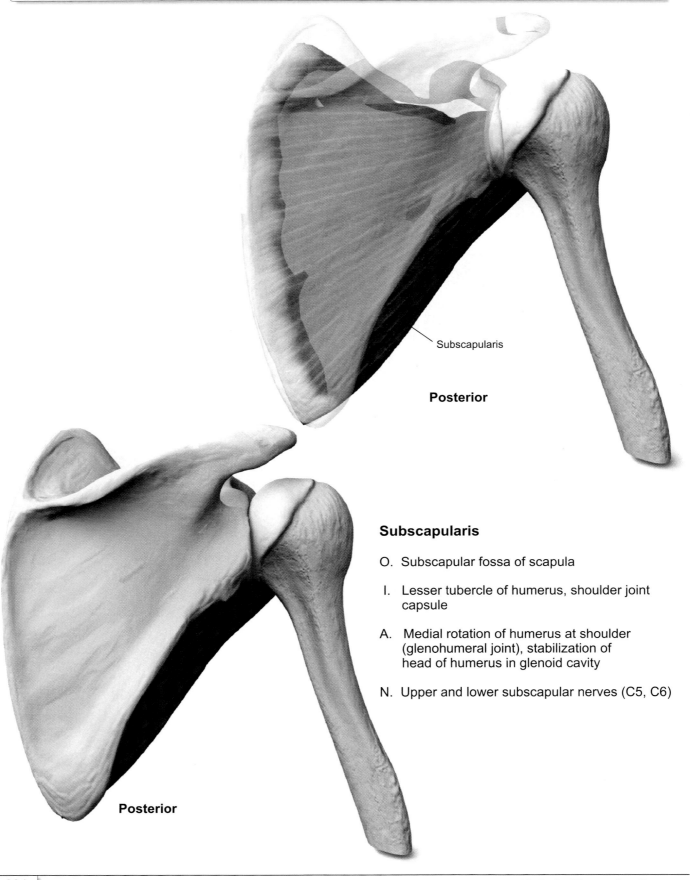

Subscapularis

Posterior

Subscapularis

O. Subscapular fossa of scapula

I. Lesser tubercle of humerus, shoulder joint
    capsule

A. Medial rotation of humerus at shoulder
    (glenohumeral joint), stabilization of
    head of humerus in glenoid cavity

N. Upper and lower subscapular nerves (C5, C6)

Posterior

Unit 3 Muscular System

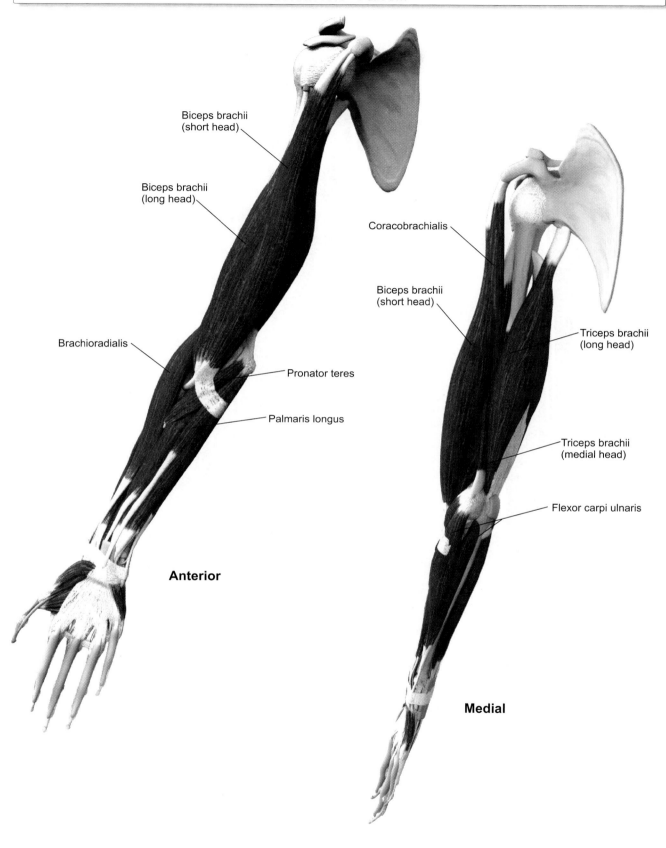

Biceps brachii
(short head)

Biceps brachii
(long head)

Coracobrachialis

Biceps brachii
(short head)

Brachioradialis

Triceps brachii
(long head)

Pronator teres

Palmaris longus

Triceps brachii
(medial head)

Anterior

Flexor carpi ulnaris

Medial

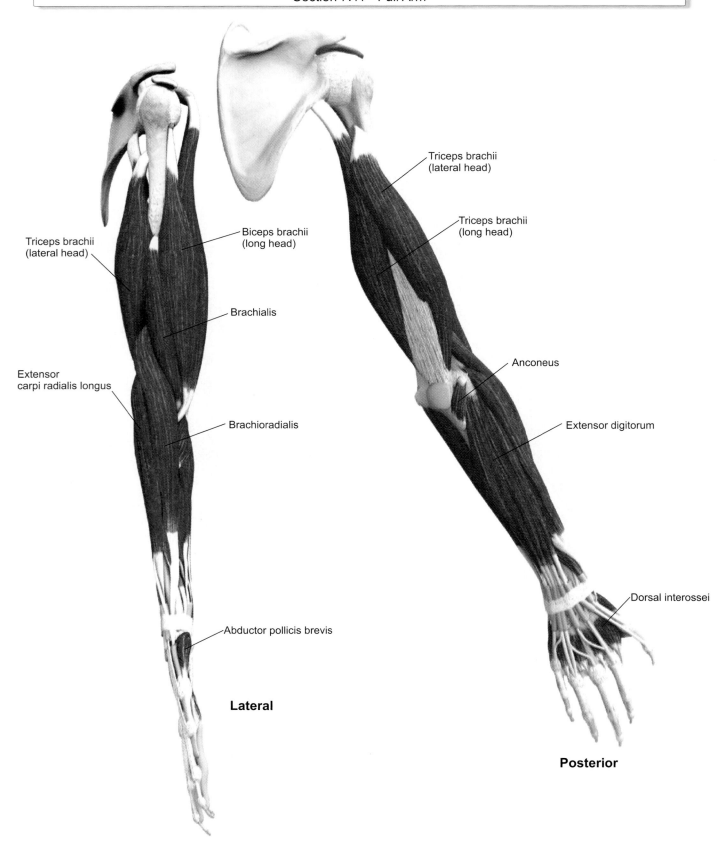

Triceps brachii
(lateral head)

Triceps brachii
(long head)

Triceps brachii
(lateral head)

Biceps brachii
(long head)

Brachialis

Anconeus

Extensor
carpi radialis longus

Brachioradialis

Extensor digitorum

Dorsal interossei

Abductor pollicis brevis

Lateral

Posterior

Unit 3 Muscular System

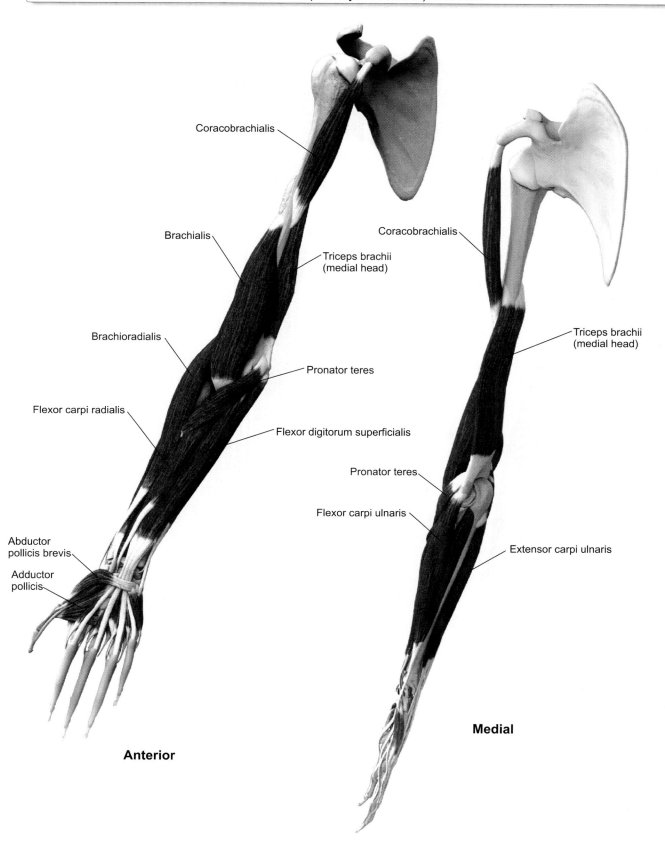

Coracobrachialis

Brachialis

Triceps brachii
(medial head)

Coracobrachialis

Brachioradialis

Triceps brachii
(medial head)

Pronator teres

Flexor carpi radialis

Flexor digitorum superficialis

Pronator teres

Flexor carpi ulnaris

Abductor
pollicis brevis

Adductor
pollicis

Extensor carpi ulnaris

Anterior

Medial

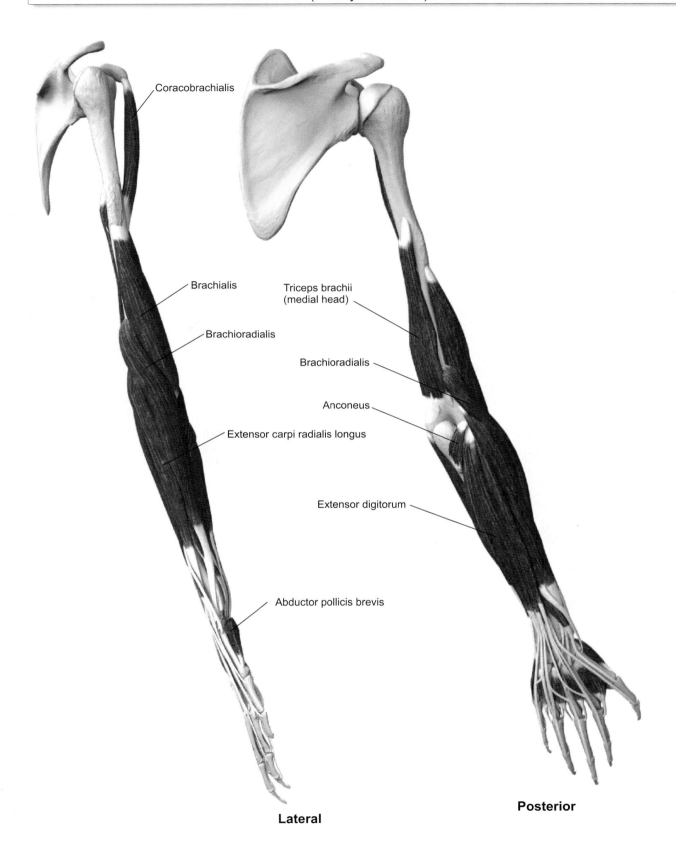

Coracobrachialis

Brachialis

Brachioradialis

Extensor carpi radialis longus

Abductor pollicis brevis

Triceps brachii
(medial head)

Brachioradialis

Anconeus

Extensor digitorum

Lateral

Posterior

Unit 3 Muscular System

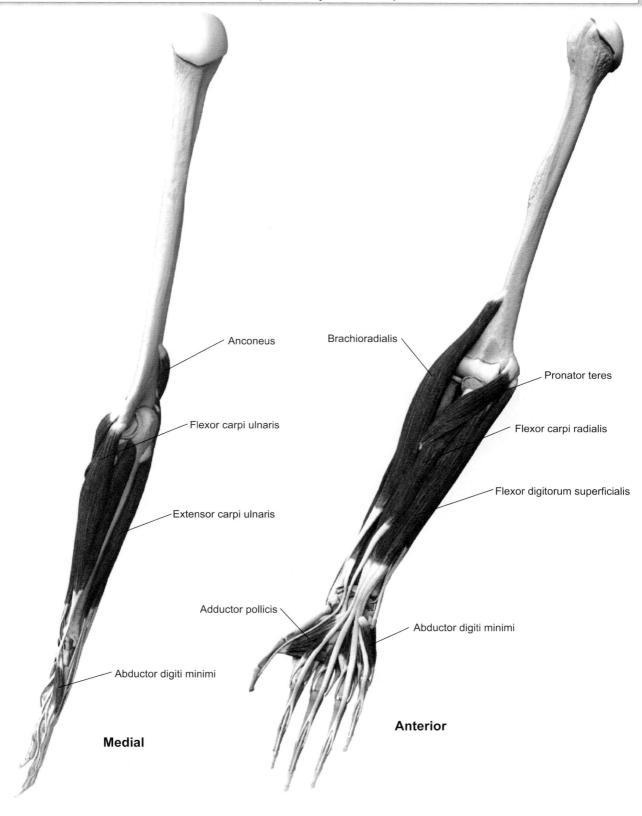

Anconeus

Brachioradialis

Pronator teres

Flexor carpi ulnaris

Flexor carpi radialis

Extensor carpi ulnaris

Flexor digitorum superficialis

Adductor pollicis

Abductor digiti minimi

Abductor digiti minimi

Medial

Anterior

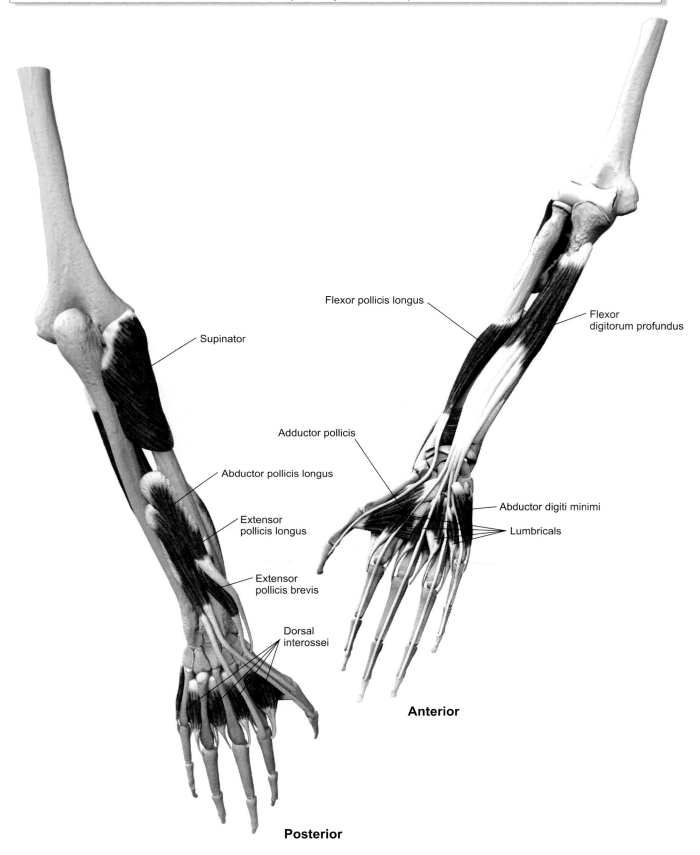

Supinator

Flexor pollicis longus

Flexor
digitorum profundus

Adductor pollicis

Abductor pollicis longus

Abductor digiti minimi

Extensor
pollicis longus

Lumbricals

Extensor
pollicis brevis

Dorsal
interossei

Anterior

Posterior

Unit 3 Muscular System

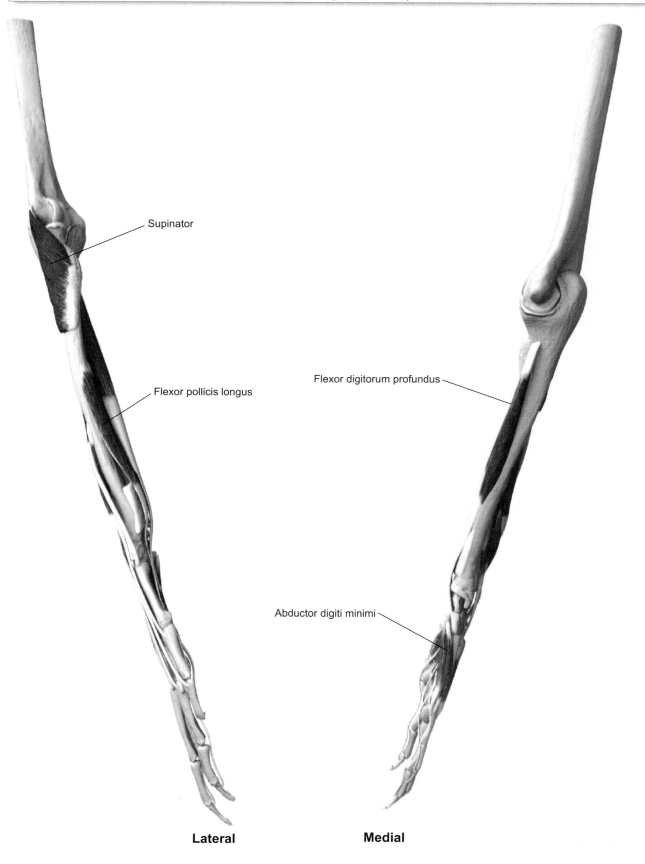

Supinator

Flexor pollicis longus

Flexor digitorum profundus

Abductor digiti minimi

Lateral

Medial

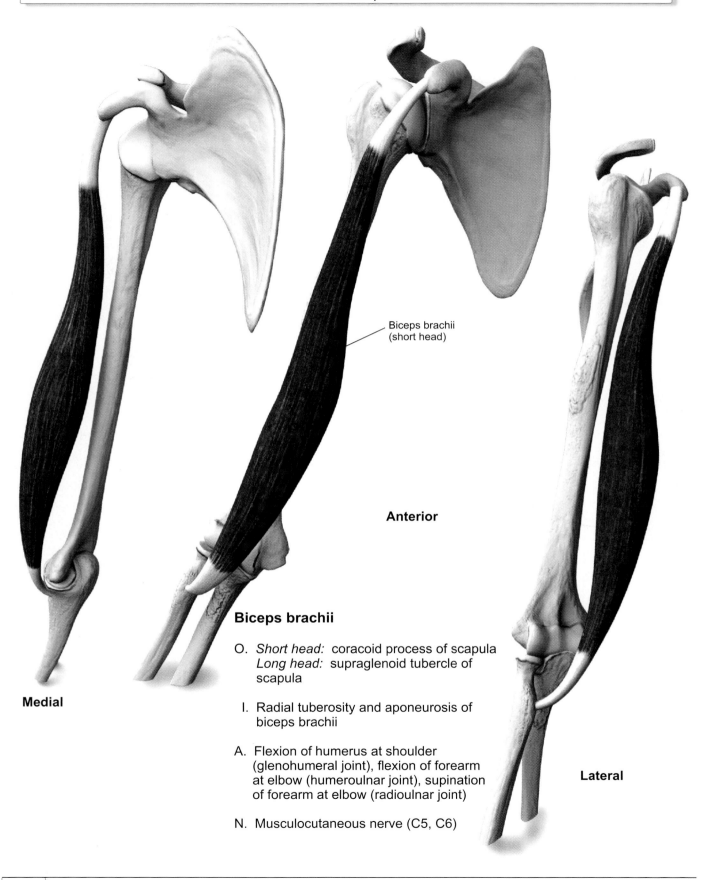

Biceps brachii
(short head)

Anterior

Medial

Lateral

Biceps brachii

O. *Short head:* coracoid process of scapula
Long head: supraglenoid tubercle of
scapula

I. Radial tuberosity and aponeurosis of
biceps brachii

A. Flexion of humerus at shoulder
(glenohumeral joint), flexion of forearm
at elbow (humeroulnar joint), supination
of forearm at elbow (radioulnar joint)

N. Musculocutaneous nerve (C5, C6)

Unit 3 Muscular System

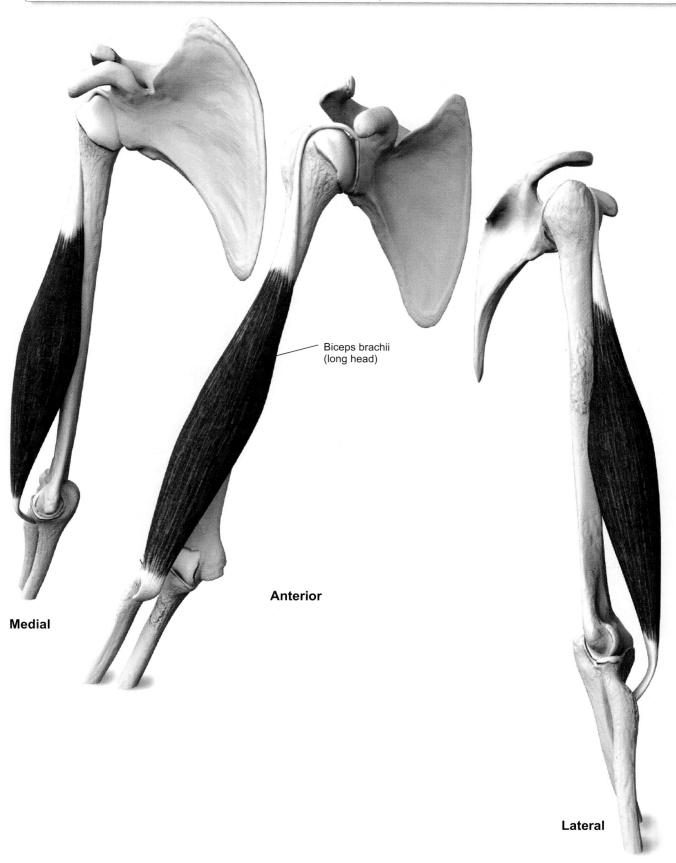

Biceps brachii
(long head)

Anterior

Medial

Lateral

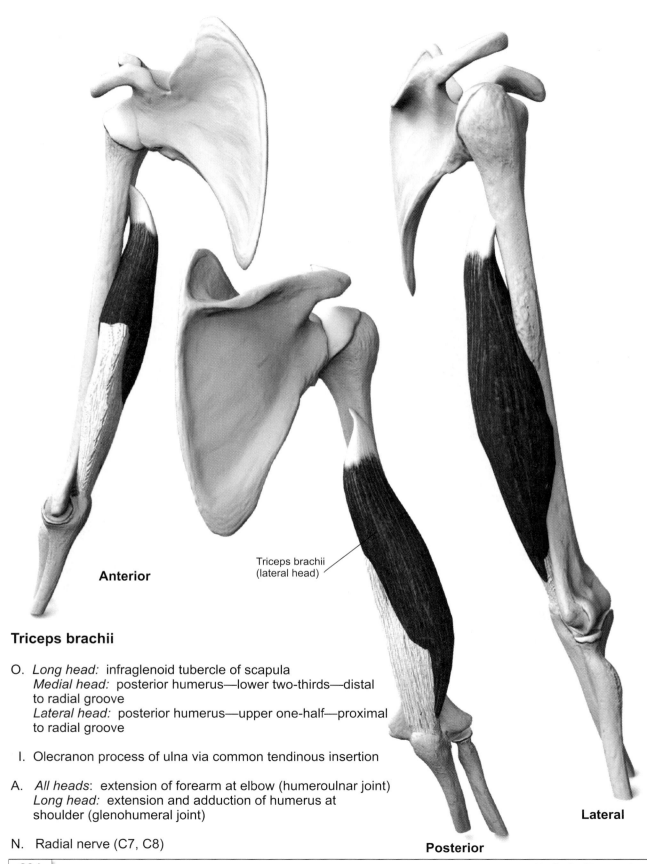

Anterior

Triceps brachii
(lateral head)

Posterior

Lateral

Triceps brachii

O. *Long head:* infraglenoid tubercle of scapula
Medial head: posterior humerus—lower two-thirds—distal
to radial groove
Lateral head: posterior humerus—upper one-half—proximal
to radial groove

I. Olecranon process of ulna via common tendinous insertion

A. *All heads:* extension of forearm at elbow (humeroulnar joint)
Long head: extension and adduction of humerus at
shoulder (glenohumeral joint)

N. Radial nerve (C7, C8)

Unit 3 Muscular System

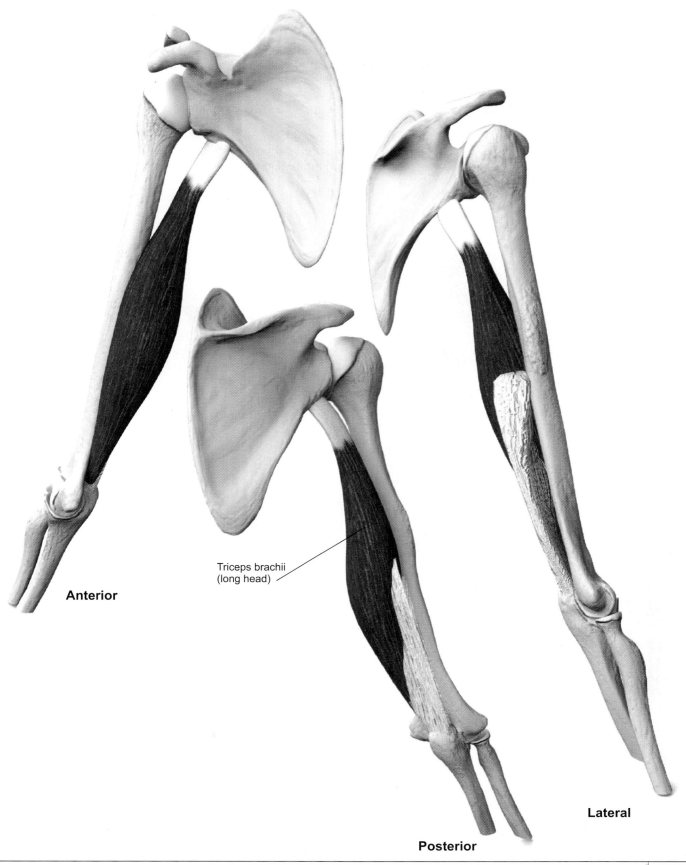

Anterior

Triceps brachii
(long head)

Posterior

Lateral

Unit 3 Muscular System

Triceps brachii

O. *Long head:* infraglenoid tubercle of scapula
Medial head: posterior humerus—distal two-thirds
Lateral head: posterior humerus—upper one-half

I. Olecranon process of ulna via common tendinous insertion

A. *All heads:* extension of forearm at elbow (humeroulnar joint)
Long head: extension and adduction of humerus
at shoulder (glenohumeral joint)

N. Radial nerve (C7, C8)

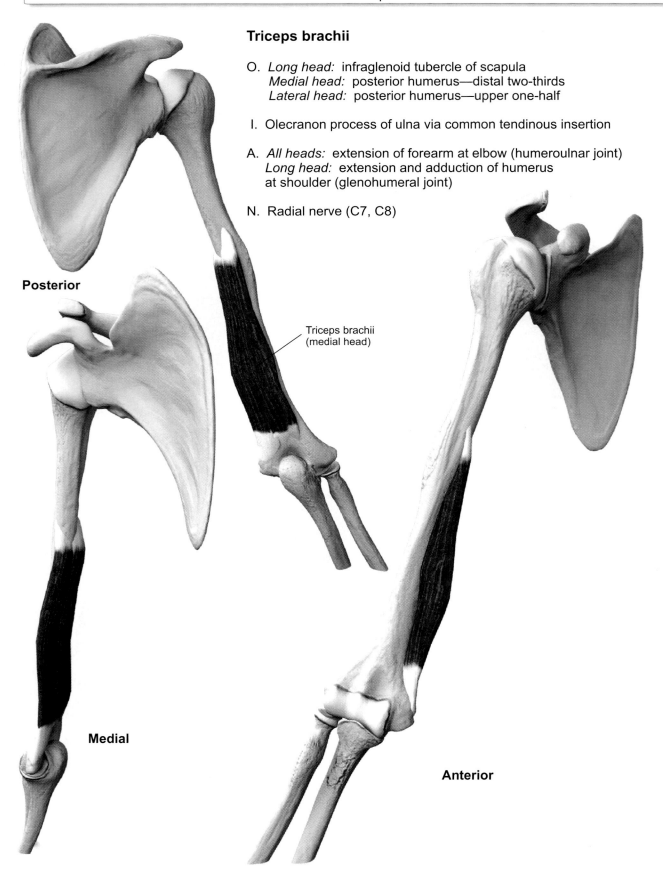

Posterior

Triceps brachii
(medial head)

Medial

Anterior

Unit 3 Muscular System

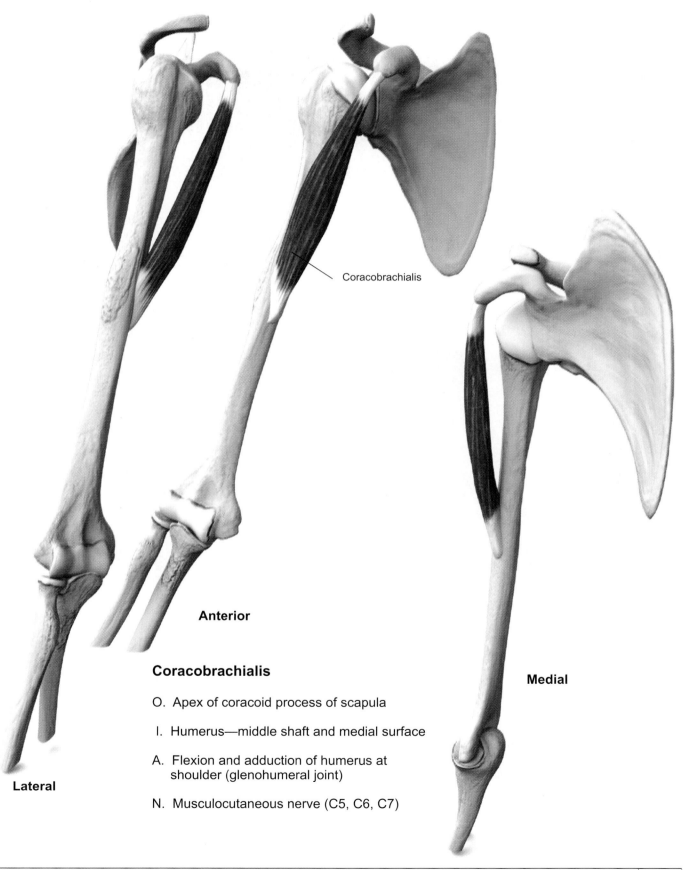

Coracobrachialis

Anterior

Coracobrachialis

O. Apex of coracoid process of scapula

I. Humerus—middle shaft and medial surface

A. Flexion and adduction of humerus at shoulder (glenohumeral joint)

N. Musculocutaneous nerve (C5, C6, C7)

Medial

Lateral

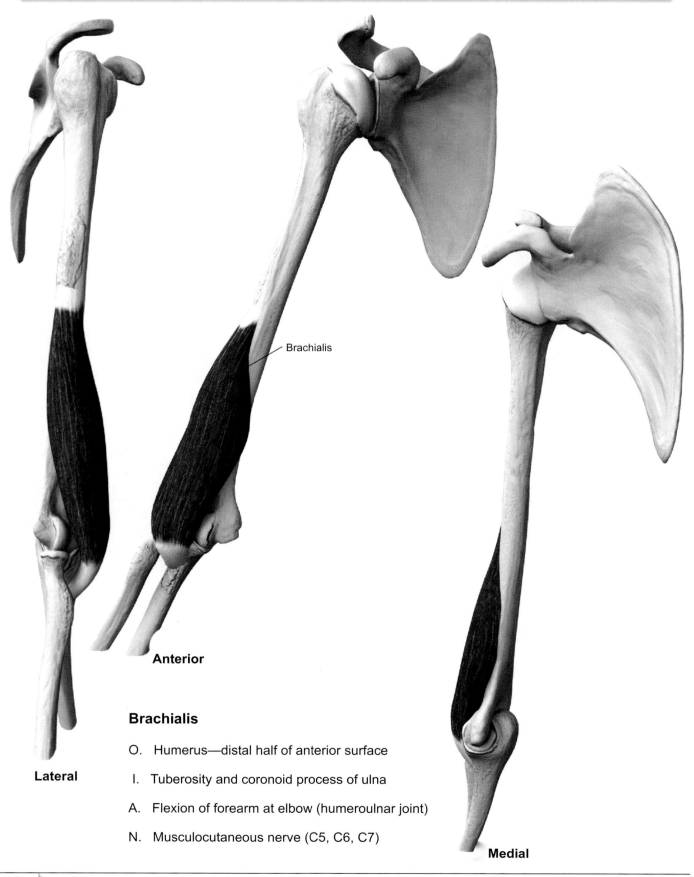

Brachialis

Anterior

Lateral

Medial

Brachialis

O. Humerus—distal half of anterior surface

I. Tuberosity and coronoid process of ulna

A. Flexion of forearm at elbow (humeroulnar joint)

N. Musculocutaneous nerve (C5, C6, C7)

Unit 3 Muscular System

Brachioradialis

O. Lateral supracondylar crest of humerus

I. Styloid process of radius

A. Flexion of forearm at elbow (humeroulnar joint), assists pronation and supination of forearm when these movements are resisted

N. Radial nerve (C5, C6)

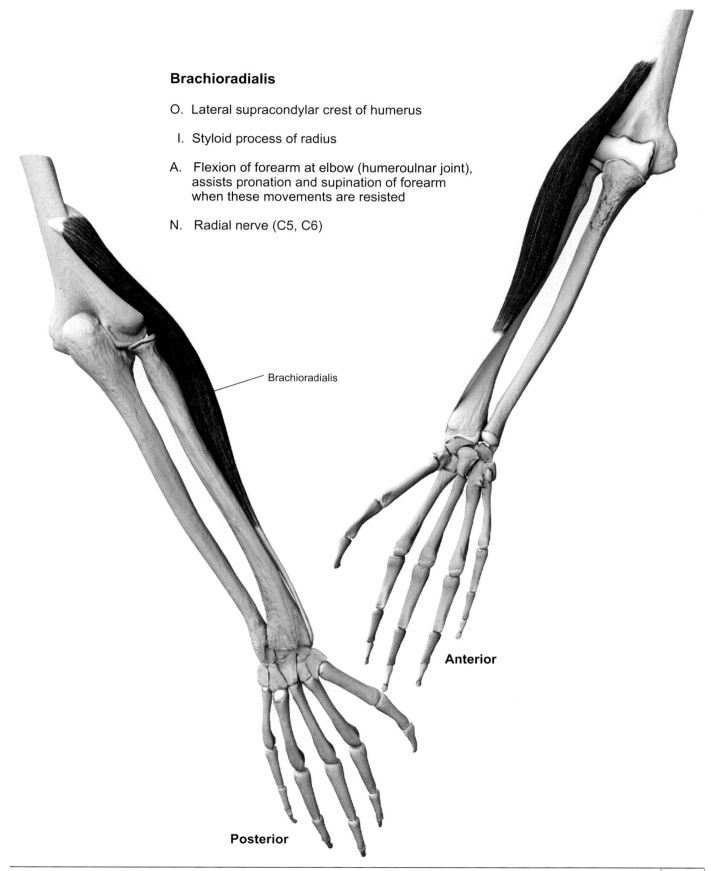

Brachioradialis

Anterior

Posterior

Brachioradialis

O. Lateral supracondylar ridge of humerus

I. Styloid process of radius

A. Flexion of forearm at elbow (humeroulnar joint), assists pronation and supination of forearm when these movements are resisted

N. Radial nerve (C5, C6)

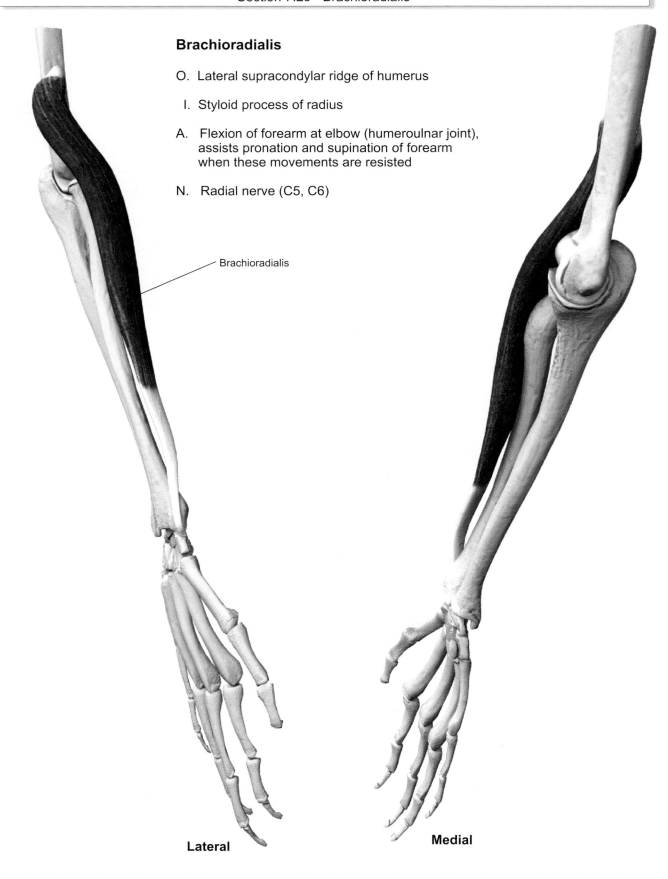

Brachioradialis

Lateral

Medial

Unit 3 Muscular System

Anconeus

O. Lateral epicondyle of posterior humerus

I. Olecranon process—lateral surface, posterior ulna—upper surface

A. Extension of forearm at elbow (humeroulnar joint), stabilization of elbow joint

N. Radial nerve (C7, C8)

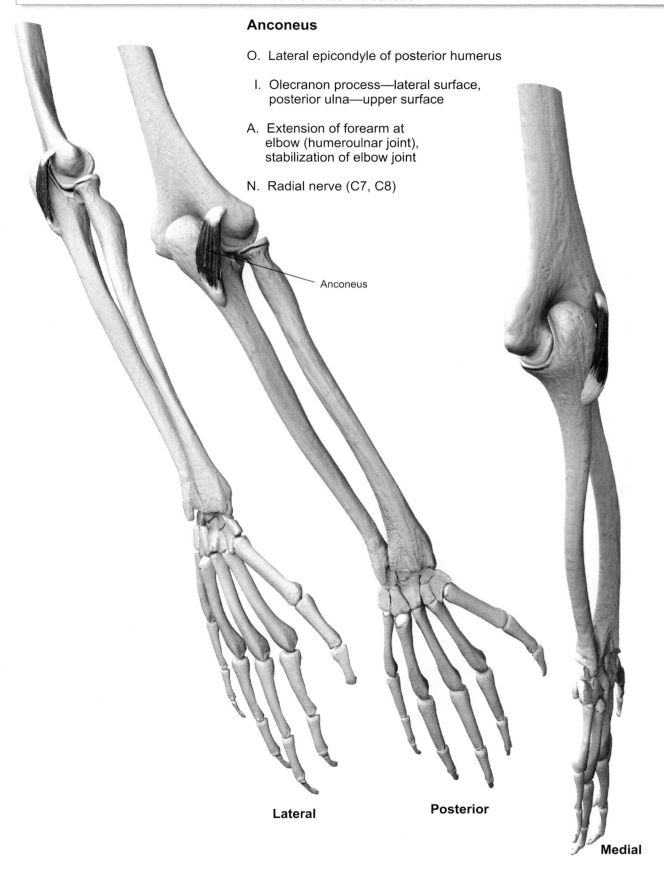

Anconeus

Lateral

Posterior

Medial

Palmaris longus

O. Medial epicondyle of humerus via common flexor tendon

I. Palmar aponeurosis and flexor retinaculum

A. Flexion of hand at wrist (radiocarpal joint), flexion of forearm at elbow (humeroulnar joint)

N. Median nerve (C6, C7, C8)

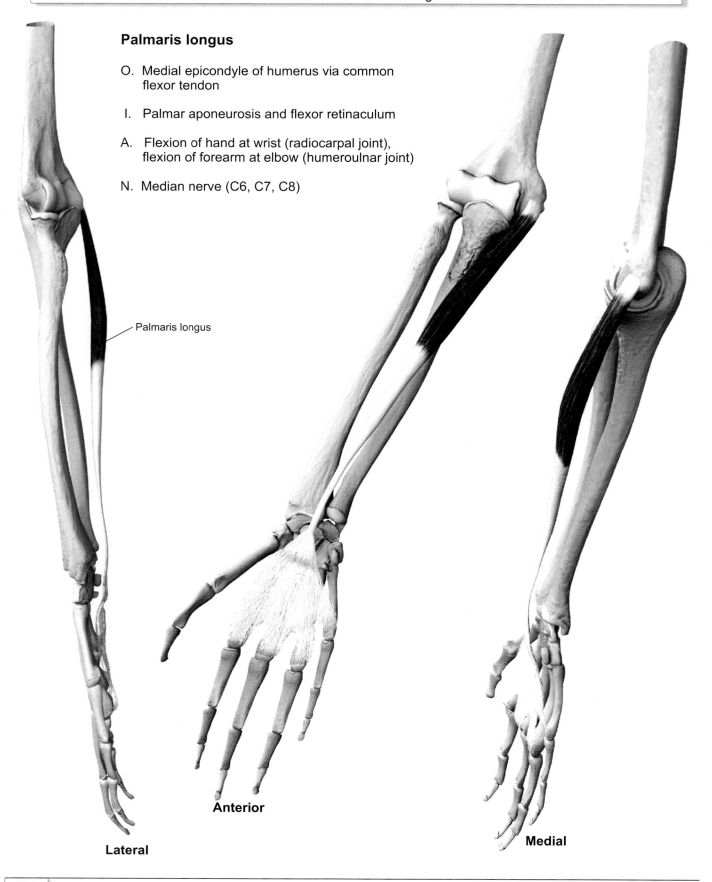

Palmaris longus

Lateral

Anterior

Medial

Unit 3 Muscular System

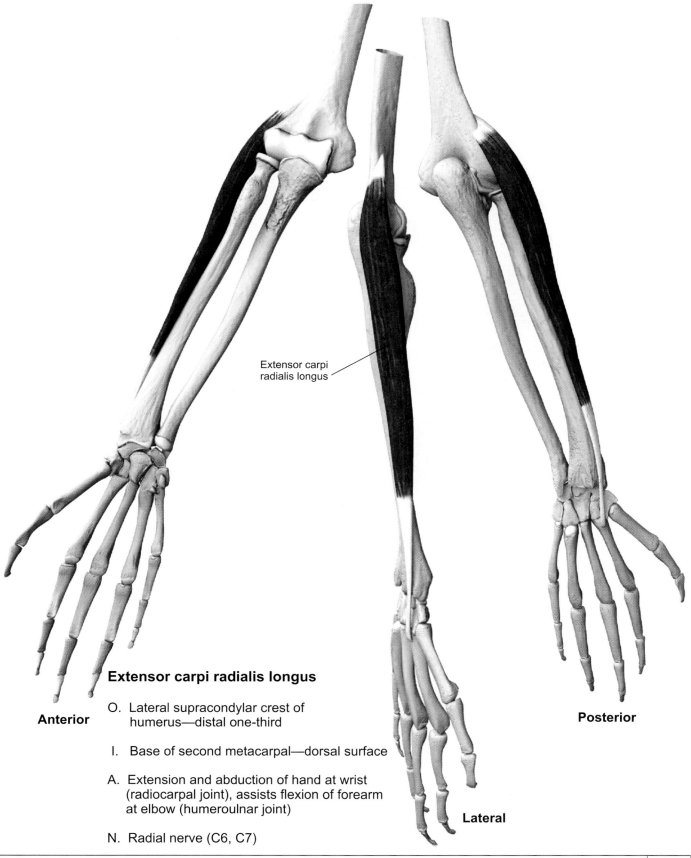

Extensor carpi
radialis longus

Extensor carpi radialis longus

O. Lateral supracondylar crest of
    humerus—distal one-third

I. Base of second metacarpal—dorsal surface

A. Extension and abduction of hand at wrist
    (radiocarpal joint), assists flexion of forearm
    at elbow (humeroulnar joint)

N. Radial nerve (C6, C7)

Anterior

Lateral

Posterior

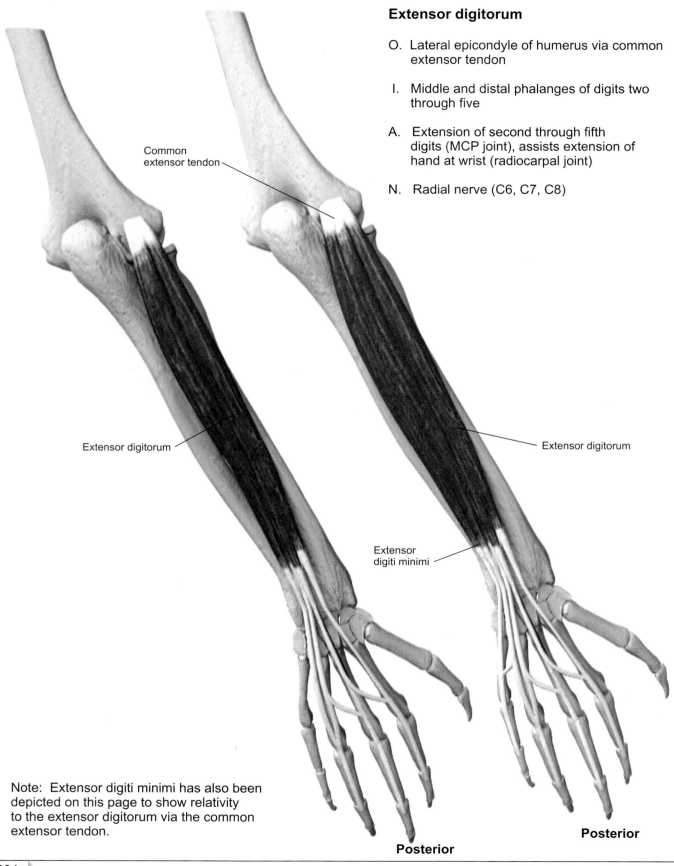

Extensor digitorum

O. Lateral epicondyle of humerus via common extensor tendon

I. Middle and distal phalanges of digits two through five

A. Extension of second through fifth digits (MCP joint), assists extension of hand at wrist (radiocarpal joint)

N. Radial nerve (C6, C7, C8)

Common extensor tendon

Extensor digitorum

Extensor digitorum

Extensor digiti minimi

Note: Extensor digiti minimi has also been depicted on this page to show relativity to the extensor digitorum via the common extensor tendon.

Posterior

Posterior

Unit 3 Muscular System

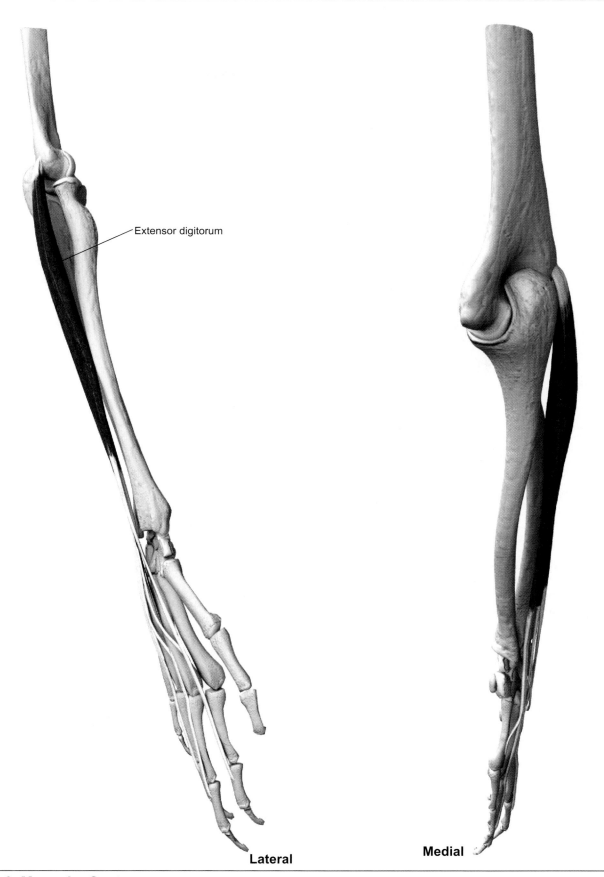

Extensor digitorum

Lateral

Medial

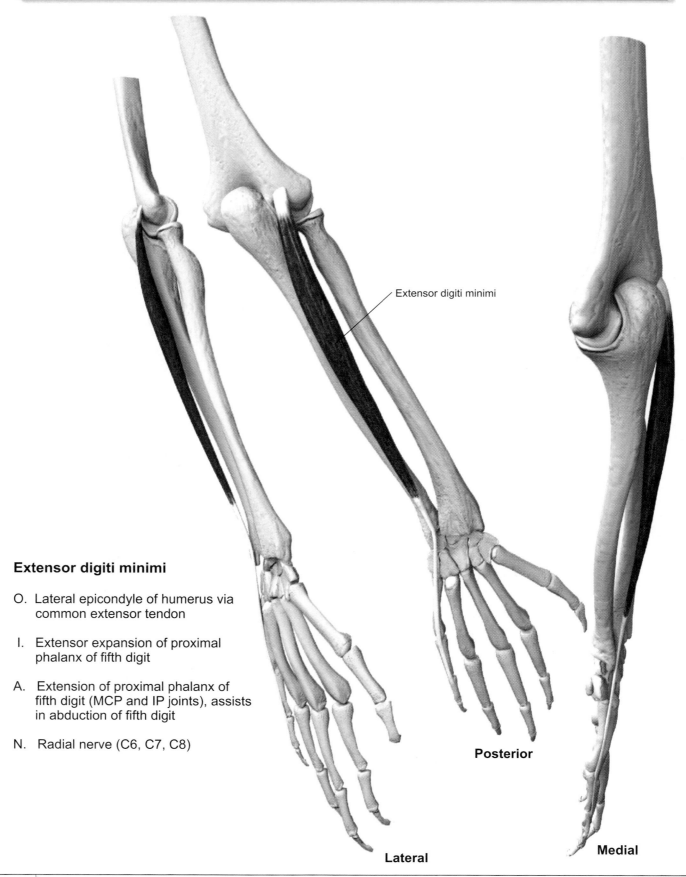

Extensor digiti minimi

Extensor digiti minimi

O. Lateral epicondyle of humerus via common extensor tendon

I. Extensor expansion of proximal phalanx of fifth digit

A. Extension of proximal phalanx of fifth digit (MCP and IP joints), assists in abduction of fifth digit

N. Radial nerve (C6, C7, C8)

Posterior

Lateral

Medial

Unit 3 Muscular System

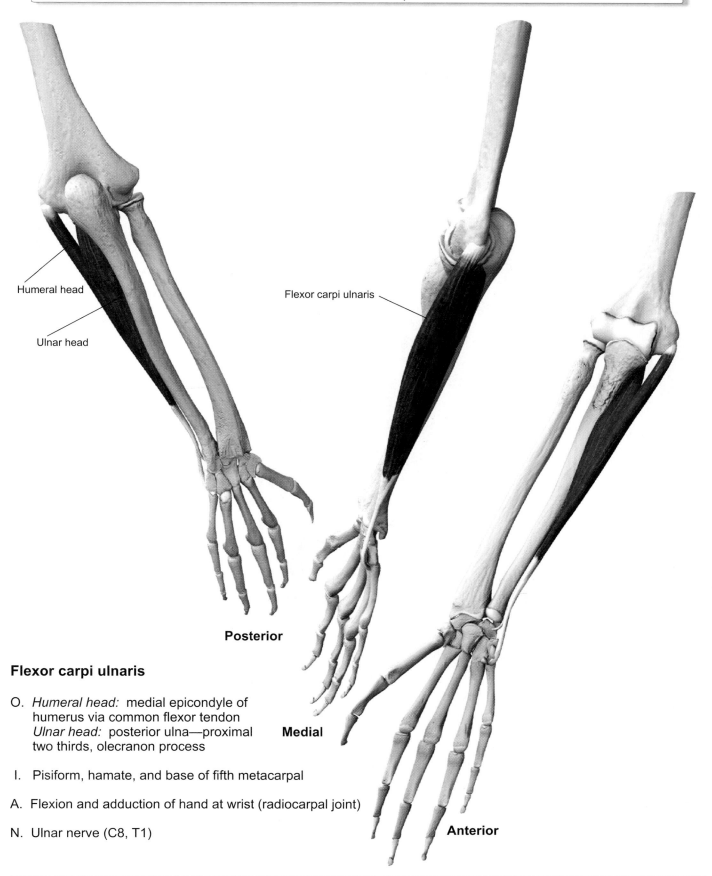

Humeral head

Ulnar head

Flexor carpi ulnaris

Posterior

Medial

Anterior

Flexor carpi ulnaris

O. *Humeral head:* medial epicondyle of
   humerus via common flexor tendon
   Ulnar head: posterior ulna—proximal
   two thirds, olecranon process

I. Pisiform, hamate, and base of fifth metacarpal

A. Flexion and adduction of hand at wrist (radiocarpal joint)

N. Ulnar nerve (C8, T1)

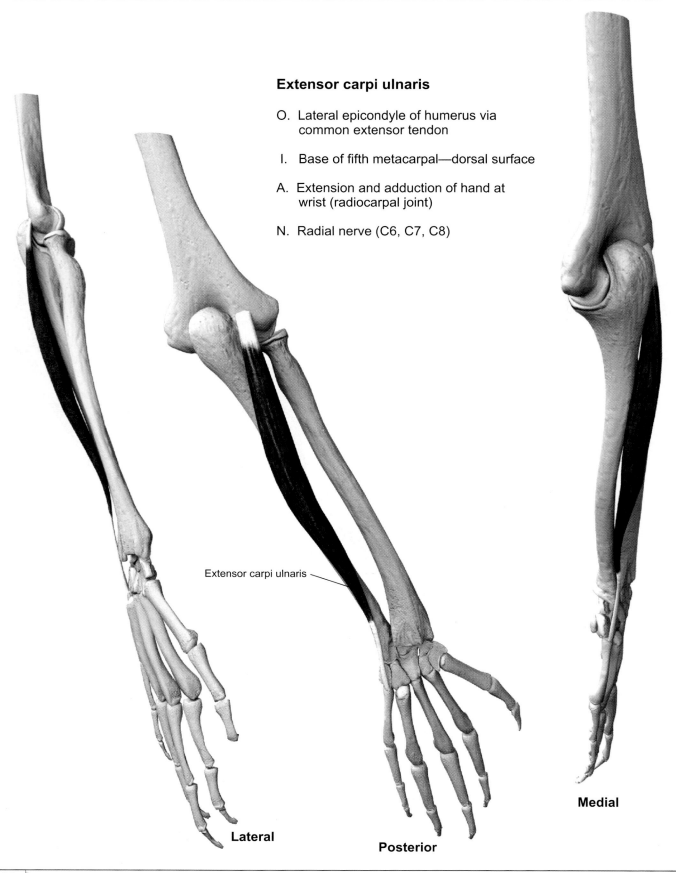

Extensor carpi ulnaris

O. Lateral epicondyle of humerus via common extensor tendon

I. Base of fifth metacarpal—dorsal surface

A. Extension and adduction of hand at wrist (radiocarpal joint)

N. Radial nerve (C6, C7, C8)

Extensor carpi ulnaris

Lateral

Posterior

Medial

Unit 3 Muscular System

Pronator teres

O. *Humeral head:* superior to medial epicondyle of humerus
Ulnar head: coranoid process of ulna—medial aspect

I. Radius—middle of lateral surface

A. Pronation of forearm at elbow (radioulnar joint), assists flexion of forearm at elbow (humeroulnar joint)

N. Median nerve (C6, C7)

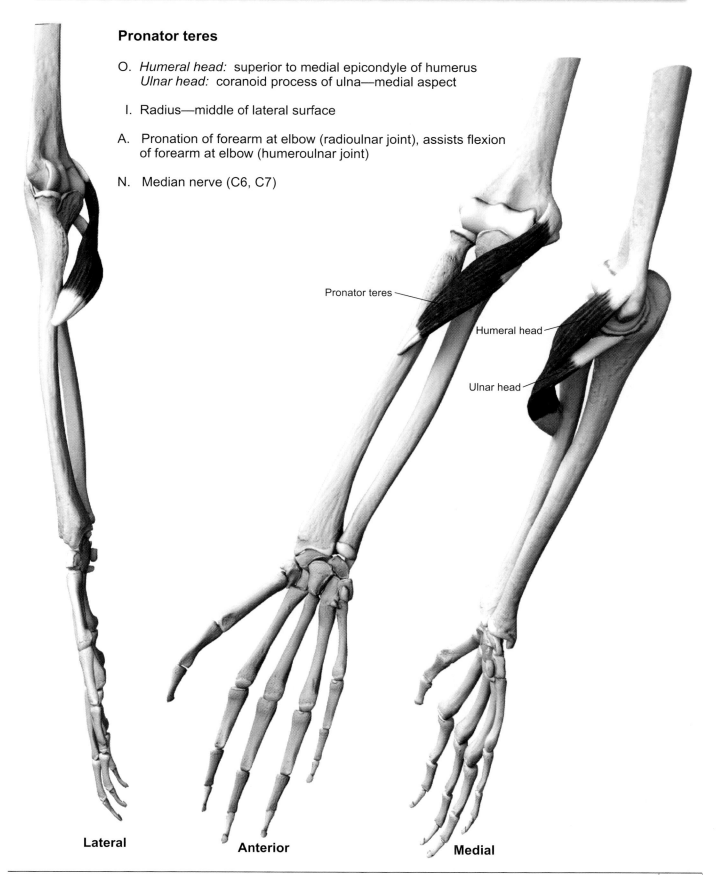

Pronator teres

Humeral head

Ulnar head

Lateral

Anterior

Medial

Unit 3 Muscular System

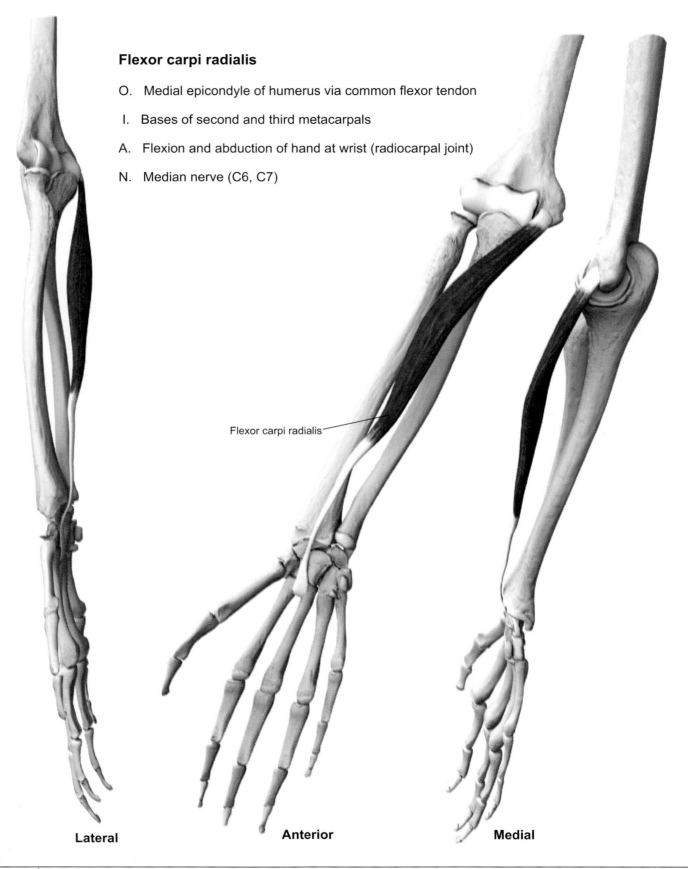

Flexor carpi radialis

O. Medial epicondyle of humerus via common flexor tendon

I. Bases of second and third metacarpals

A. Flexion and abduction of hand at wrist (radiocarpal joint)

N. Median nerve (C6, C7)

Flexor carpi radialis

Lateral

Anterior

Medial

Unit 3 Muscular System

Flexor digitorum superficialis

O. *Humeral head:* medial epicondyle of humerus via common flexor tendon
Ulnar head: coronoid process of ulna
Radial head: anterior oblique line of radius

I. Middle phalanges of second through fifth digits via individual tendons

A. Flexion of second through fifth digits (MCP and PIP joints), flexion of hand at wrist (radiocarpal joint)

N. Median nerve (C7, C8, T1)

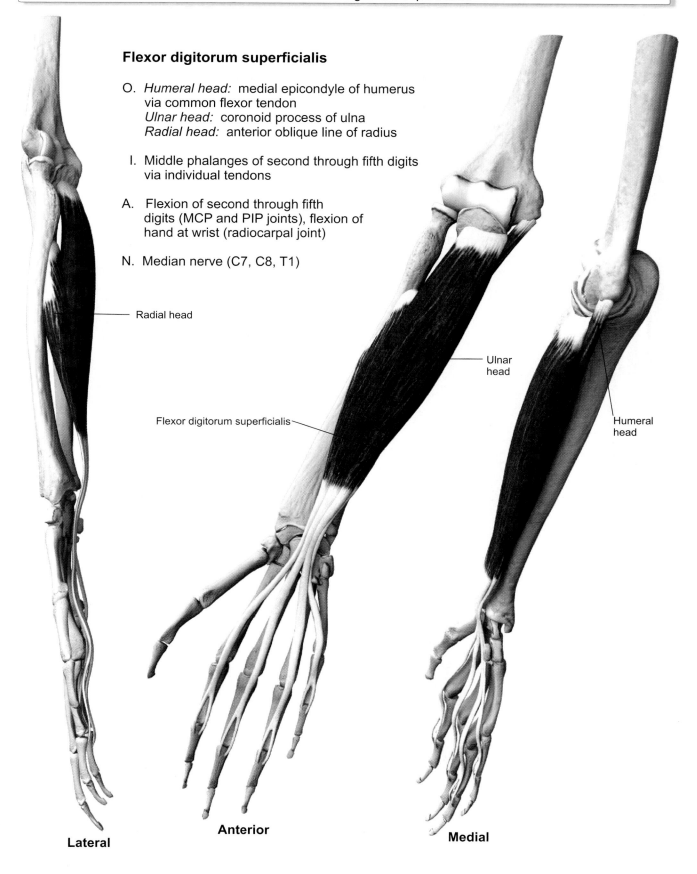

Radial head

Ulnar head

Humeral head

Flexor digitorum superficialis

Lateral

Anterior

Medial

Flexor digitorum profundus

O. Proximal three-fourths of ulna—anterior and medial surfaces, interosseous membrane

I. Bases of distal phalanges of digits two through five—anterior surfaces via individual tendons

A. Flexion of digits two through five (DIP joints), assists flexion of digits two through five (PIP joints and MCP joints)

N. Median nerve—second and third digits (C8, T1)
   Ulnar nerve—fourth and fifth digits (C8, T1)

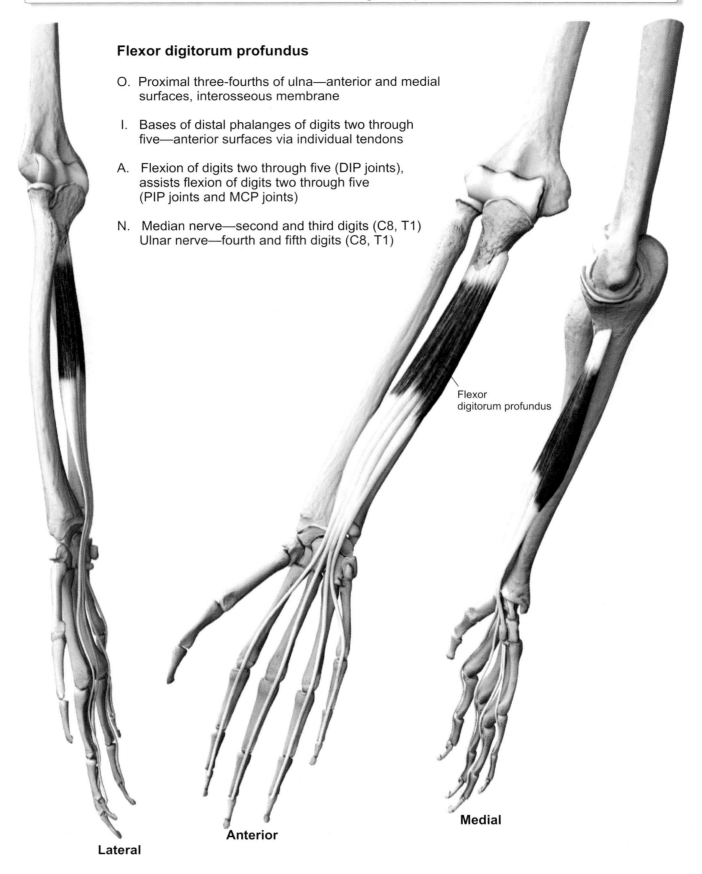

Flexor digitorum profundus

Lateral

Anterior

Medial

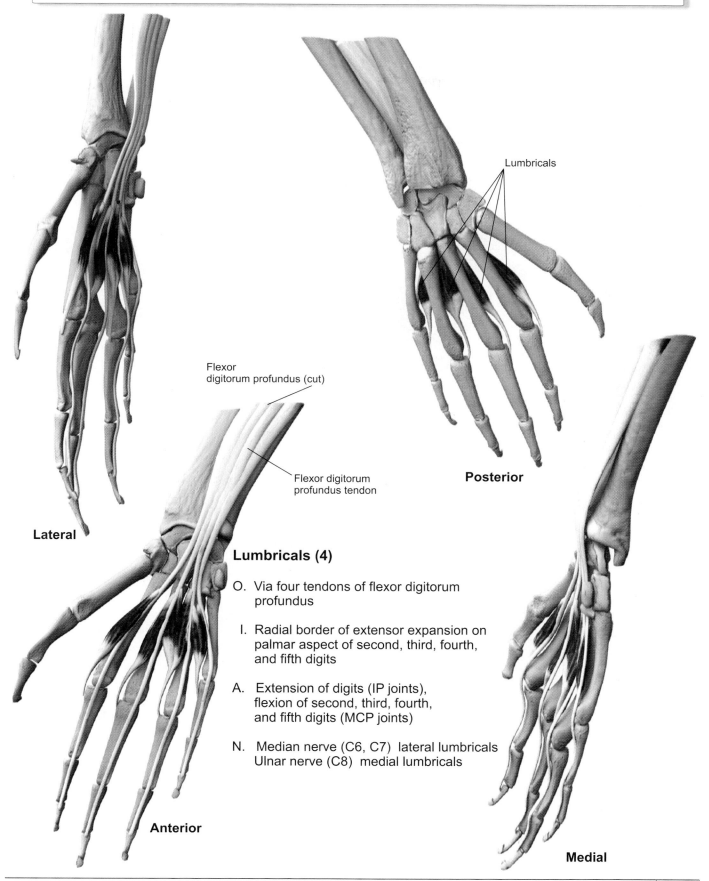

Lumbricals

Flexor
digitorum profundus (cut)

Flexor digitorum
profundus tendon

Lateral

Posterior

Lumbricals (4)

O. Via four tendons of flexor digitorum
profundus

I. Radial border of extensor expansion on
palmar aspect of second, third, fourth,
and fifth digits

A. Extension of digits (IP joints),
flexion of second, third, fourth,
and fifth digits (MCP joints)

N. Median nerve (C6, C7) lateral lumbricals
Ulnar nerve (C8) medial lumbricals

Anterior

Medial

Extensor carpi radialis brevis

O. Lateral epicondyle of humerus

I. Base of third metacarpal—dorsal surface

A. Extension of hand at wrist, assists in abduction of hand at wrist (radiocarpal joint)

N. Radial nerve (C6, C7)

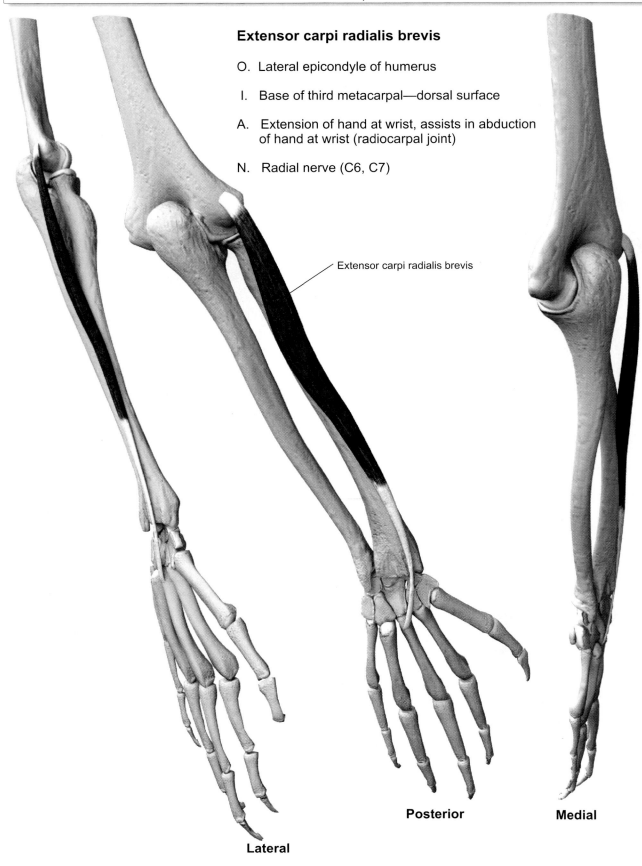

Extensor carpi radialis brevis

Lateral

Posterior

Medial

Unit 3 Muscular System

Supinator

O. Lateral epicondyle of humerus, annular, and radiocollateral ligaments, supinator crest of ulna

I. Anterior radius—upper one-third and lateral surface

A. Supination of forearm at elbow (radioulnar joint)

N. Radial nerve (C6)

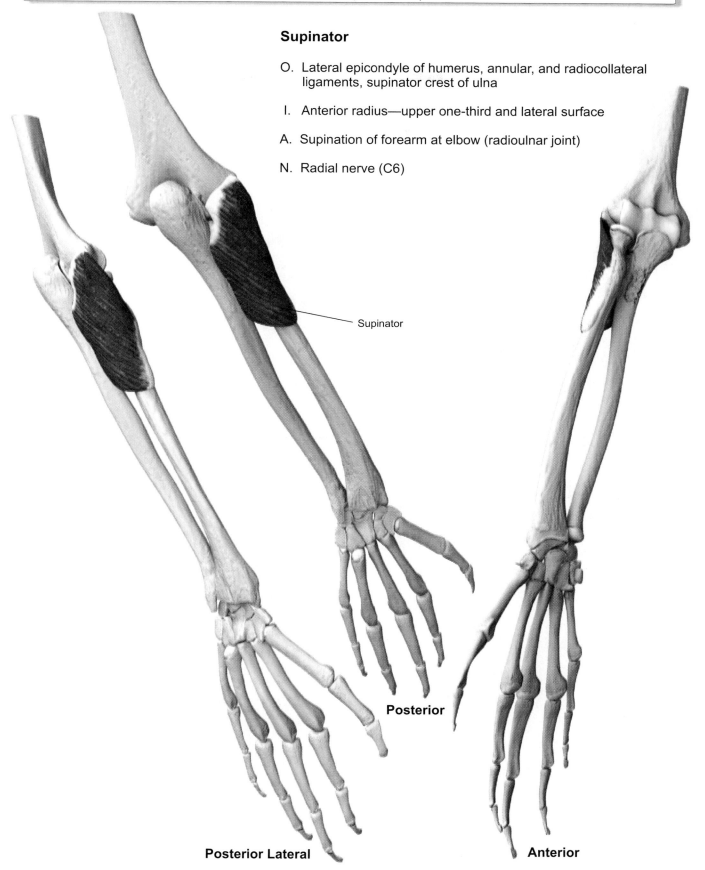

Supinator

Posterior

Posterior Lateral

Anterior

Abductor pollicis brevis

O. Tubercle of trapezium, tubercle of scaphoid, flexor retinaculum

I. Base of proximal phalanx of thumb—radial side

A. Abduction of thumb, assists opposition of thumb (CM joint)

N. Median nerve (C8, T1)

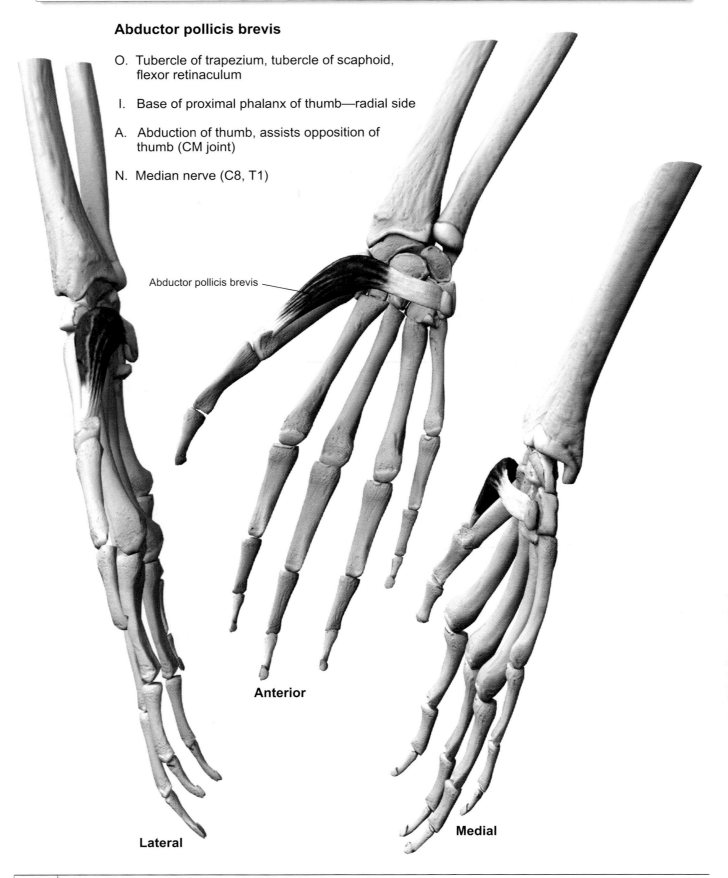

Abductor pollicis brevis

Anterior

Lateral

Medial

Unit 3 Muscular System

Abductor pollicis longus

O. Ulna—distal and posterior surface, interosseous membrane, posterior radius—middle one-third

I. Base of first metacarpal—radial side

A. Abduction and extension of first digit (MCP joint), abduction of hand at wrist (radioulnar joint)

N. Radial nerve (C6, C7, C8)

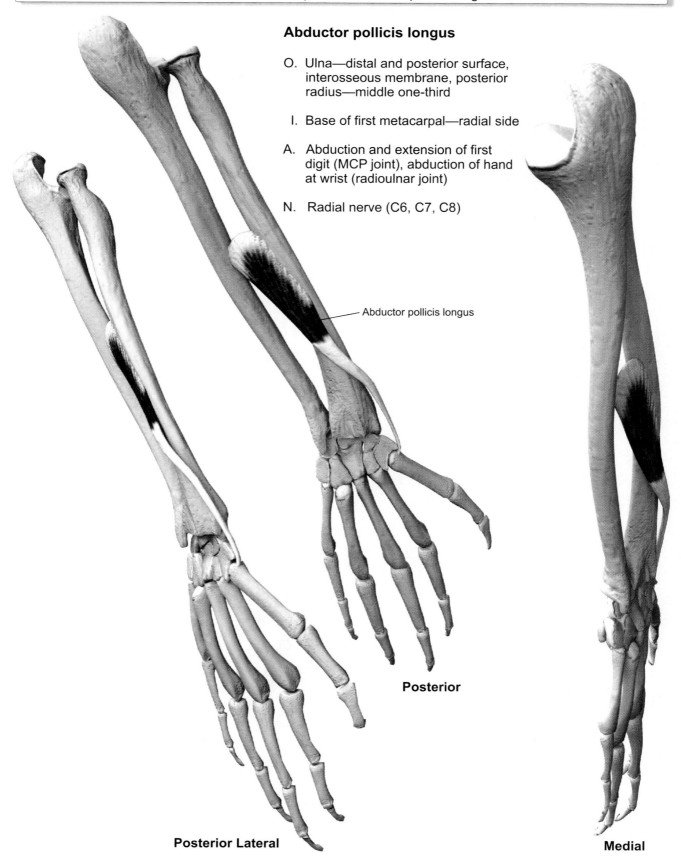

— Abductor pollicis longus

Posterior

Posterior Lateral

Medial

Extensor pollicis longus

O. Posterior ulna—middle one-third, interosseous membrane

I. Base of distal phalanx of first digit—dorsal surface

A. Extension of first digit (IP joint), assists abduction and extension of hand at wrist

N. Radial nerve (C6, C7, C8)

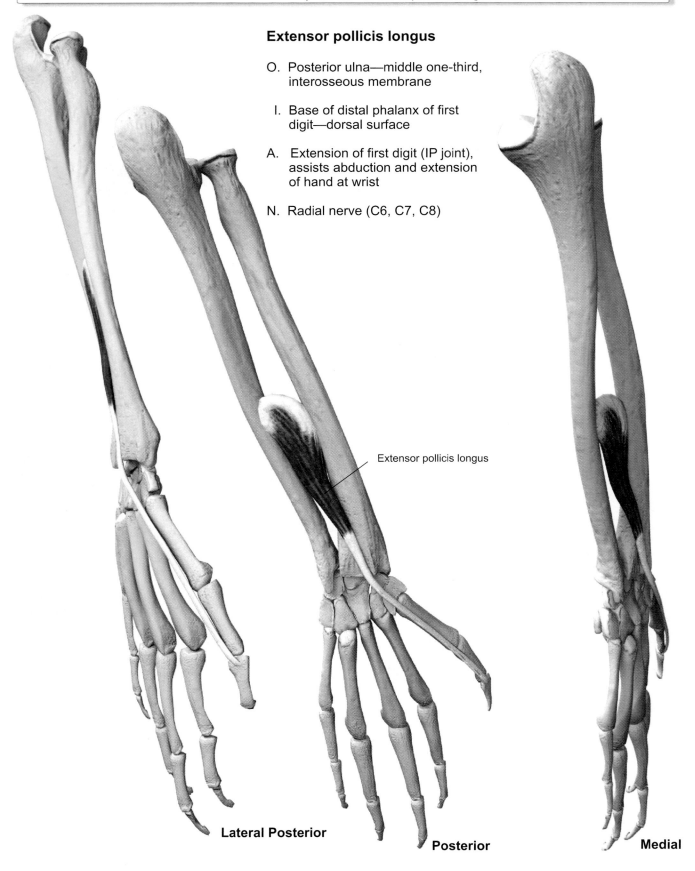

Extensor pollicis longus

Lateral Posterior

Posterior

Medial

Unit 3 Muscular System

Extensor indicis

O. Ulna—posterior surface and interosseous membrane

I. Extensor expansion of proximal phalanx of second digit

A. Extension of second digit (MCP joint)

N. Radial nerve (C6, C7, C8)

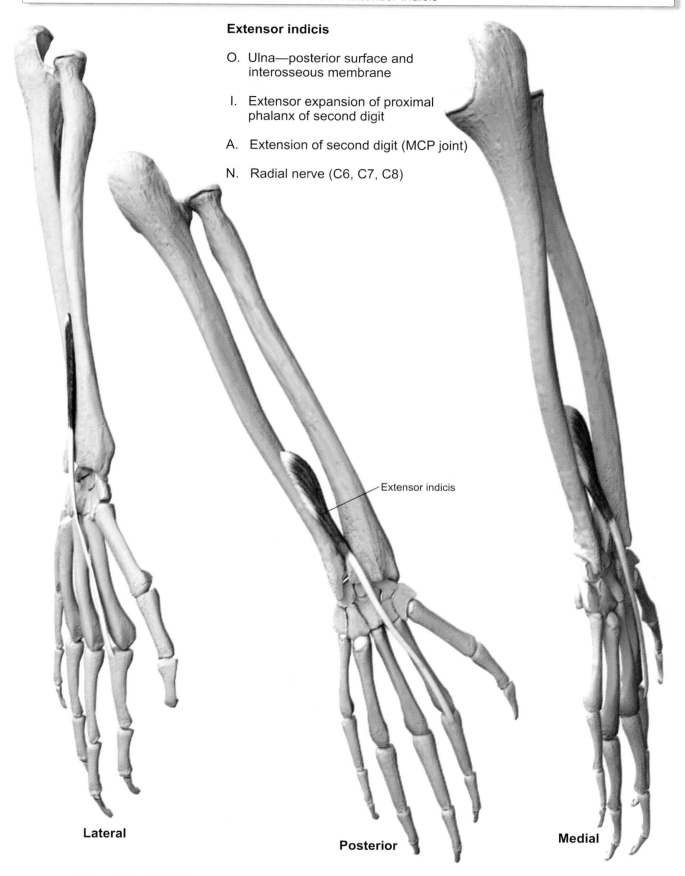

Extensor indicis

Lateral

Posterior

Medial

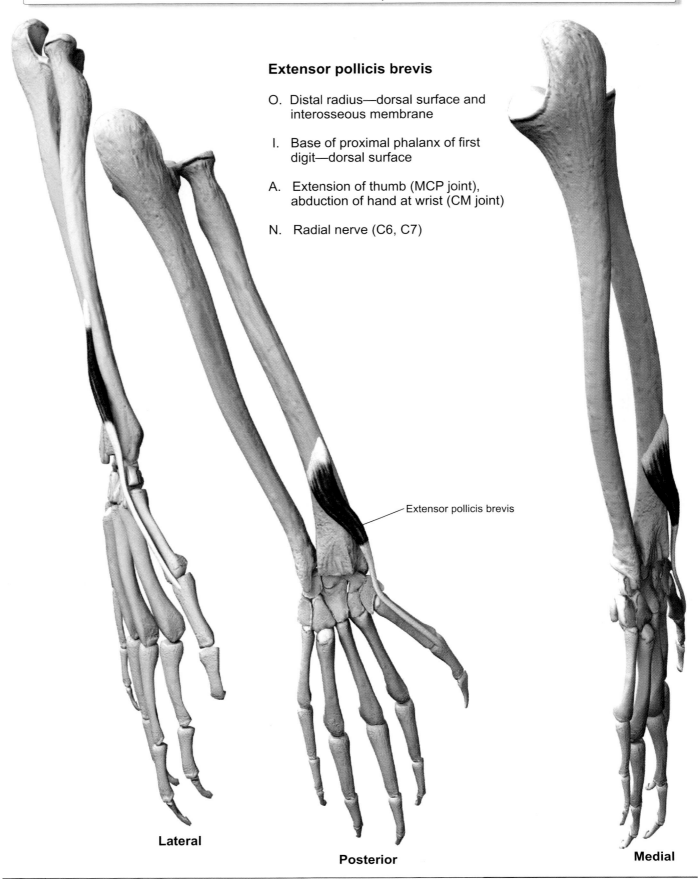

Extensor pollicis brevis

O. Distal radius—dorsal surface and interosseous membrane

I. Base of proximal phalanx of first digit—dorsal surface

A. Extension of thumb (MCP joint), abduction of hand at wrist (CM joint)

N. Radial nerve (C6, C7)

Extensor pollicis brevis

Lateral

Posterior

Medial

Unit 3 Muscular System

Flexor pollicis brevis

O. *Superficial head:* trapezium and flexor retinaculum
    Deep head: trapezoid and capitate

I. Base of proximal phalanx of thumb—radial side

A. Flexion of proximal phalanx of thumb (MP joint)

N. Median nerve (C6, C7), superficial head
    Ulnar nerve (C8, T1), deep head

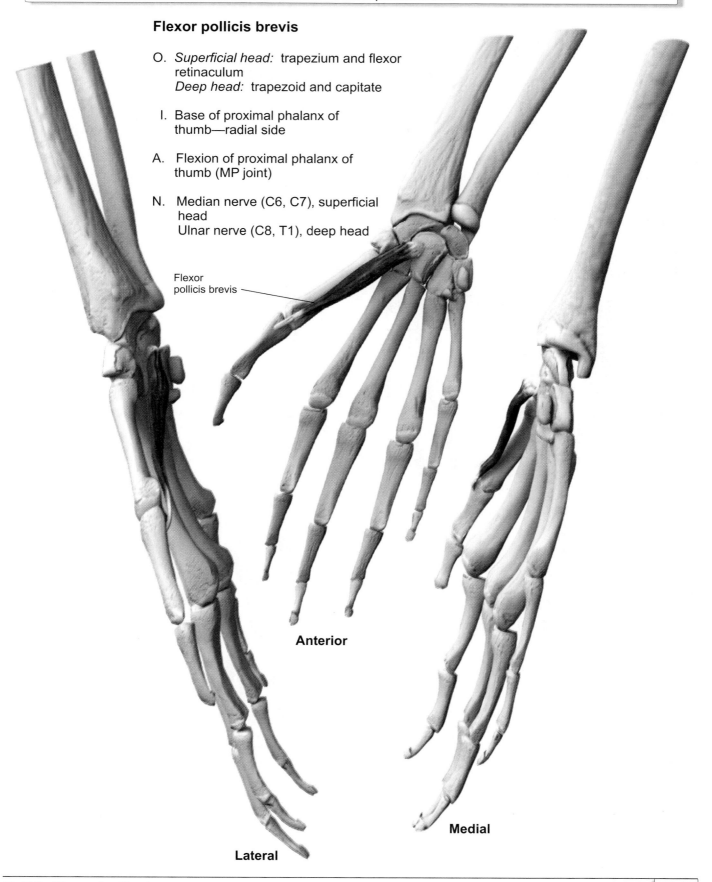

Flexor pollicis brevis

Anterior

Medial

Lateral

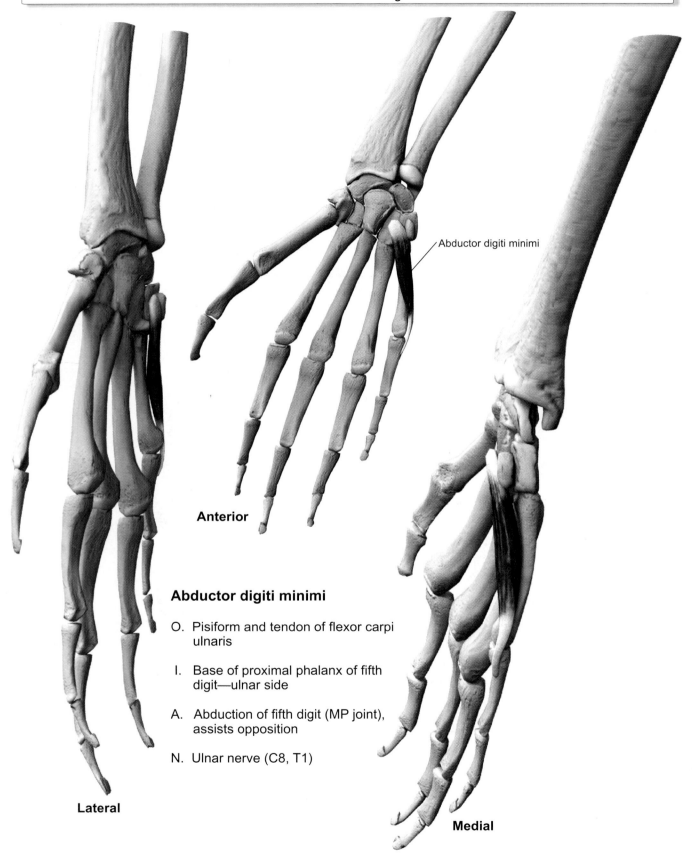

Abductor digiti minimi

Anterior

Lateral

Medial

Abductor digiti minimi

O. Pisiform and tendon of flexor carpi ulnaris

I. Base of proximal phalanx of fifth digit—ulnar side

A. Abduction of fifth digit (MP joint), assists opposition

N. Ulnar nerve (C8, T1)

Unit 3 Muscular System

Flexor digiti minimi

O. Hook of hamate and flexor retinaculum

I. Base of proximal phalanx of fifth digit—ulnar side

A. Flexion of fifth digit (MCP joint)

N. Ulnar nerve (C8, T1)

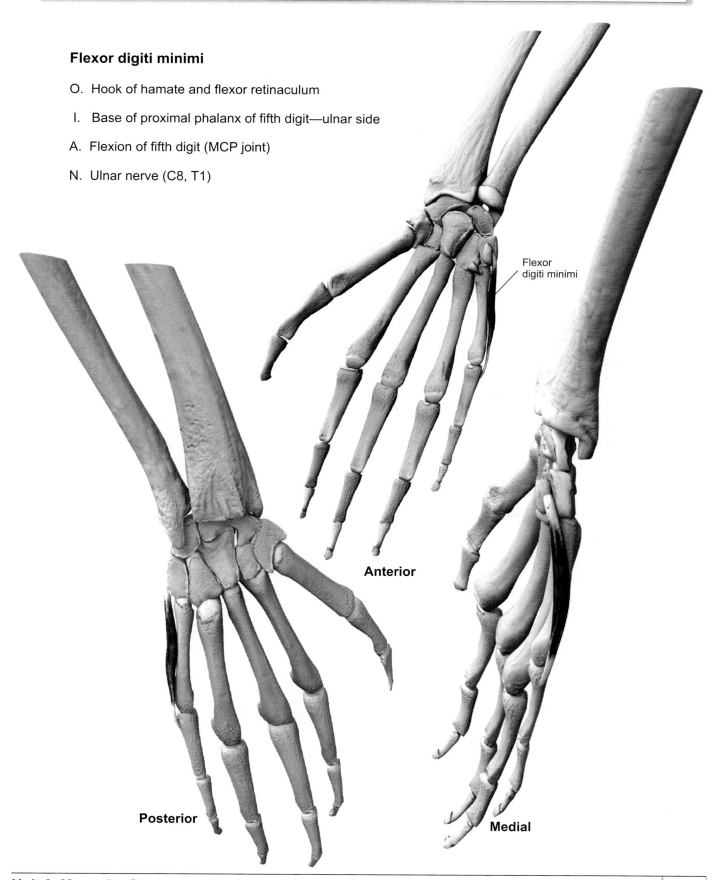

Flexor digiti minimi

Anterior

Posterior

Medial

Opponens digiti minimi

O. Hook of hamate and flexor retinaculum

I. Shaft of fifth metacarpal—ulnar side

A. Rotation of fifth metacarpal into
opposition with thumb

N. Ulnar nerve (C8, T1)

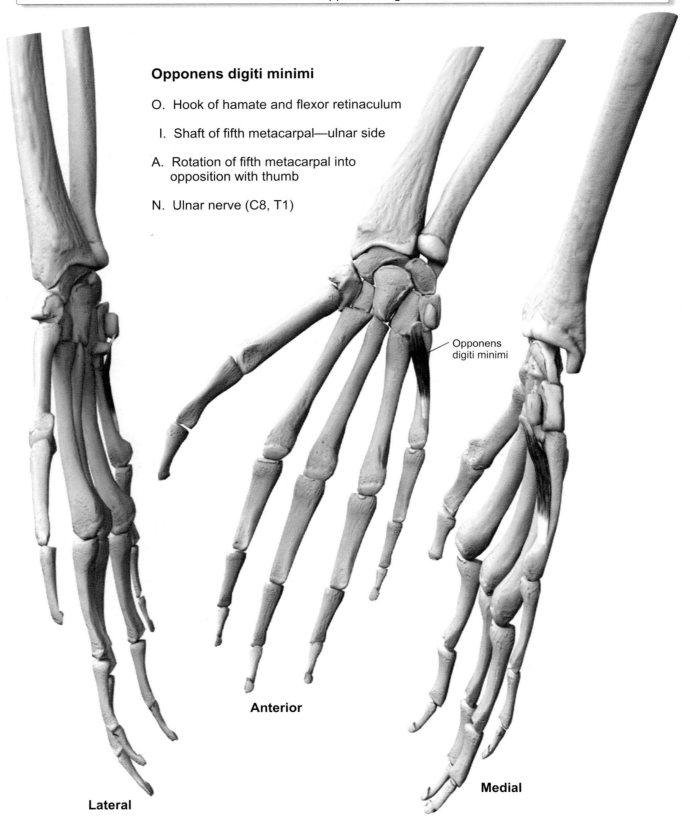

Opponens
digiti minimi

Anterior

Lateral

Medial

Unit 3 Muscular System

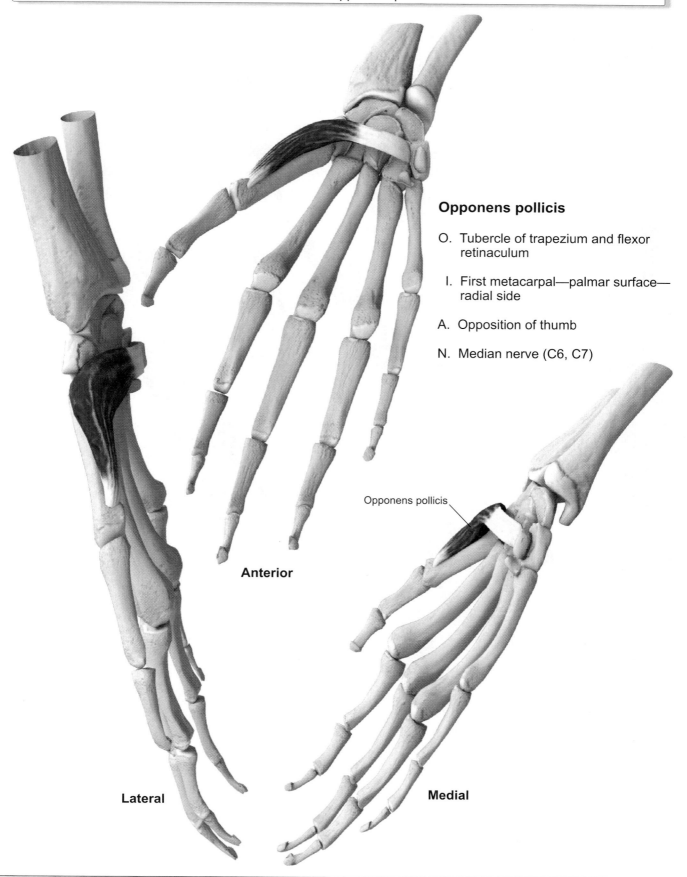

Opponens pollicis

O. Tubercle of trapezium and flexor retinaculum

I. First metacarpal—palmar surface—radial side

A. Opposition of thumb

N. Median nerve (C6, C7)

Opponens pollicis

Anterior

Lateral

Medial

Flexor pollicis longus

O. Anterior radius—middle surface, interosseous membrane

I. Base of distal phalanx of thumb—palmar surface

A. Flexion of distal phalanx of thumb (IP joint), assists flexion and abduction of hand at wrist (MCP and CM joints)

N. Median nerve (C8, T1)

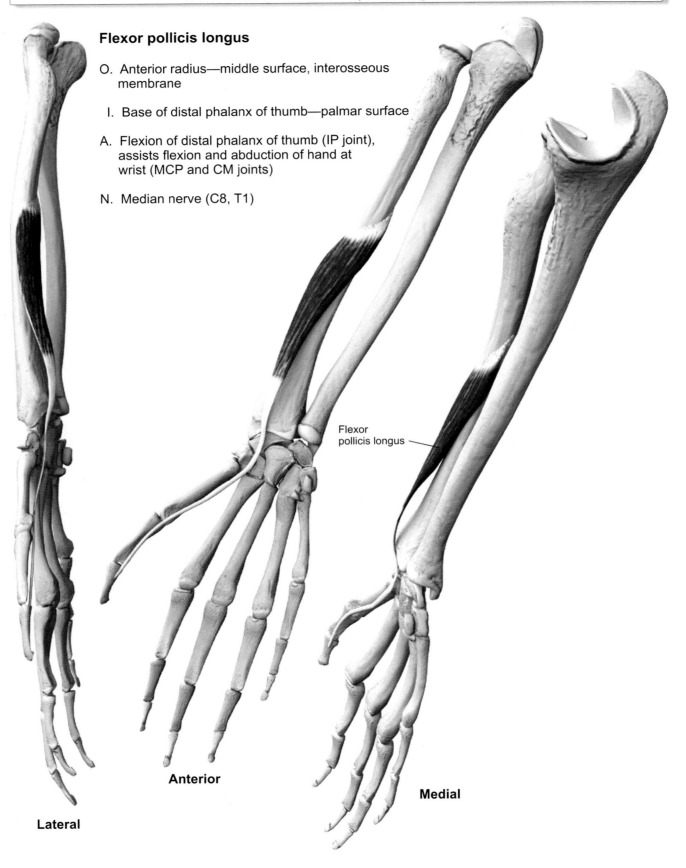

Flexor pollicis longus

Lateral

Anterior

Medial

Unit 3 Muscular System

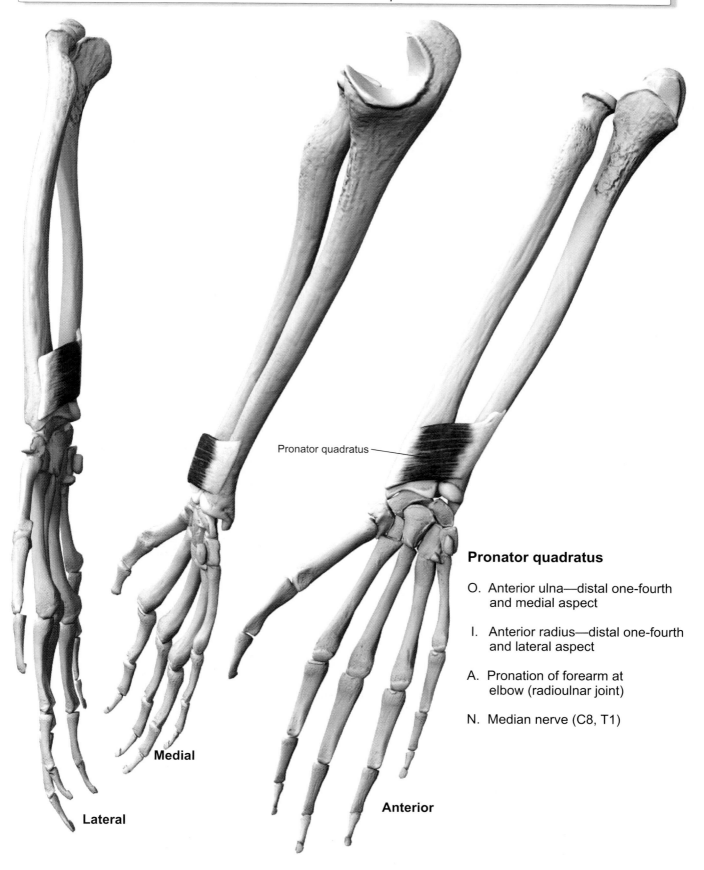

Pronator quadratus

Pronator quadratus

O. Anterior ulna—distal one-fourth
   and medial aspect

I. Anterior radius—distal one-fourth
   and lateral aspect

A. Pronation of forearm at
   elbow (radioulnar joint)

N. Median nerve (C8, T1)

Medial

Lateral

Anterior

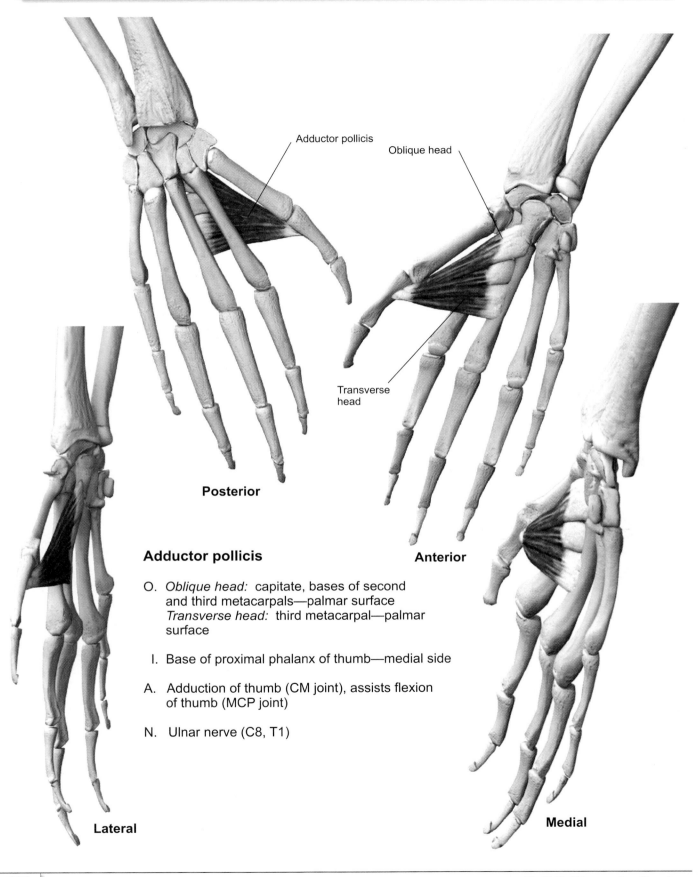

Adductor pollicis

Oblique head

Transverse head

Posterior

Anterior

Lateral

Medial

Adductor pollicis

O. *Oblique head:* capitate, bases of second and third metacarpals—palmar surface
Transverse head: third metacarpal—palmar surface

I. Base of proximal phalanx of thumb—medial side

A. Adduction of thumb (CM joint), assists flexion of thumb (MCP joint)

N. Ulnar nerve (C8, T1)

Unit 3 Muscular System

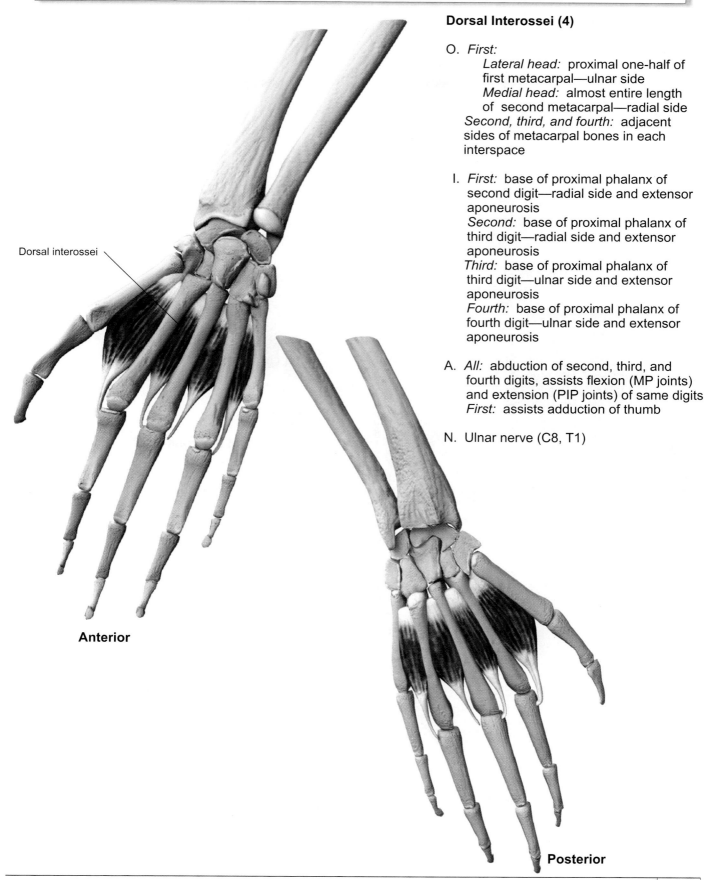

Dorsal Interossei (4)

O. *First:*
   Lateral head: proximal one-half of first metacarpal—ulnar side
   Medial head: almost entire length of second metacarpal—radial side
   Second, third, and fourth: adjacent sides of metacarpal bones in each interspace

I. *First:* base of proximal phalanx of second digit—radial side and extensor aponeurosis
   Second: base of proximal phalanx of third digit—radial side and extensor aponeurosis
   Third: base of proximal phalanx of third digit—ulnar side and extensor aponeurosis
   Fourth: base of proximal phalanx of fourth digit—ulnar side and extensor aponeurosis

A. *All:* abduction of second, third, and fourth digits, assists flexion (MP joints) and extension (PIP joints) of same digits
   First: assists adduction of thumb

N. Ulnar nerve (C8, T1)

Dorsal interossei

Anterior

Posterior

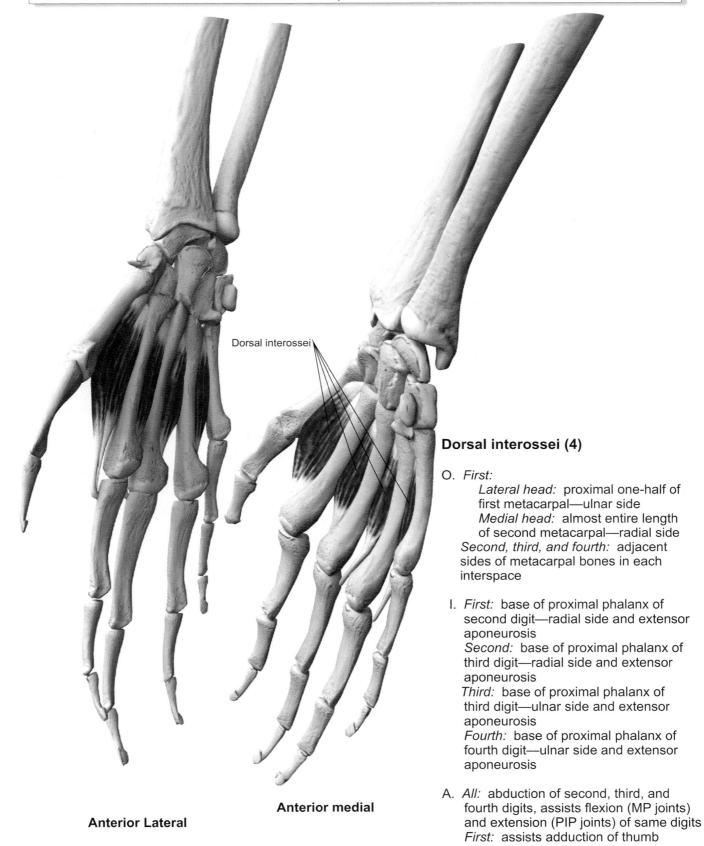

Dorsal interossei

Anterior Lateral

Anterior medial

Dorsal interossei (4)

O. *First:*
    Lateral head: proximal one-half of
    first metacarpal—ulnar side
    Medial head: almost entire length
    of second metacarpal—radial side
    Second, third, and fourth: adjacent
    sides of metacarpal bones in each
    interspace

I. *First:* base of proximal phalanx of
    second digit—radial side and extensor
    aponeurosis
    Second: base of proximal phalanx of
    third digit—radial side and extensor
    aponeurosis
    Third: base of proximal phalanx of
    third digit—ulnar side and extensor
    aponeurosis
    Fourth: base of proximal phalanx of
    fourth digit—ulnar side and extensor
    aponeurosis

A. *All:* abduction of second, third, and
    fourth digits, assists flexion (MP joints)
    and extension (PIP joints) of same digits
    First: assists adduction of thumb

N. Ulnar nerve (C8, T1)

Unit 3 Muscular System

Palmar interossei (3)

O. Anterior surfaces of second, fourth, and fifth metacarpals—palmar side

I. Bases of proximal phalanges of second, fourth, and fifth digits and extensor aponeurosis

A. Adduction of second, fourth, and fifth digits, assists in flexion (MCP joints) and extension (IP joints) of second, fourth, and fifth digits

N. Ulnar nerve (C8, T1)

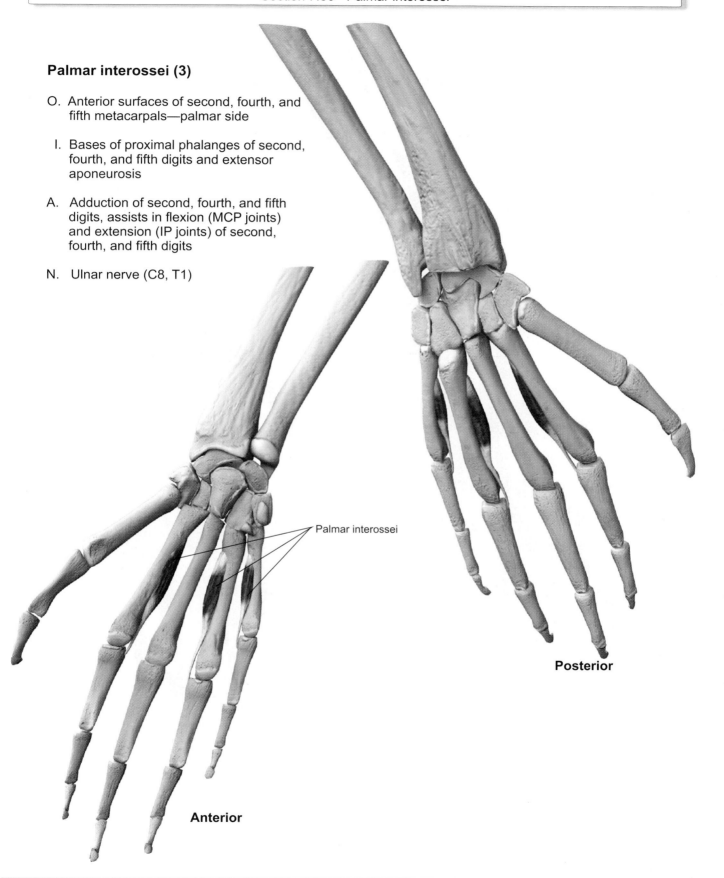

Palmar interossei

Anterior

Posterior

Palmar interossei (3)

O. Surfaces of second, fourth, and fifth metacarpals—palmar side

I. Bases of proximal phalanges of second, fourth, and fifth digits and extensor aponeurosis

A. Adduction of second, fourth, and fifth digits, assists in flexion (MCP joints) and extension (IP joints) of second, fourth, and fifth digits

N. Ulnar nerve (C8, T1)

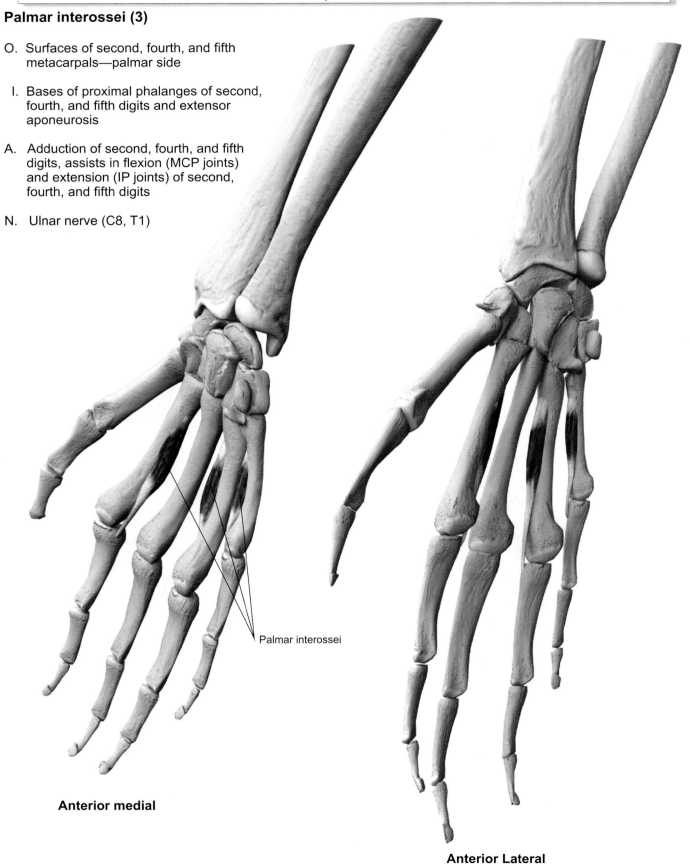

Palmar interossei

Anterior medial

Anterior Lateral

Unit 3 Muscular System

Section 1 - Muscle Group Movements, 336–408

Realism   *a study in human structural anatomy*

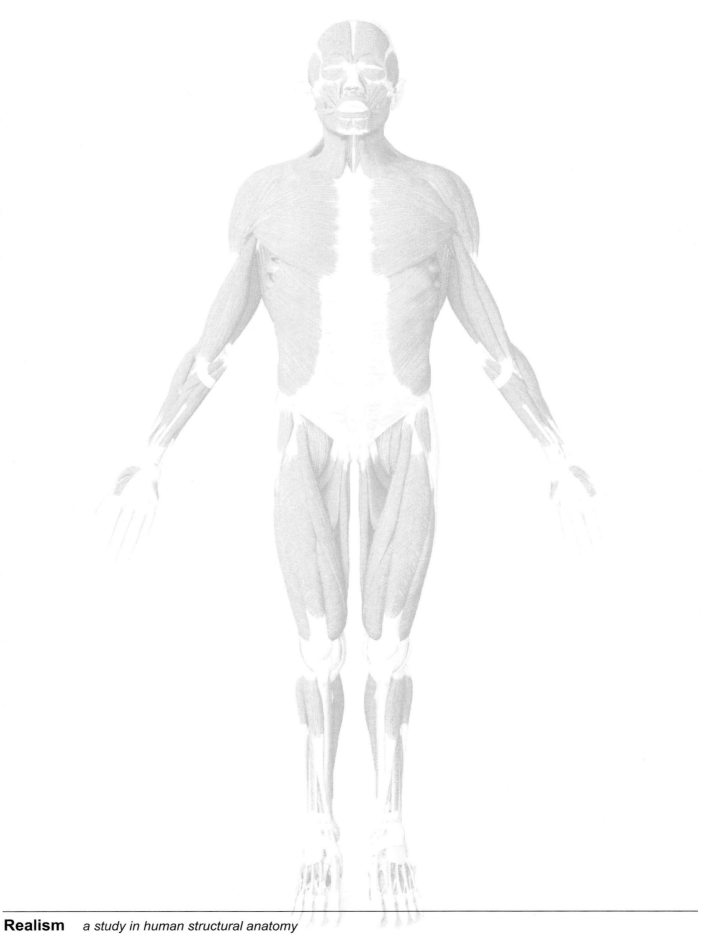

Realism   *a study in human structural anatomy*

Muscle Group Terms

Epicranius

Occipitalis and Frontalis are sometimes considered one muscle, the Occipitofrontalis, and are part of the Epicranius

Suboccipitals (6)

(Located immediately below the occipital bone)

Rectus capitis anterior
Rectus capitis posterior major
Rectus capitis posterior minor
Rectus capitis lateralis
Oblique capitis superior
Oblique capitis inferior

Rotator Cuff Muscles (4)

Supraspinatus
Infraspinatus
Teres minor
Subscapularis

Erector Spinae (Superficial) (9)

Iliocostalis cervicis
Iliocostalis thoracis
Iliocostalis lumborum
Longissimus cervicis
Longissimus capitis
Longissimus thoracis
Spinalis capitis
Spinalis cervicis
Spinalis thoracis

Transversospinalis (Deep) (5)

Semispinalis (first layer) most superficial
     Semispinalis capitis
     Semispinalis cervicis
     Semispinalis thoracis
Multifidi (second layer)
Rotatores (third layer)

Segmentals (2)

Interspinales
Intertransversarii

Intercostals (3)

1. External—first layer and most superficial; eleven pairs
2. Internal—second layer, middle; eleven pairs
3. Innermost—third layer and deepest consisting of transverse thoracis and subcostals

Iliopsoas

The combination of two muscles, the "psoas major" and the "iliacus," sometimes considered a single muscle, the iliopsoas

Deep Lateral Rotators of the Hip (6)

Piriformis
Gemellus superior
Obturator internus
Gemellus inferior
Obturator externus
Quadratus femoris

Quadriceps (4)

Rectus femoris
Vastus intermedius
Vastus medialis
Vastus lateralis

Hamstrings (3)

Biceps femoris
Semimembranosus
Semitendinosus

Suprahyoid Group (4)

Mylohyoid
Digastric
Geniohyoid
Stylohyoid

Infrahyoid Group (4)

Thyrohyoid
Sternothyroid
Sternohyoid
Omohyoid

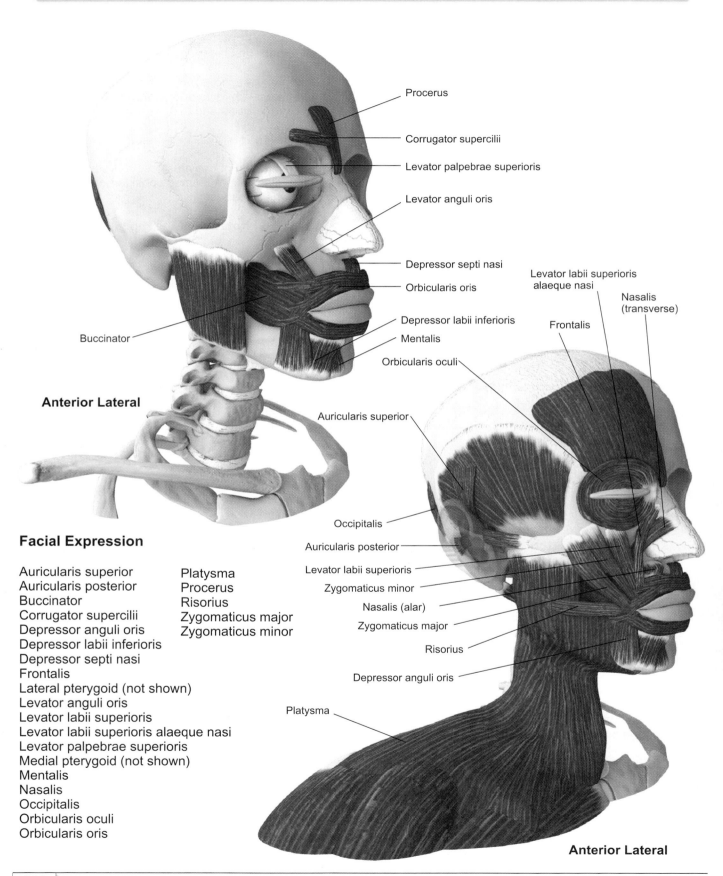

Procerus

Corrugator supercilii

Levator palpebrae superioris

Levator anguli oris

Depressor septi nasi

Orbicularis oris

Buccinator

Depressor labii inferioris

Mentalis

Orbicularis oculi

Levator labii superioris alaeque nasi

Nasalis (transverse)

Frontalis

Anterior Lateral

Auricularis superior

Occipitalis

Auricularis posterior

Levator labii superioris

Zygomaticus minor

Nasalis (alar)

Zygomaticus major

Risorius

Depressor anguli oris

Platysma

Anterior Lateral

Facial Expression

Auricularis superior
Auricularis posterior
Buccinator
Corrugator supercilii
Depressor anguli oris
Depressor labii inferioris
Depressor septi nasi
Frontalis
Lateral pterygoid (not shown)
Levator anguli oris
Levator labii superioris
Levator labii superioris alaeque nasi
Levator palpebrae superioris
Medial pterygoid (not shown)
Mentalis
Nasalis
Occipitalis
Orbicularis oculi
Orbicularis oris

Platysma
Procerus
Risorius
Zygomaticus major
Zygomaticus minor

Unit 4 Muscle Group Movements

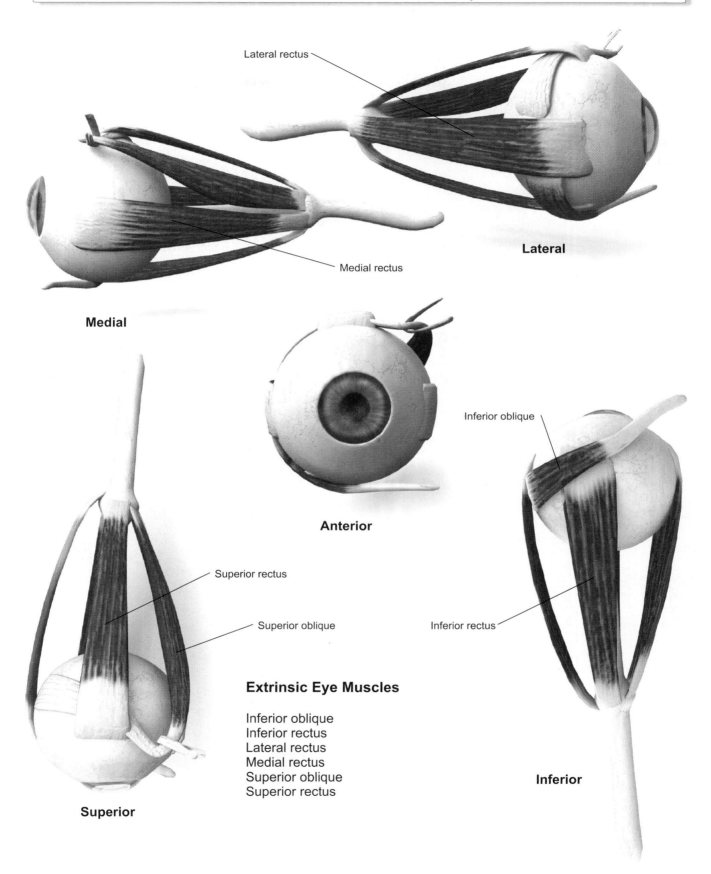

Lateral rectus

Medial rectus

Lateral

Medial

Anterior

Inferior oblique

Superior rectus

Superior oblique

Inferior rectus

Extrinsic Eye Muscles

Inferior oblique
Inferior rectus
Lateral rectus
Medial rectus
Superior oblique
Superior rectus

Superior

Inferior

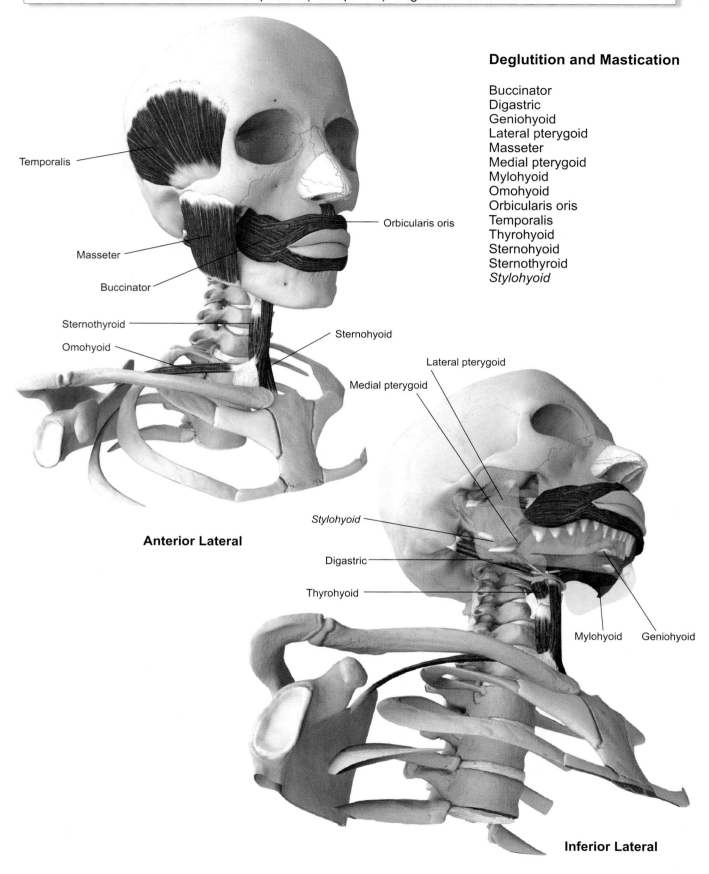

Deglutition and Mastication

Buccinator
Digastric
Geniohyoid
Lateral pterygoid
Masseter
Medial pterygoid
Mylohyoid
Omohyoid
Orbicularis oris
Temporalis
Thyrohyoid
Sternohyoid
Sternothyroid
Stylohyoid

Temporalis

Orbicularis oris

Masseter

Buccinator

Sternothyroid

Sternohyoid

Omohyoid

Anterior Lateral

Lateral pterygoid

Medial pterygoid

Stylohyoid

Digastric

Thyrohyoid

Mylohyoid   Geniohyoid

Inferior Lateral

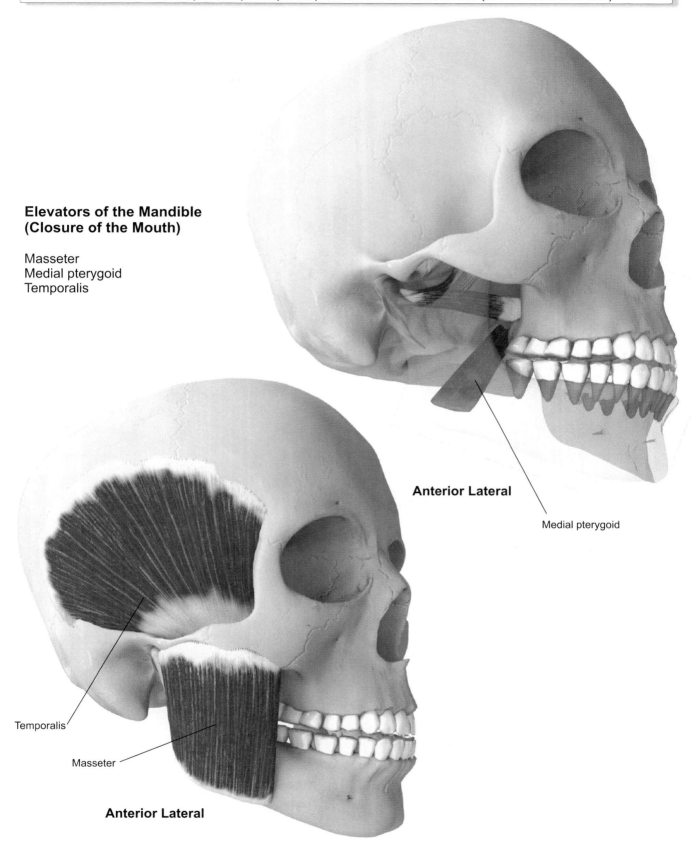

**Elevators of the Mandible
(Closure of the Mouth)**

Masseter
Medial pterygoid
Temporalis

Anterior Lateral

Medial pterygoid

Temporalis

Masseter

Anterior Lateral

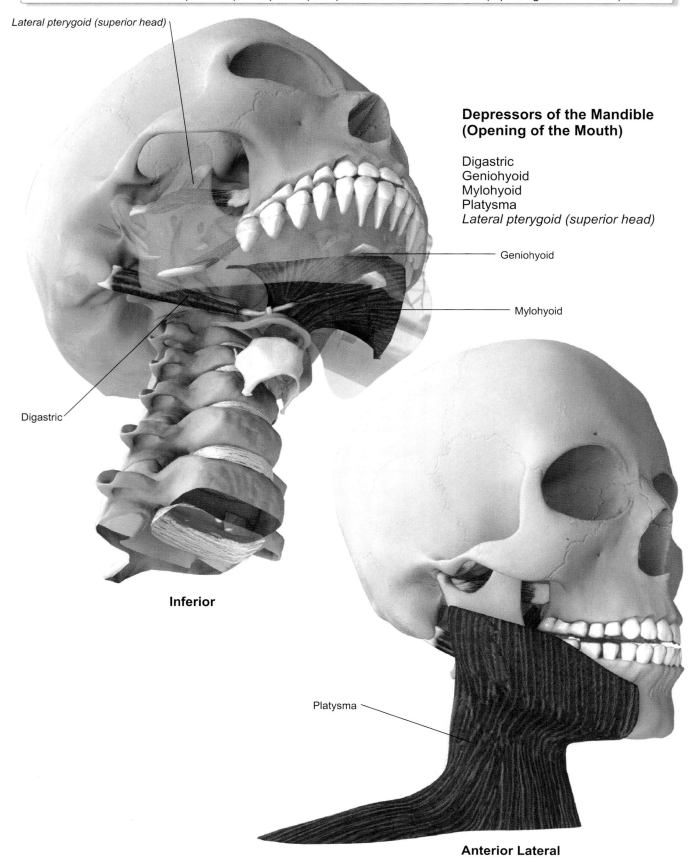

Lateral pterygoid (superior head)

Depressors of the Mandible (Opening of the Mouth)

Digastric
Geniohyoid
Mylohyoid
Platysma
Lateral pterygoid (superior head)

Geniohyoid

Mylohyoid

Digastric

Inferior

Platysma

Anterior Lateral

Unit 4 Muscle Group Movements

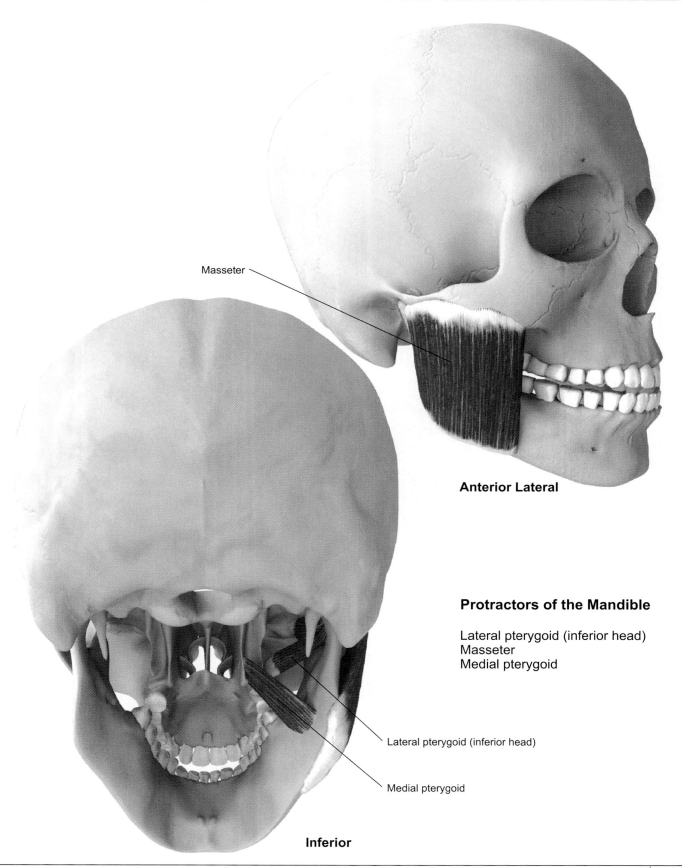

Masseter

Anterior Lateral

Protractors of the Mandible

Lateral pterygoid (inferior head)
Masseter
Medial pterygoid

Lateral pterygoid (inferior head)

Medial pterygoid

Inferior

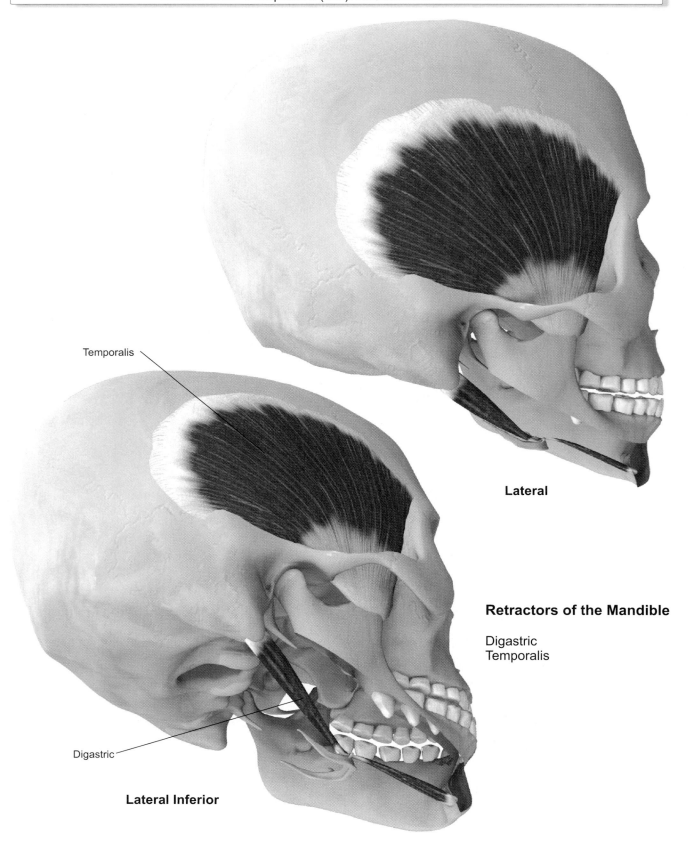

Temporalis

Lateral

Retractors of the Mandible

Digastric
Temporalis

Digastric

Lateral Inferior

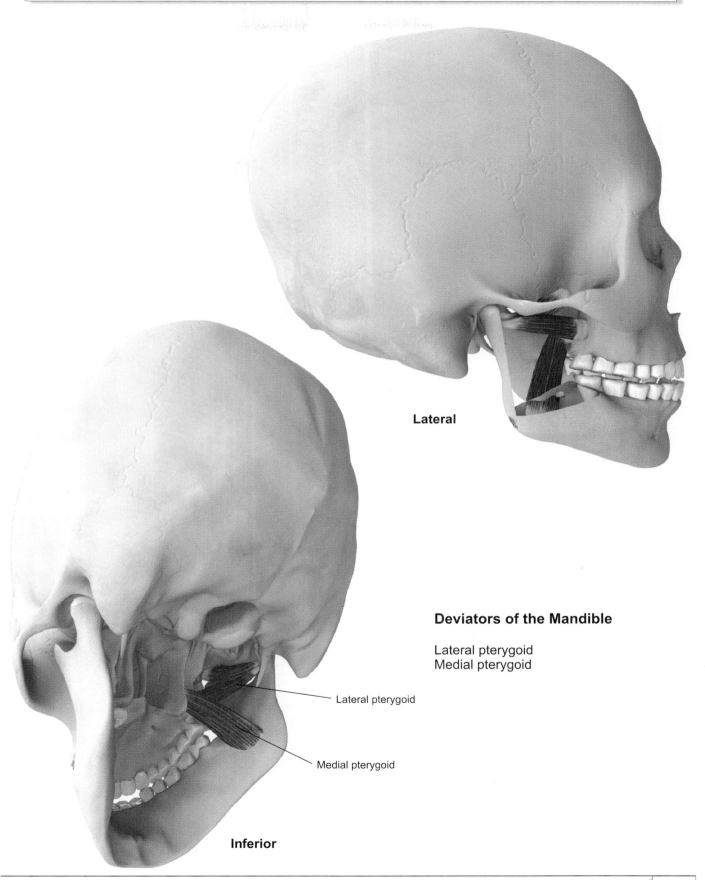

Lateral

Deviators of the Mandible

Lateral pterygoid
Medial pterygoid

Lateral pterygoid

Medial pterygoid

Inferior

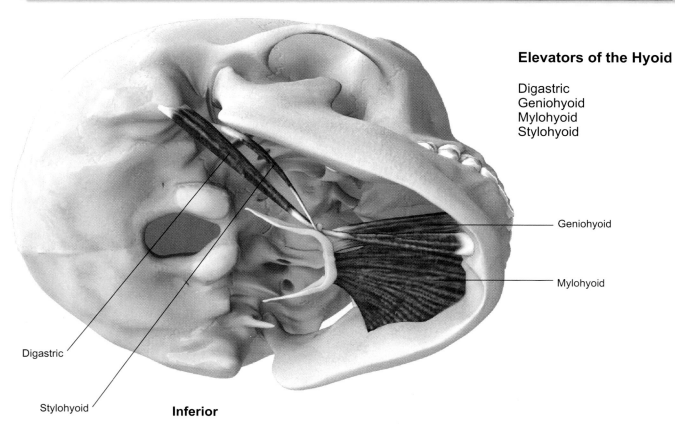

Elevators of the Hyoid

Digastric
Geniohyoid
Mylohyoid
Stylohyoid

Geniohyoid

Mylohyoid

Digastric

Stylohyoid

Inferior

Protractors of the Hyoid

Geniohyoid

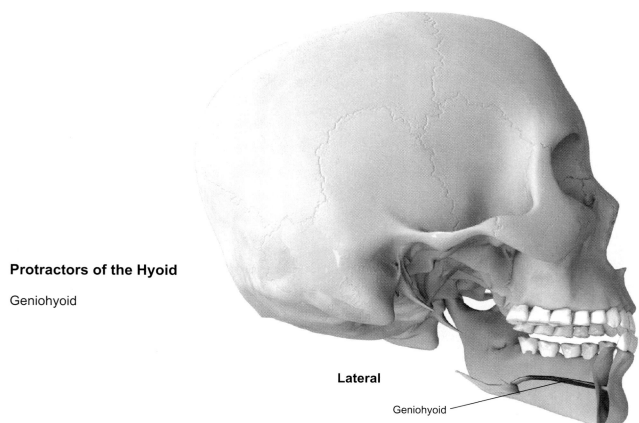

Lateral

Geniohyoid

Unit 4 Muscle Group Movements

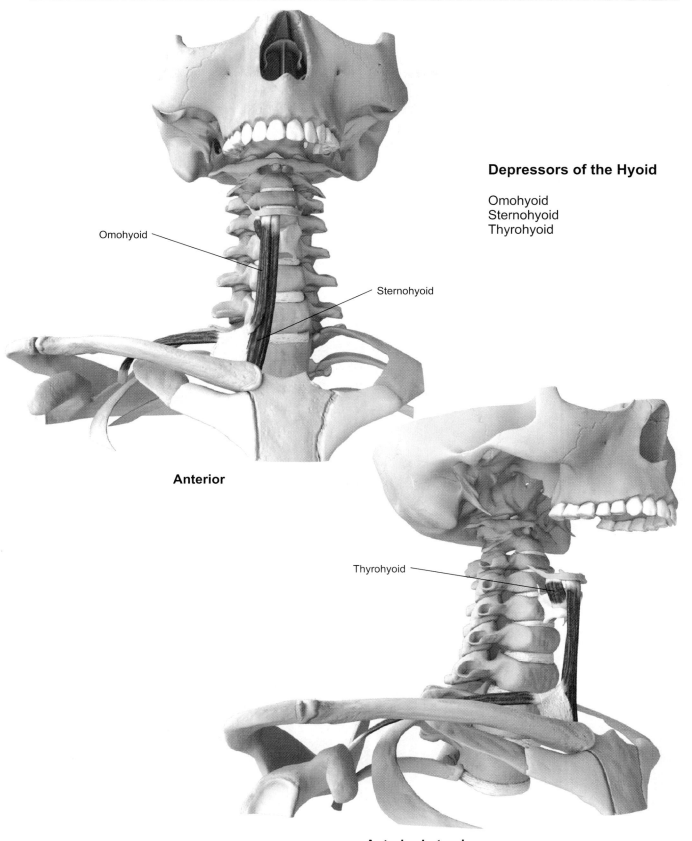

Depressors of the Hyoid

Omohyoid
Sternohyoid
Thyrohyoid

Omohyoid

Sternohyoid

Anterior

Thyrohyoid

Anterior Lateral

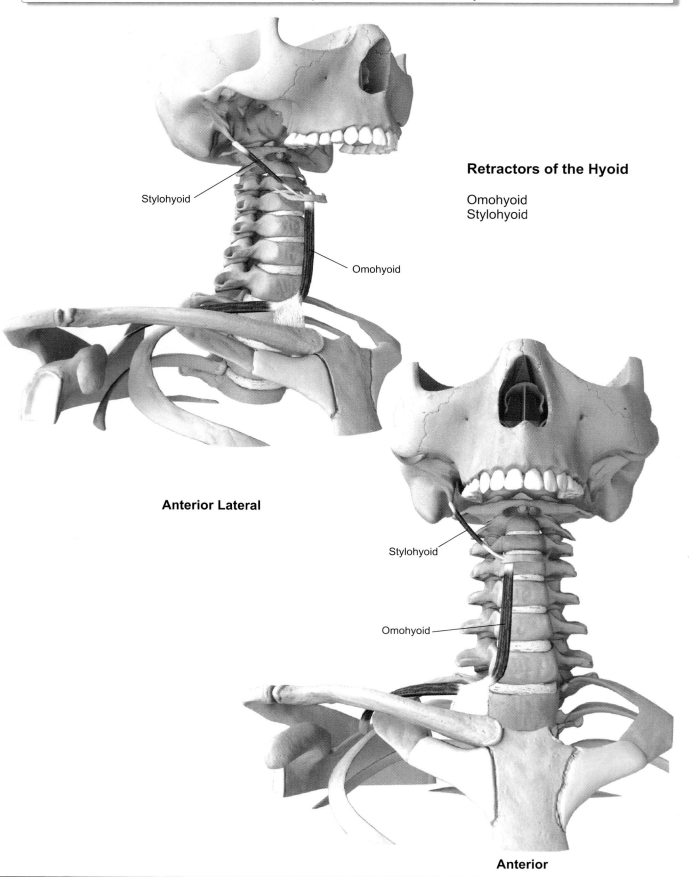

Stylohyoid

Omohyoid

Retractors of the Hyoid

Omohyoid
Stylohyoid

Anterior Lateral

Stylohyoid

Omohyoid

Anterior

**Flexors of the Head and/or Neck—
Cervical Spine (Part 1)**

Longus coli
Longus capitis
Rectus capitis anterior
Sternocleidomastoid
Anterior scalenes

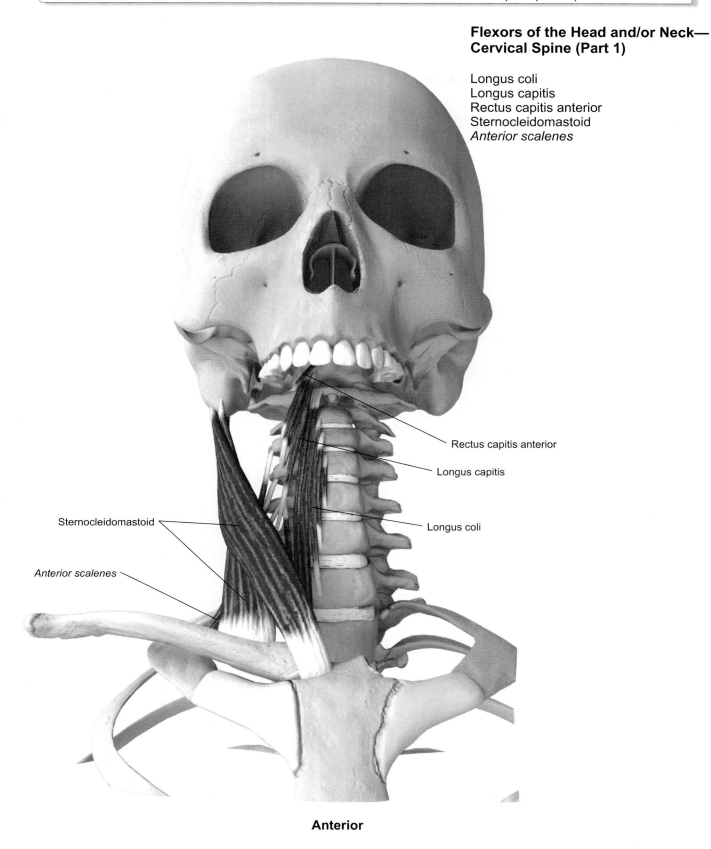

Rectus capitis anterior

Longus capitis

Longus coli

Sternocleidomastoid

Anterior scalenes

Anterior

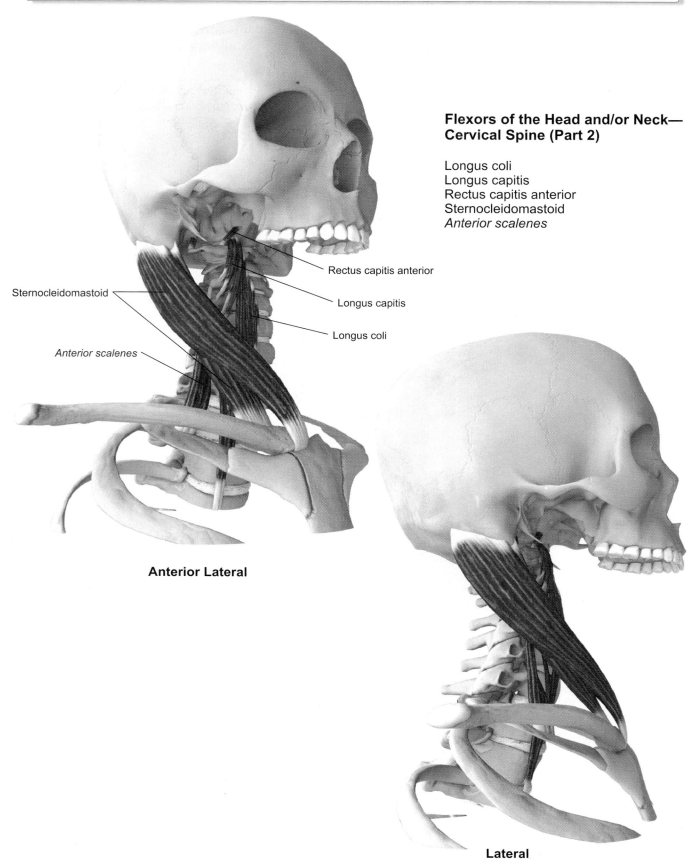

**Flexors of the Head and/or Neck—
Cervical Spine (Part 2)**

Longus coli
Longus capitis
Rectus capitis anterior
Sternocleidomastoid
Anterior scalenes

Rectus capitis anterior

Sternocleidomastoid

Longus capitis

Longus coli

Anterior scalenes

Anterior Lateral

Lateral

Unit 4   Muscle Group Movements

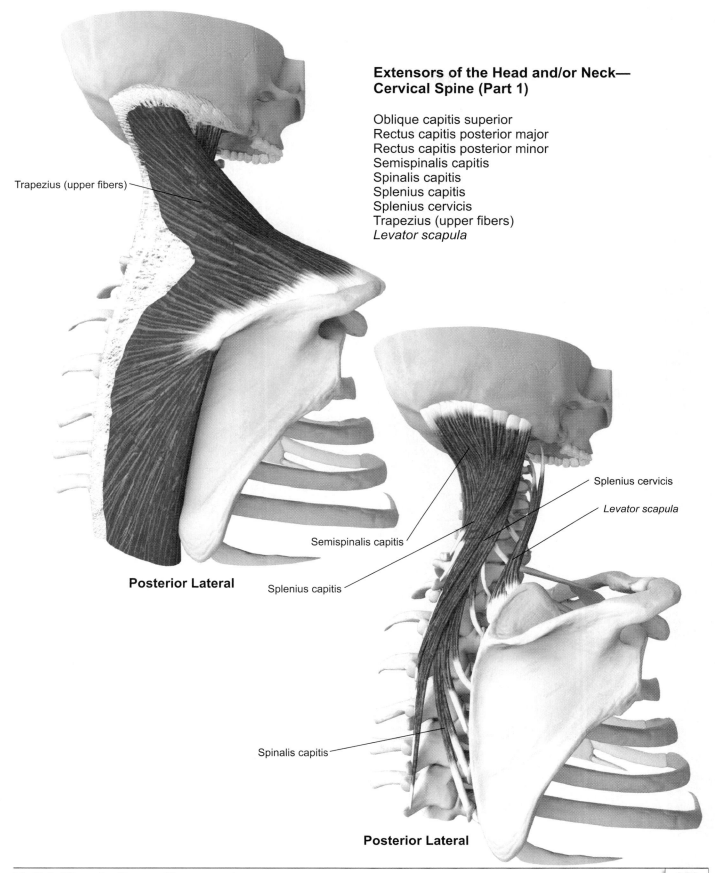

**Extensors of the Head and/or Neck—
Cervical Spine (Part 1)**

Oblique capitis superior
Rectus capitis posterior major
Rectus capitis posterior minor
Semispinalis capitis
Spinalis capitis
Splenius capitis
Splenius cervicis
Trapezius (upper fibers)
Levator scapula

Trapezius (upper fibers)

Posterior Lateral

Semispinalis capitis

Splenius capitis

Splenius cervicis

Levator scapula

Spinalis capitis

Posterior Lateral

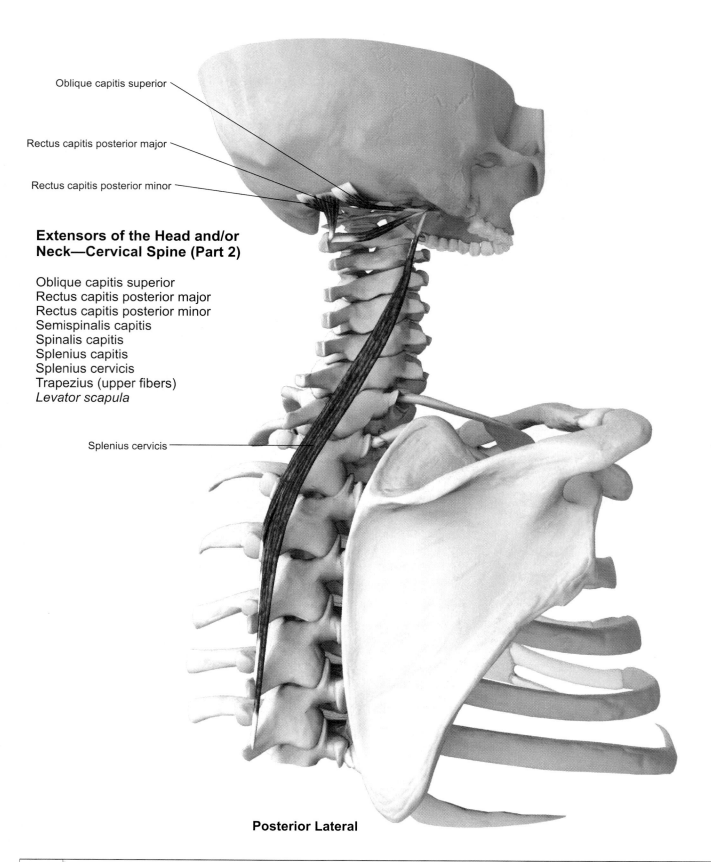

Oblique capitis superior

Rectus capitis posterior major

Rectus capitis posterior minor

Extensors of the Head and/or Neck—Cervical Spine (Part 2)

Oblique capitis superior
Rectus capitis posterior major
Rectus capitis posterior minor
Semispinalis capitis
Spinalis capitis
Splenius capitis
Splenius cervicis
Trapezius (upper fibers)
Levator scapula

Splenius cervicis

Posterior Lateral

Unit 4 Muscle Group Movements

Lateral Flexors of the Head and/or Neck—Cervical Spine (Part 1)

Levator scapula
Longus coli (oblique portions)
Oblique capitis superior
Rectus capitis lateralis
Scalenes
Sternocleidomastoid
Trapezius (upper fibers)

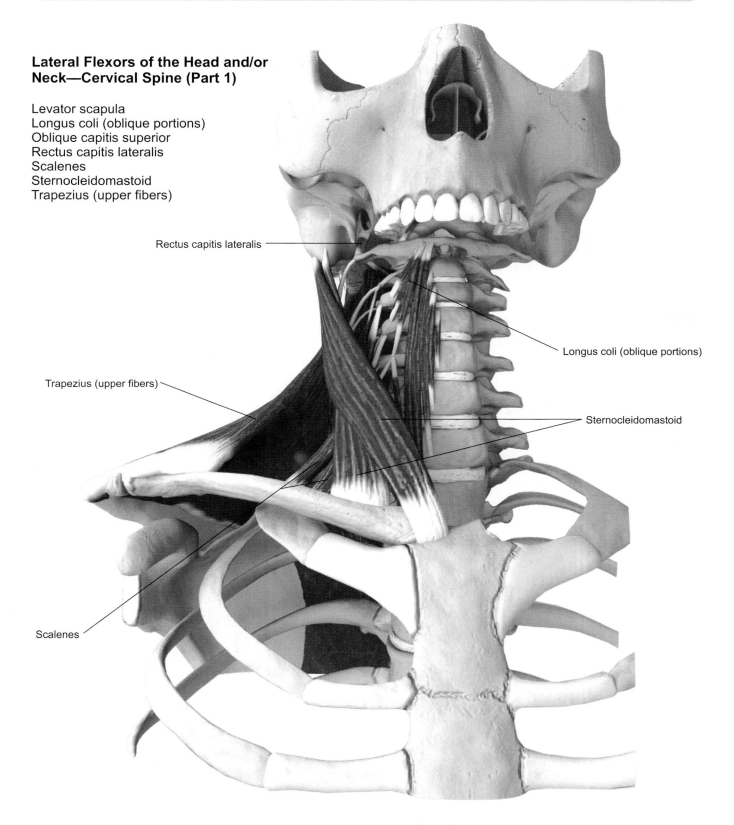

Rectus capitis lateralis

Longus coli (oblique portions)

Trapezius (upper fibers)

Sternocleidomastoid

Scalenes

Anterior

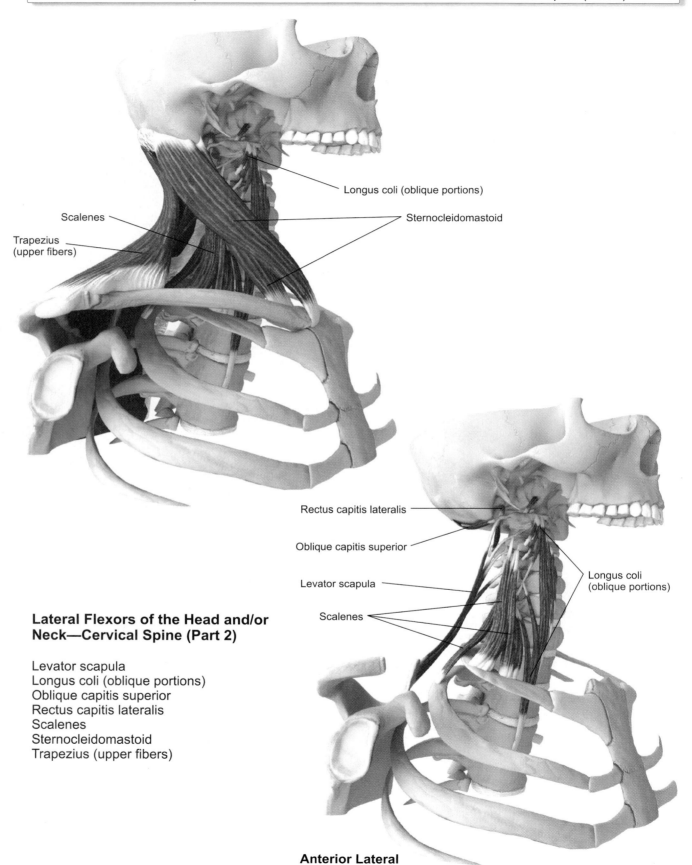

Longus coli (oblique portions)

Scalenes

Trapezius
(upper fibers)

Sternocleidomastoid

Rectus capitis lateralis

Oblique capitis superior

Levator scapula

Scalenes

Longus coli
(oblique portions)

**Lateral Flexors of the Head and/or
Neck—Cervical Spine (Part 2)**

Levator scapula
Longus coli (oblique portions)
Oblique capitis superior
Rectus capitis lateralis
Scalenes
Sternocleidomastoid
Trapezius (upper fibers)

Anterior Lateral

Rotators of the Head and/or Neck—Cervical Spine (Part 1)

Levator scapula
Longissimus capitis
Longus coli (inferior obliques)
Oblique capitis inferior
Rectus capitis posterior major
Scalenes
Semispinalis capitis
Splenius capitis
Splenius cervicis
Sternocleidomastoid
Trapezius (upper fibers)

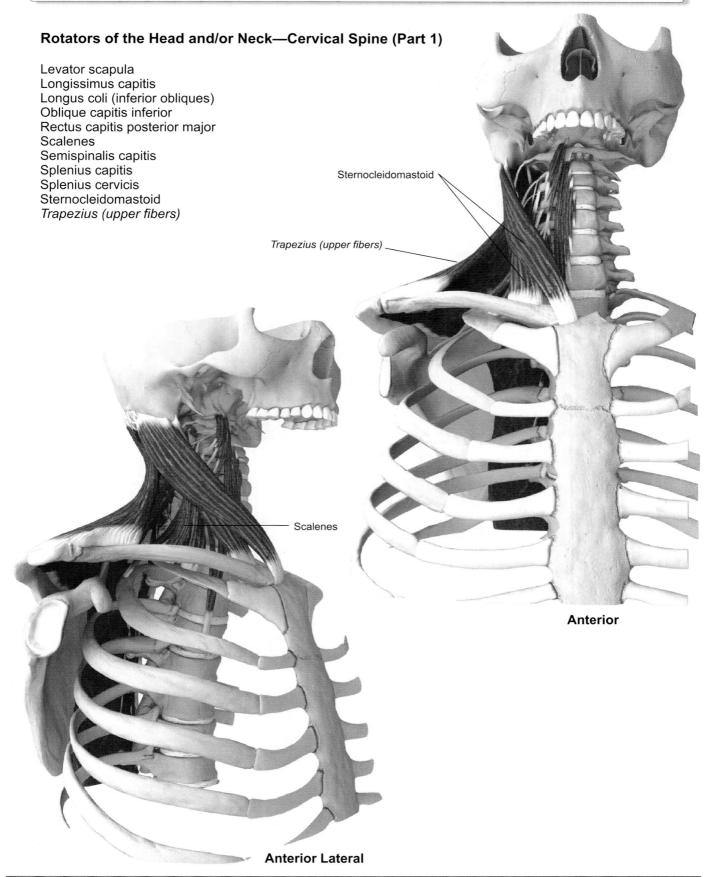

Sternocleidomastoid

Trapezius (upper fibers)

Scalenes

Anterior

Anterior Lateral

Rotators of the Head and/or Neck—Cervical Spine (Part 2)

Levator scapula
Longissimus capitis
Longus coli (inferior obliques)
Oblique capitis inferior
Rectus capitis posterior major
Scalenes
Semispinalis capitis
Splenius capitis
Splenius cervicis
Sternocleidomastoid
Trapezius (upper fibers)

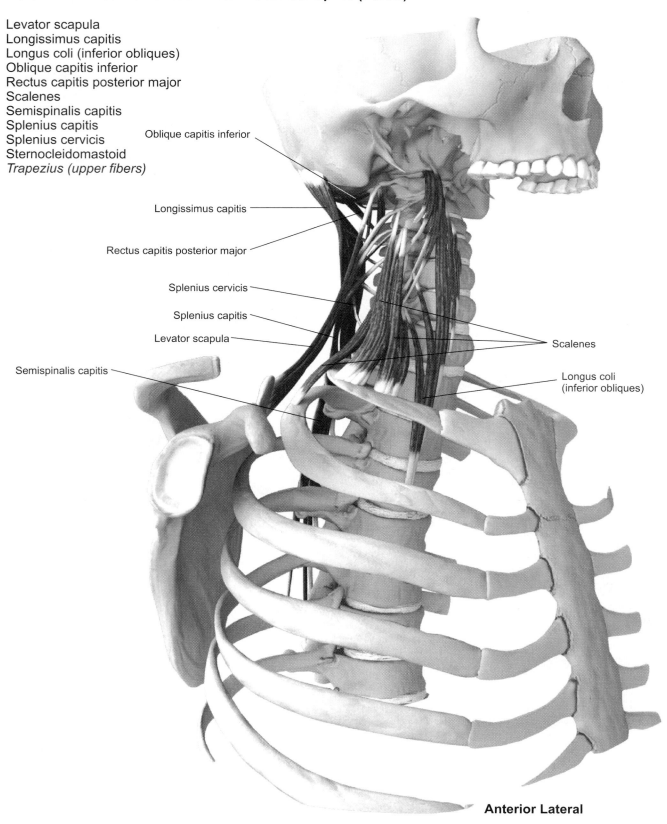

Oblique capitis inferior

Longissimus capitis

Rectus capitis posterior major

Splenius cervicis

Splenius capitis

Levator scapula

Semispinalis capitis

Scalenes

Longus coli
(inferior obliques)

Anterior Lateral

Unit 4 Muscle Group Movements

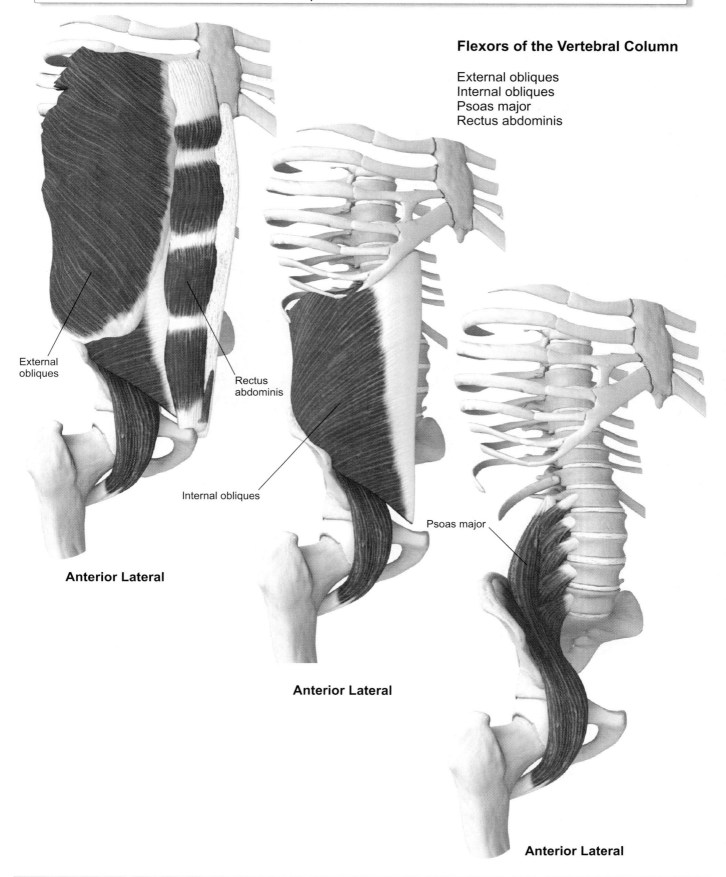

Flexors of the Vertebral Column

External obliques
Internal obliques
Psoas major
Rectus abdominis

External
obliques

Rectus
abdominis

Internal obliques

Psoas major

Anterior Lateral

Anterior Lateral

Anterior Lateral

Extensors of the Vertebral Column (Part 1)

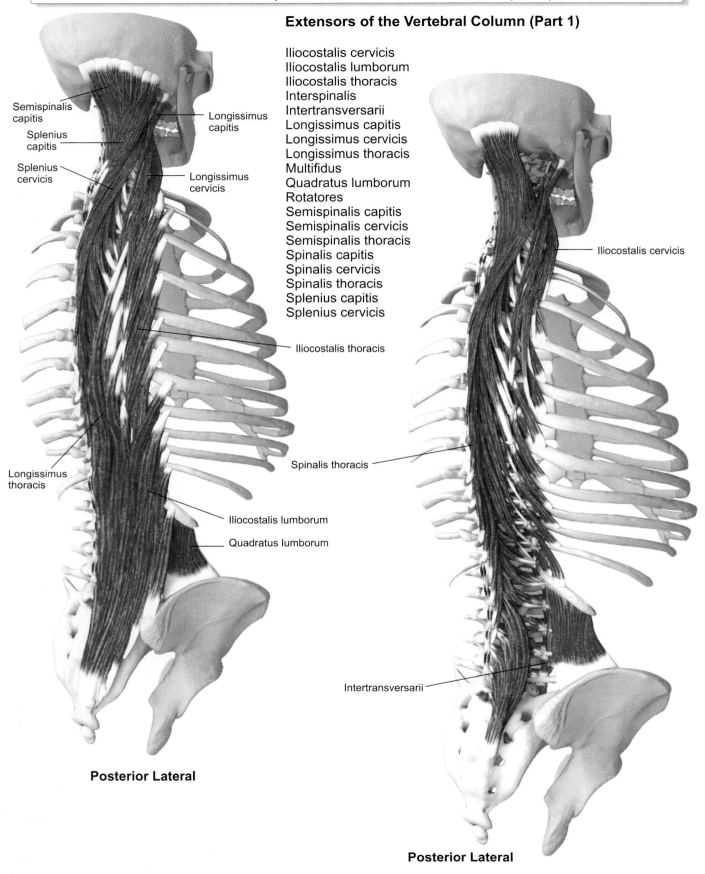

Iliocostalis cervicis
Iliocostalis lumborum
Iliocostalis thoracis
Interspinalis
Intertransversarii
Longissimus capitis
Longissimus cervicis
Longissimus thoracis
Multifidus
Quadratus lumborum
Rotatores
Semispinalis capitis
Semispinalis cervicis
Semispinalis thoracis
Spinalis capitis
Spinalis cervicis
Spinalis thoracis
Splenius capitis
Splenius cervicis

Semispinalis capitis

Splenius capitis

Splenius cervicis

Longissimus capitis

Longissimus cervicis

Iliocostalis thoracis

Longissimus thoracis

Iliocostalis lumborum

Quadratus lumborum

Iliocostalis cervicis

Spinalis thoracis

Intertransversarii

Posterior Lateral

Posterior Lateral

Extensors of the Vertebral Column (Part 2)

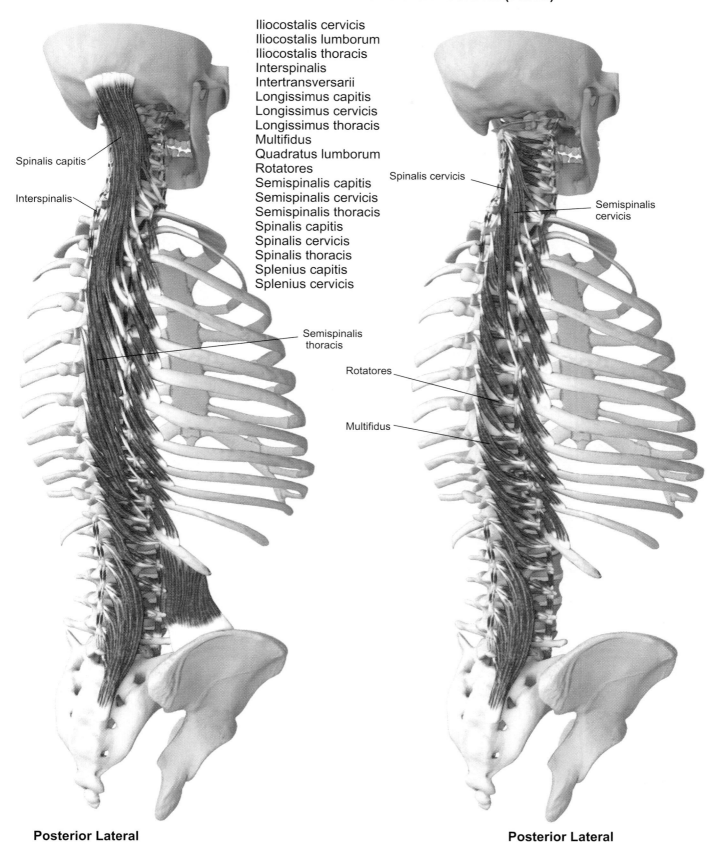

Iliocostalis cervicis
Iliocostalis lumborum
Iliocostalis thoracis
Interspinalis
Intertransversarii
Longissimus capitis
Longissimus cervicis
Longissimus thoracis
Multifidus
Quadratus lumborum
Rotatores
Semispinalis capitis
Semispinalis cervicis
Semispinalis thoracis
Spinalis capitis
Spinalis cervicis
Spinalis thoracis
Splenius capitis
Splenius cervicis

Spinalis capitis

Interspinalis

Semispinalis
thoracis

Spinalis cervicis

Semispinalis
cervicis

Rotatores

Multifidus

Posterior Lateral

Posterior Lateral

Lateral Flexors of the Vertebral Column

External obliques
Internal obliques
Iliocostalis cervicis
Iliocostalis lumborum
Iliocostalis thoracis
Intertransversarii
Levator costarum
Longissimus cervicis
Longissimus thoracis
Psoas minor (not shown)
Quadratus lumborum

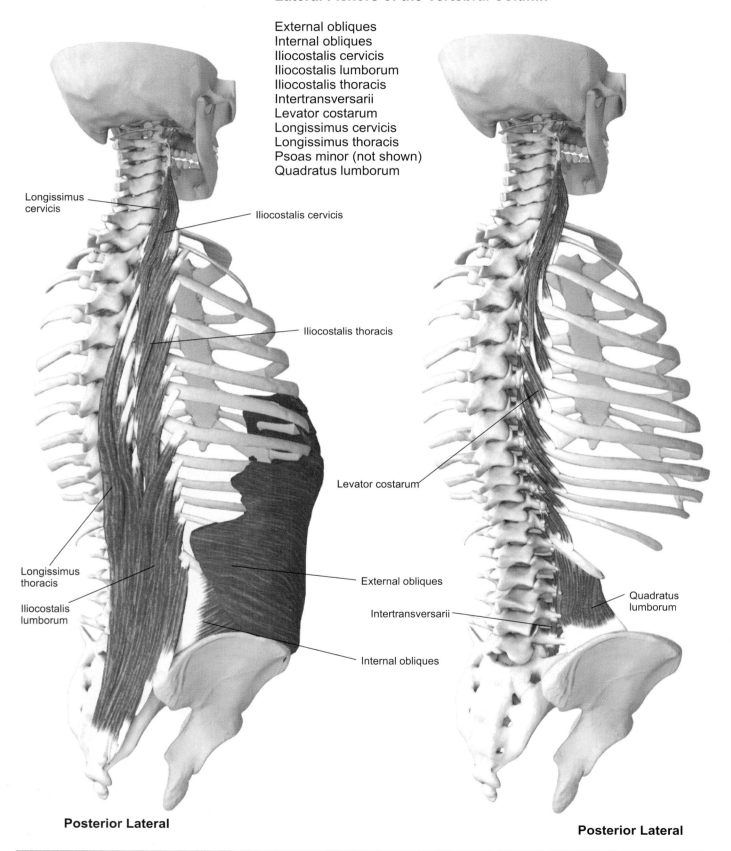

Longissimus cervicis

Iliocostalis cervicis

Iliocostalis thoracis

Levator costarum

Longissimus thoracis

Iliocostalis lumborum

External obliques

Intertransversarii

Internal obliques

Quadratus lumborum

Posterior Lateral

Posterior Lateral

Unit 4 Muscle Group Movements

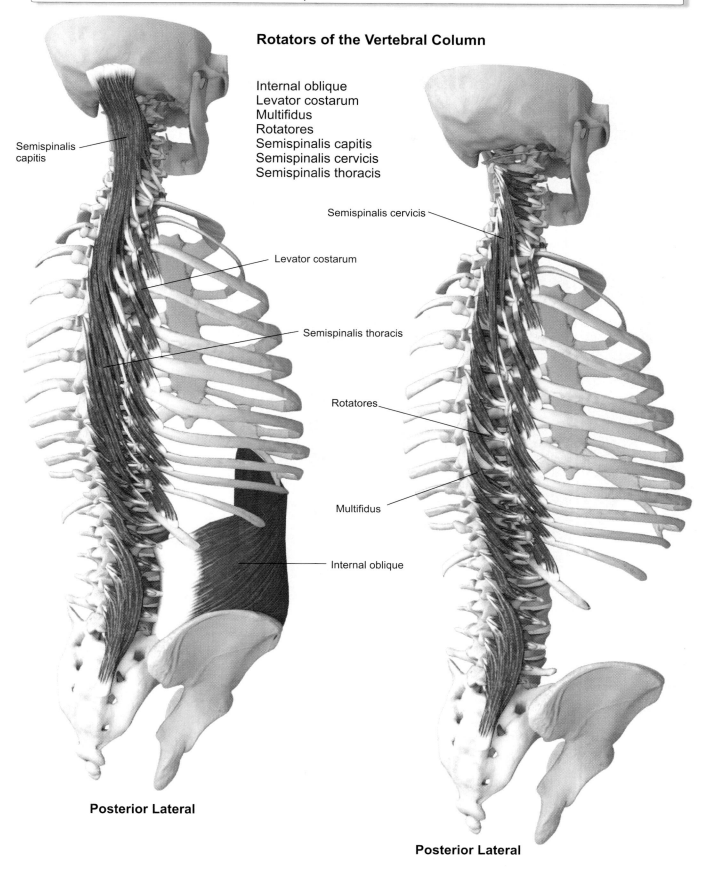

Rotators of the Vertebral Column

Internal oblique
Levator costarum
Multifidus
Rotatores
Semispinalis capitis
Semispinalis cervicis
Semispinalis thoracis

Semispinalis capitis

Semispinalis cervicis

Levator costarum

Semispinalis thoracis

Rotatores

Multifidus

Internal oblique

Posterior Lateral

Posterior Lateral

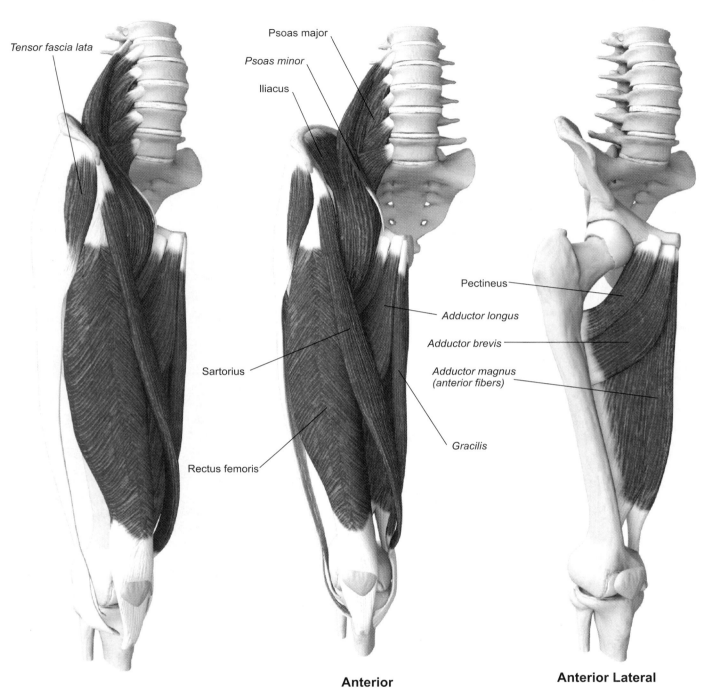

Tensor fascia lata

Psoas major

Psoas minor

Iliacus

Sartorius

Rectus femoris

Pectineus

Adductor longus

Adductor brevis

Adductor magnus
(anterior fibers)

Gracilis

Anterior Lateral

Anterior

Anterior Lateral

Flexors of the Femur at Hip

Iliacus
Pectineus
Psoas major
Rectus femoris
Sartorius
Adductor brevis
Adductor longus

Adductor magnus (anterior fibers)
Gracilis
Psoas minor
Tensor fascia lata

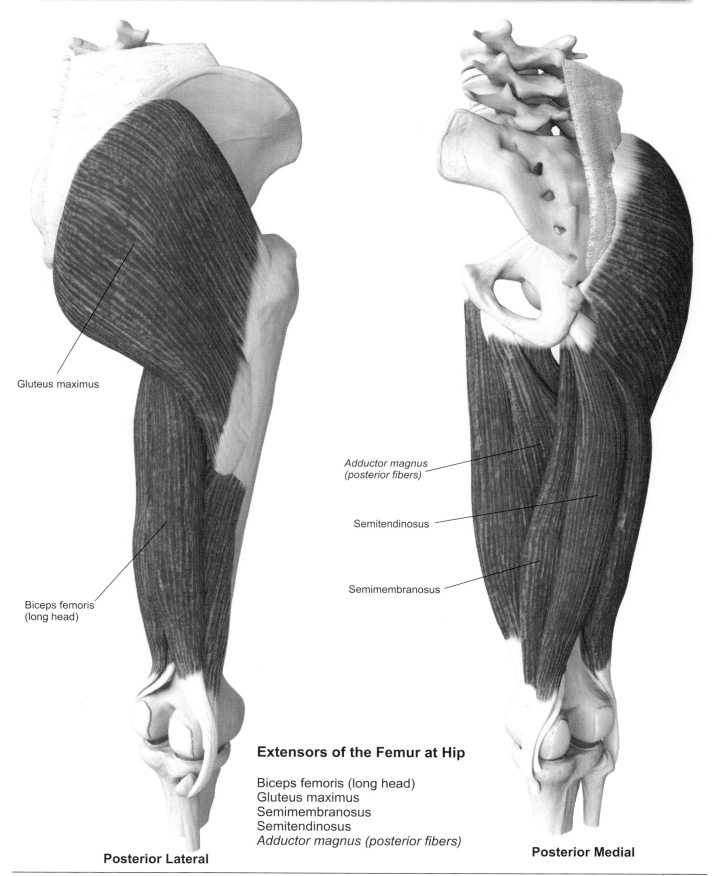

Gluteus maximus

Biceps femoris
(long head)

Adductor magnus
(posterior fibers)

Semitendinosus

Semimembranosus

Extensors of the Femur at Hip

Biceps femoris (long head)
Gluteus maximus
Semimembranosus
Semitendinosus
Adductor magnus (posterior fibers)

Posterior Lateral

Posterior Medial

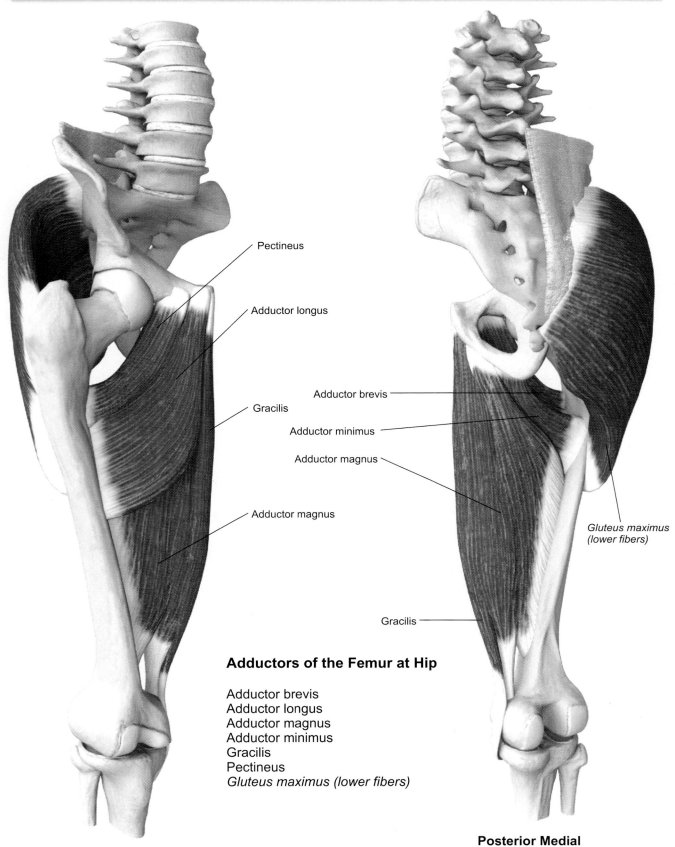

Pectineus

Adductor longus

Gracilis

Adductor magnus

Adductor brevis

Adductor minimus

Adductor magnus

Gluteus maximus
(lower fibers)

Gracilis

Adductors of the Femur at Hip

Adductor brevis
Adductor longus
Adductor magnus
Adductor minimus
Gracilis
Pectineus
Gluteus maximus (lower fibers)

Anterior Lateral

Posterior Medial

Unit 4 Muscle Group Movements

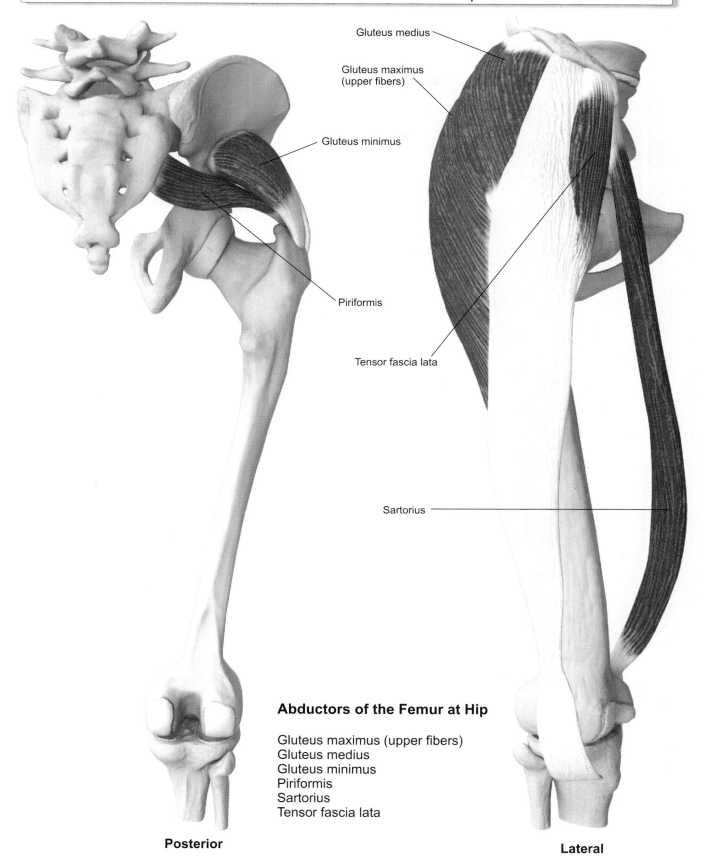

Gluteus medius

Gluteus maximus
(upper fibers)

Gluteus minimus

Piriformis

Tensor fascia lata

Sartorius

Abductors of the Femur at Hip

Gluteus maximus (upper fibers)
Gluteus medius
Gluteus minimus
Piriformis
Sartorius
Tensor fascia lata

Posterior

Lateral

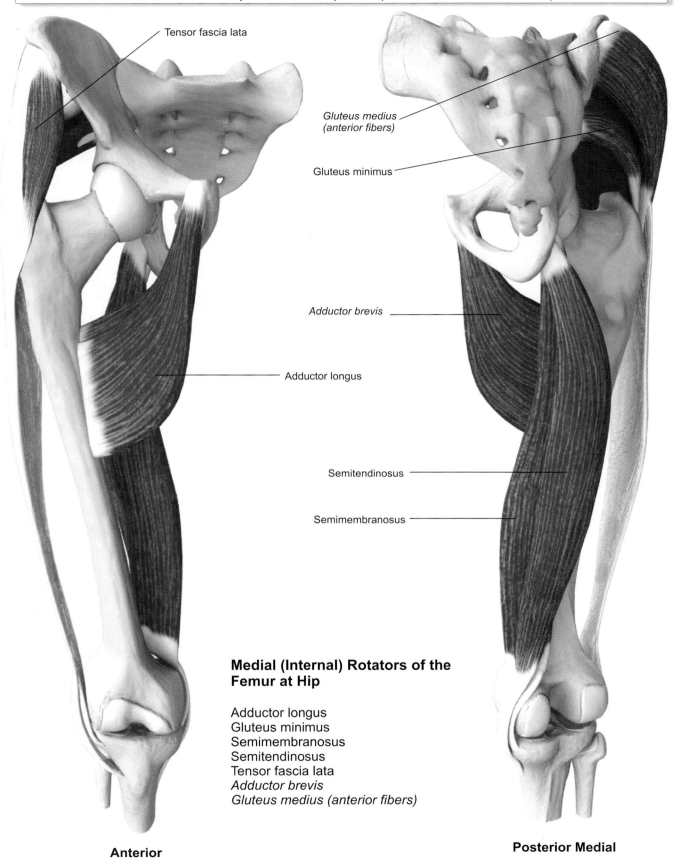

Tensor fascia lata

Gluteus medius
(anterior fibers)

Gluteus minimus

Adductor brevis

Adductor longus

Semitendinosus

Semimembranosus

Medial (Internal) Rotators of the Femur at Hip

Adductor longus
Gluteus minimus
Semimembranosus
Semitendinosus
Tensor fascia lata
Adductor brevis
Gluteus medius (anterior fibers)

Anterior

Posterior Medial

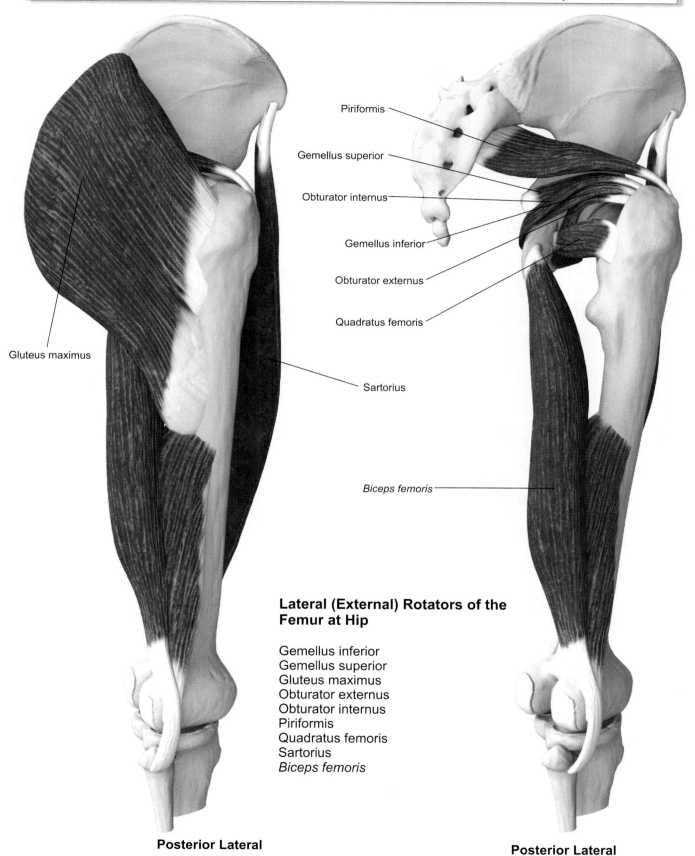

Piriformis

Gemellus superior

Obturator internus

Gemellus inferior

Obturator externus

Quadratus femoris

Gluteus maximus

Sartorius

Biceps femoris

Lateral (External) Rotators of the Femur at Hip

Gemellus inferior
Gemellus superior
Gluteus maximus
Obturator externus
Obturator internus
Piriformis
Quadratus femoris
Sartorius
Biceps femoris

Posterior Lateral

Posterior Lateral

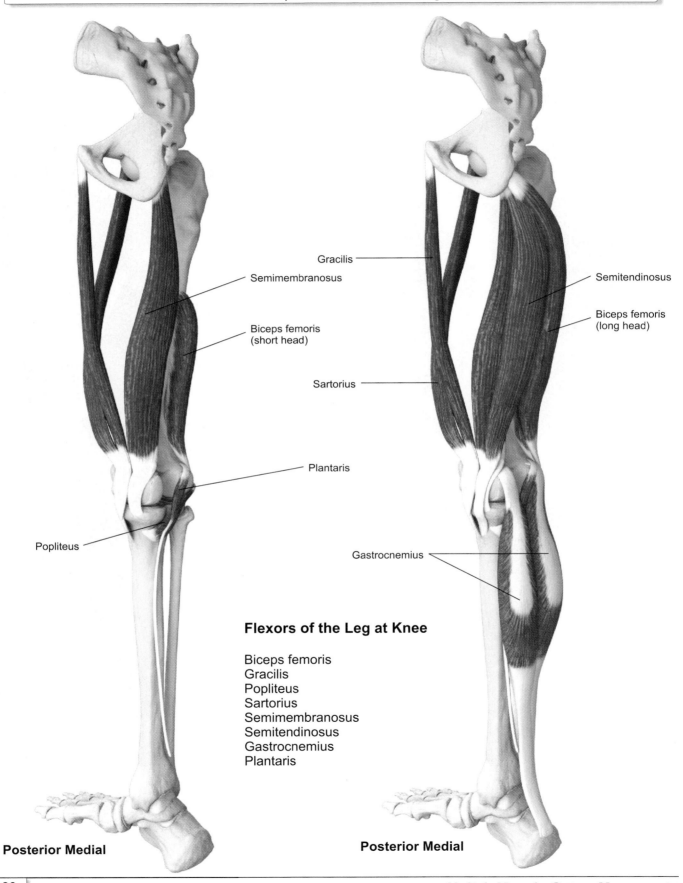

Gracilis

Semimembranosus

Semitendinosus

Biceps femoris
(short head)

Biceps femoris
(long head)

Sartorius

Plantaris

Popliteus

Gastrocnemius

Flexors of the Leg at Knee

Biceps femoris
Gracilis
Popliteus
Sartorius
Semimembranosus
Semitendinosus
Gastrocnemius
Plantaris

Posterior Medial

Posterior Medial

Unit 4 Muscle Group Movements

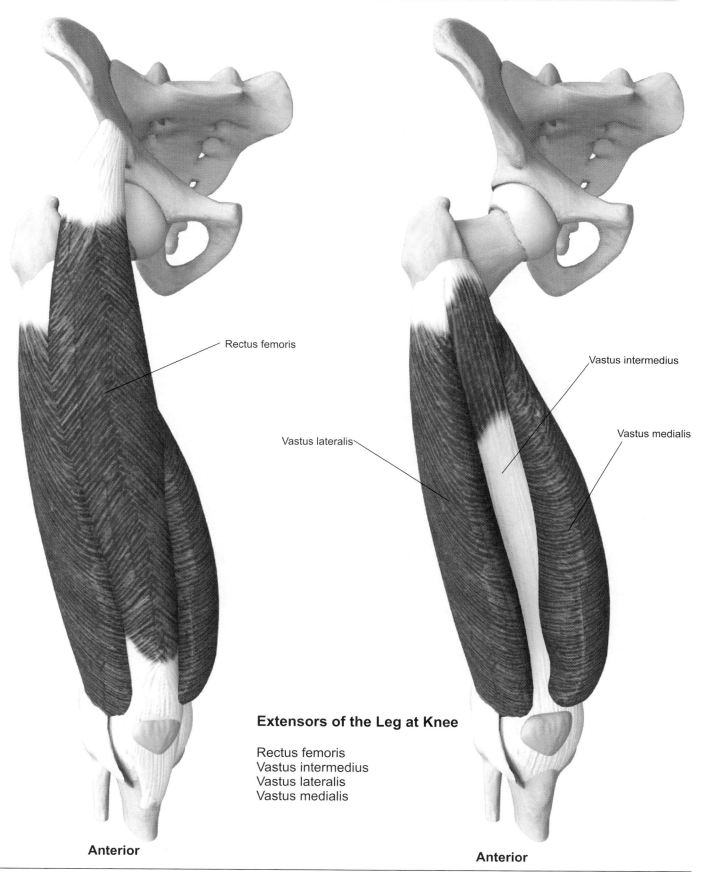

Rectus femoris

Vastus intermedius

Vastus lateralis

Vastus medialis

Extensors of the Leg at Knee

Rectus femoris
Vastus intermedius
Vastus lateralis
Vastus medialis

Anterior

Anterior

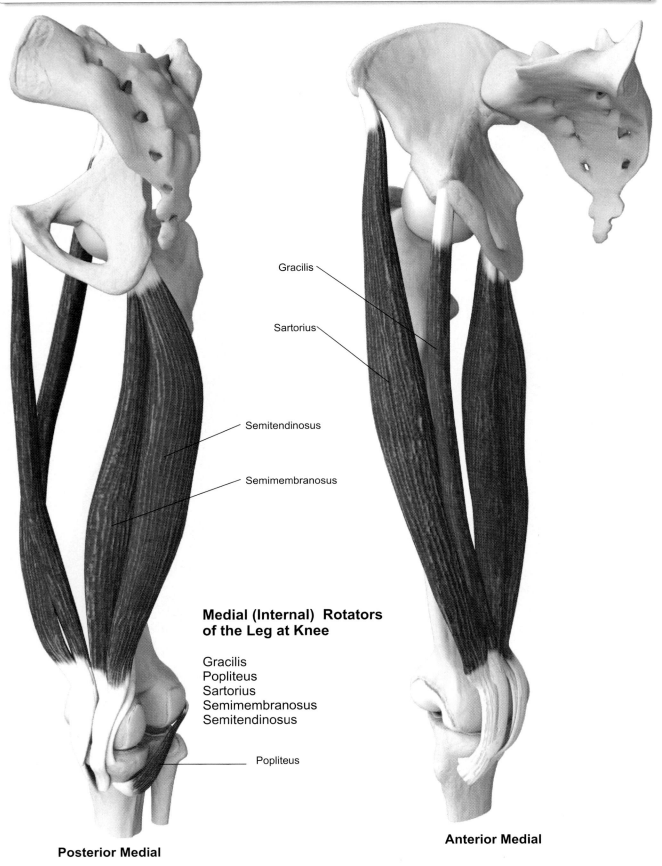

Gracilis

Sartorius

Semitendinosus

Semimembranosus

**Medial (Internal) Rotators
of the Leg at Knee**

Gracilis
Popliteus
Sartorius
Semimembranosus
Semitendinosus

Popliteus

Posterior Medial

Anterior Medial

Unit 4 Muscle Group Movements

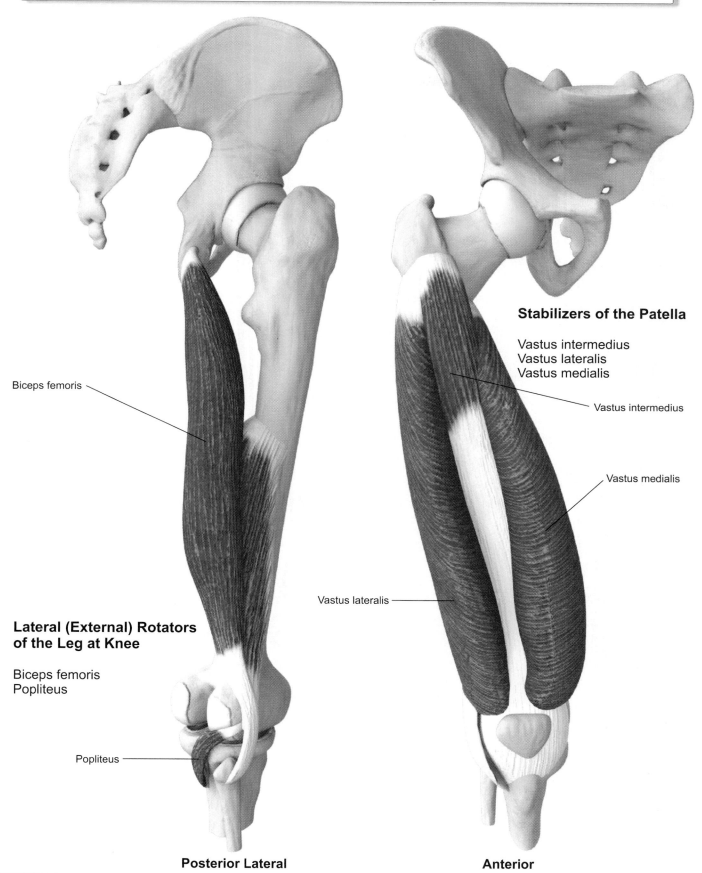

Biceps femoris

Stabilizers of the Patella

Vastus intermedius
Vastus lateralis
Vastus medialis

Vastus intermedius

Vastus medialis

**Lateral (External) Rotators
of the Leg at Knee**

Biceps femoris
Popliteus

Vastus lateralis

Popliteus

Posterior Lateral

Anterior

Unit 4 Muscle Group Movements

369

Plantarflexors of the Ankle/Foot

Flexor digitorum longus
Gastrocnemius
Peroneus brevis
Peroneus longus
Plantaris
Soleus
Tibialis posterior
Flexor hallucis longus

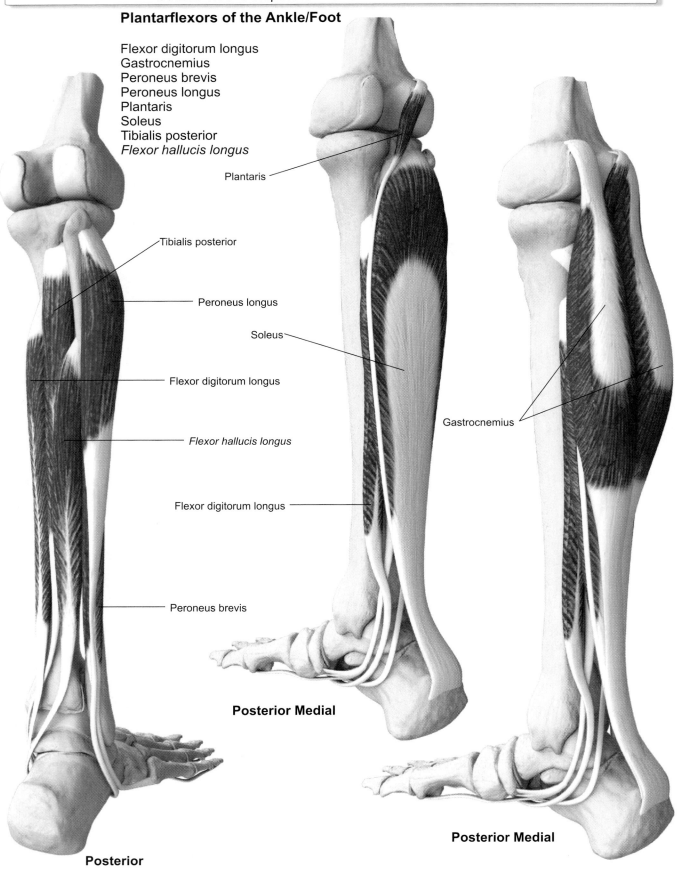

Plantaris

Tibialis posterior

Peroneus longus

Soleus

Flexor digitorum longus

Flexor hallucis longus

Flexor digitorum longus

Gastrocnemius

Peroneus brevis

Posterior Medial

Posterior

Posterior Medial

Unit 4 Muscle Group Movements

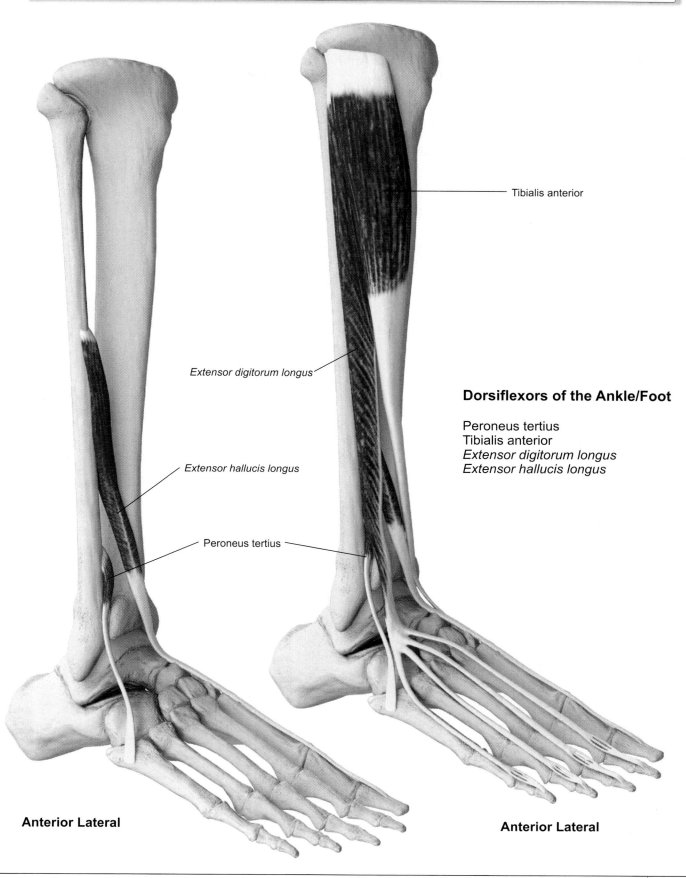

Tibialis anterior

Extensor digitorum longus

Extensor hallucis longus

Peroneus tertius

Dorsiflexors of the Ankle/Foot

Peroneus tertius
Tibialis anterior
Extensor digitorum longus
Extensor hallucis longus

Anterior Lateral

Anterior Lateral

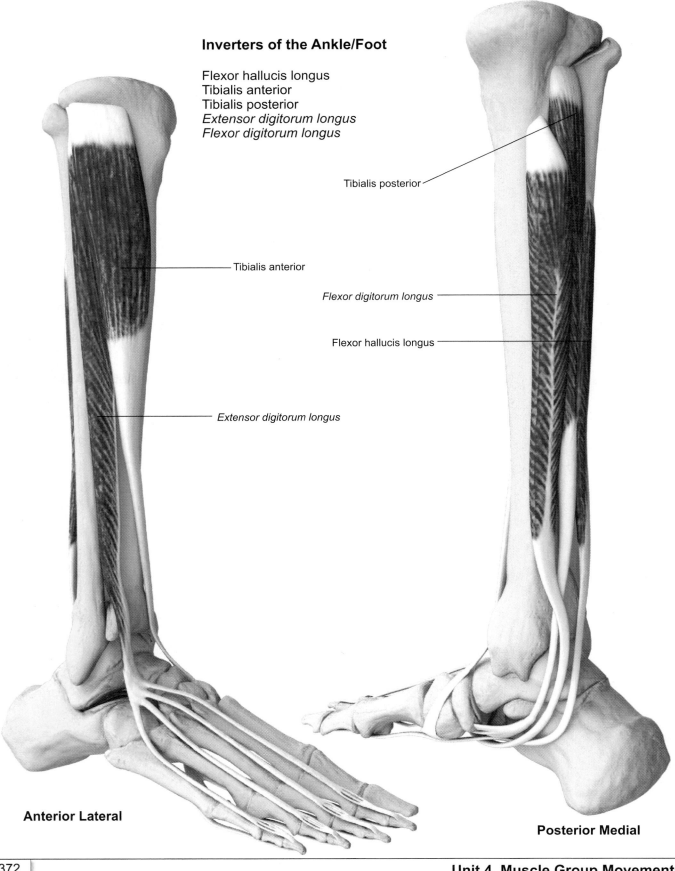

Inverters of the Ankle/Foot

Flexor hallucis longus
Tibialis anterior
Tibialis posterior
Extensor digitorum longus
Flexor digitorum longus

Tibialis posterior

Tibialis anterior

Flexor digitorum longus

Flexor hallucis longus

Extensor digitorum longus

Anterior Lateral

Posterior Medial

Unit 4 Muscle Group Movements

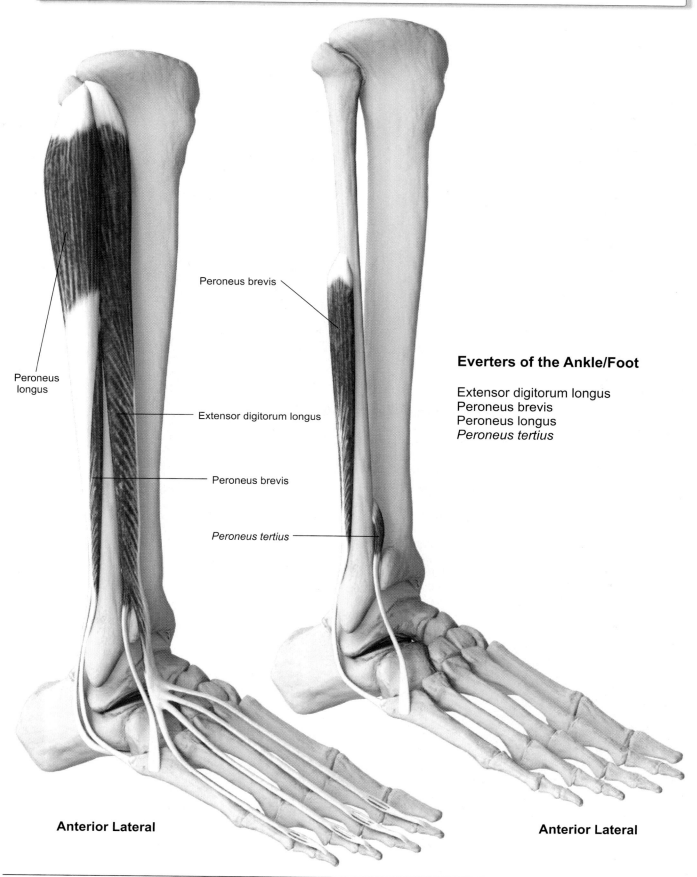

Peroneus brevis

Peroneus longus

Extensor digitorum longus

Peroneus brevis

Peroneus tertius

Everters of the Ankle/Foot

Extensor digitorum longus
Peroneus brevis
Peroneus longus
Peroneus tertius

Anterior Lateral

Anterior Lateral

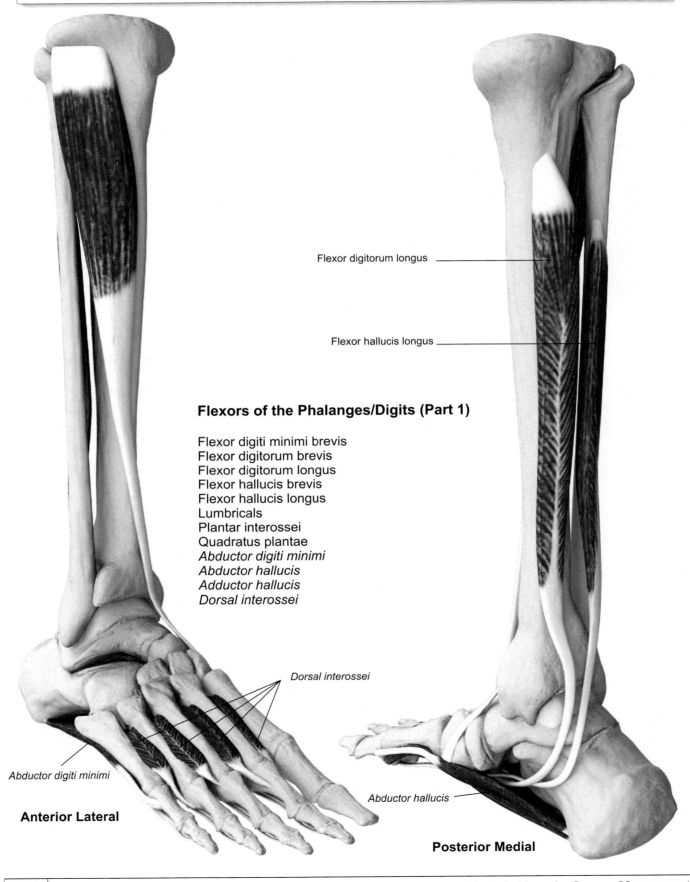

Flexor digitorum longus

Flexor hallucis longus

Flexors of the Phalanges/Digits (Part 1)

Flexor digiti minimi brevis
Flexor digitorum brevis
Flexor digitorum longus
Flexor hallucis brevis
Flexor hallucis longus
Lumbricals
Plantar interossei
Quadratus plantae
Abductor digiti minimi
Abductor hallucis
Adductor hallucis
Dorsal interossei

Dorsal interossei

Abductor digiti minimi

Anterior Lateral

Abductor hallucis

Posterior Medial

Unit 4 Muscle Group Movements

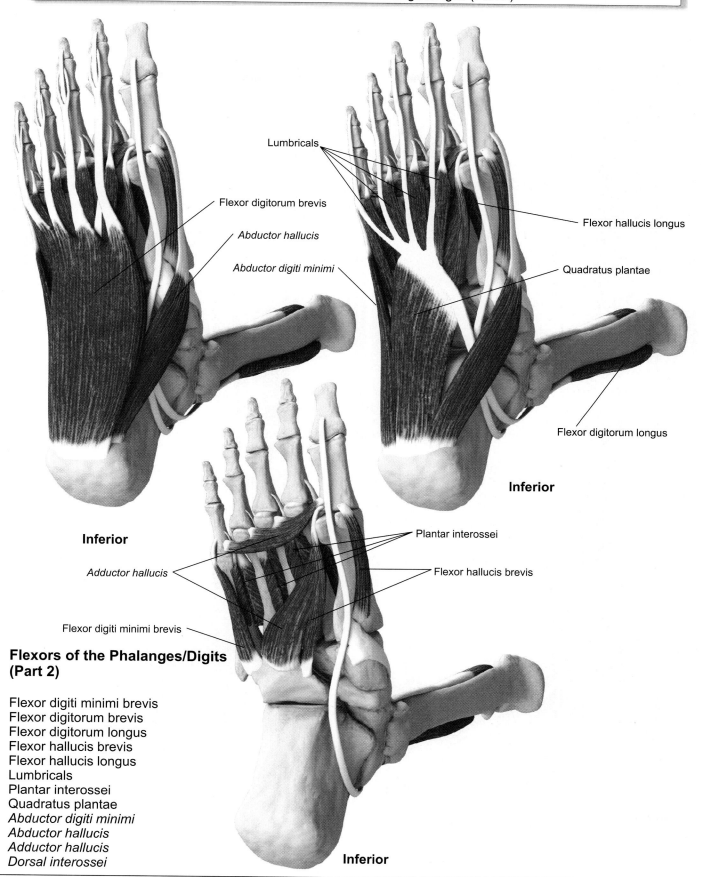

Lumbricals

Flexor digitorum brevis

Abductor hallucis

Abductor digiti minimi

Flexor hallucis longus

Quadratus plantae

Flexor digitorum longus

Inferior

Inferior

Plantar interossei

Adductor hallucis

Flexor hallucis brevis

Flexor digiti minimi brevis

Inferior

Flexors of the Phalanges/Digits (Part 2)

Flexor digiti minimi brevis
Flexor digitorum brevis
Flexor digitorum longus
Flexor hallucis brevis
Flexor hallucis longus
Lumbricals
Plantar interossei
Quadratus plantae
Abductor digiti minimi
Abductor hallucis
Adductor hallucis
Dorsal interossei

Unit 4 Muscle Group Movements

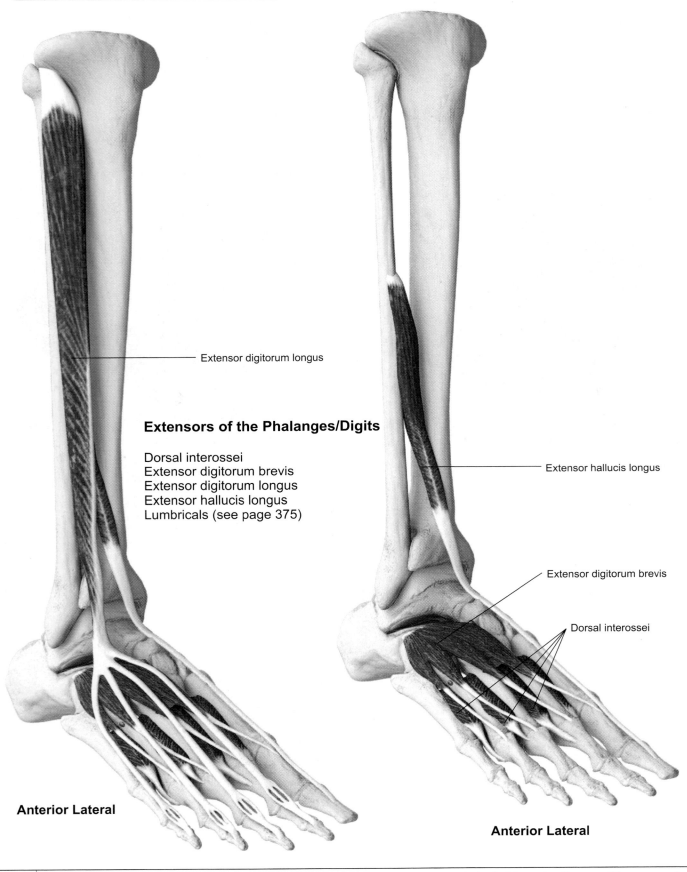

Extensor digitorum longus

Extensors of the Phalanges/Digits

Dorsal interossei
Extensor digitorum brevis
Extensor digitorum longus
Extensor hallucis longus
Lumbricals (see page 375)

Extensor hallucis longus

Extensor digitorum brevis

Dorsal interossei

Anterior Lateral

Anterior Lateral

Unit 4 Muscle Group Movements

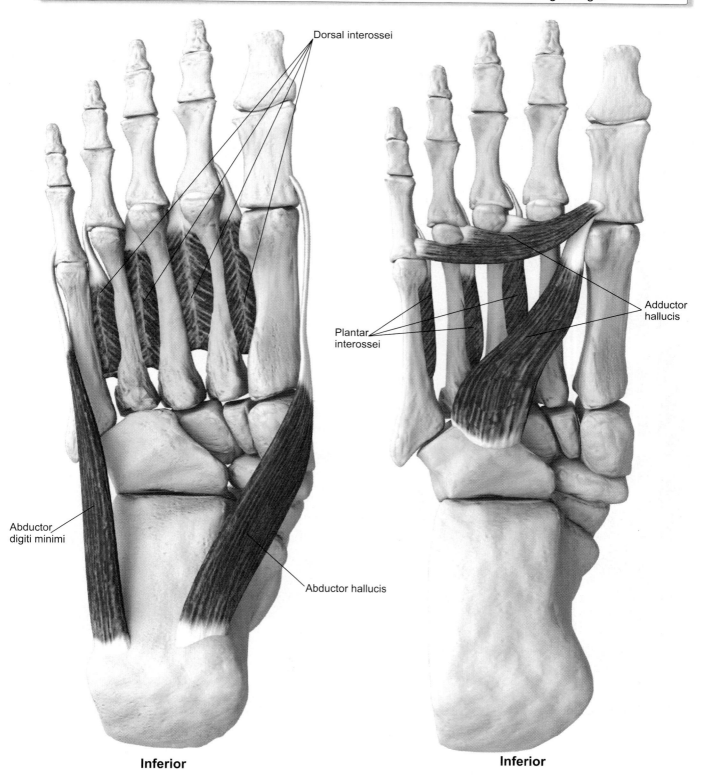

Dorsal interossei

Plantar interossei

Adductor hallucis

Abductor digiti minimi

Abductor hallucis

Inferior

Inferior

Abductors of the Phalanges/Digits

Abductor digiti minimi
Abductor hallucis
Dorsal interossei

Adductors of the Phalanges/Digits

Adductor hallucis
Plantar interossei

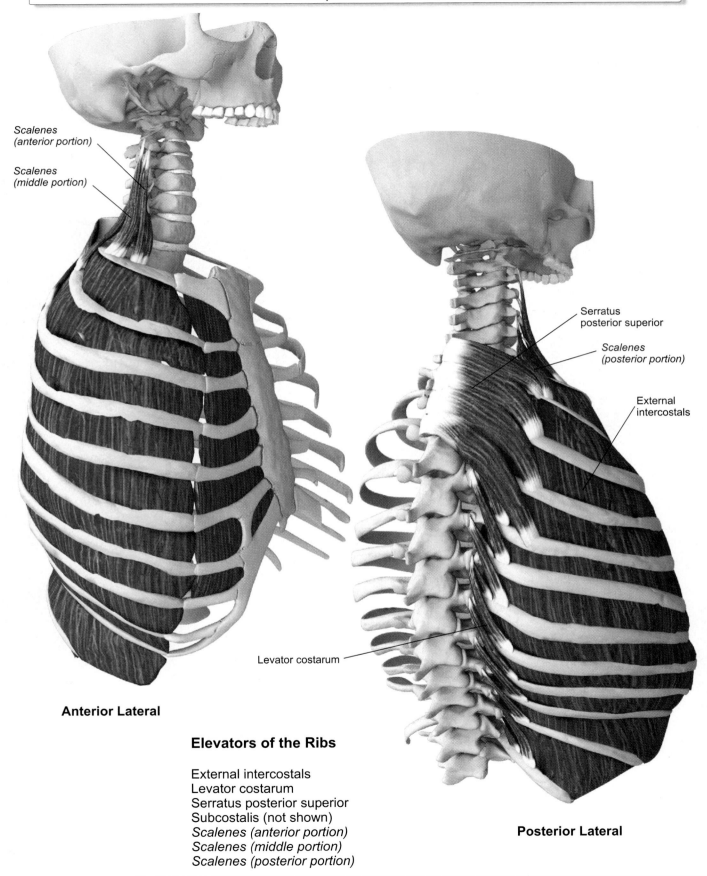

Scalenes (anterior portion)

Scalenes (middle portion)

Serratus posterior superior

Scalenes (posterior portion)

External intercostals

Levator costarum

Anterior Lateral

Posterior Lateral

Elevators of the Ribs

External intercostals
Levator costarum
Serratus posterior superior
Subcostalis (not shown)
Scalenes (anterior portion)
Scalenes (middle portion)
Scalenes (posterior portion)

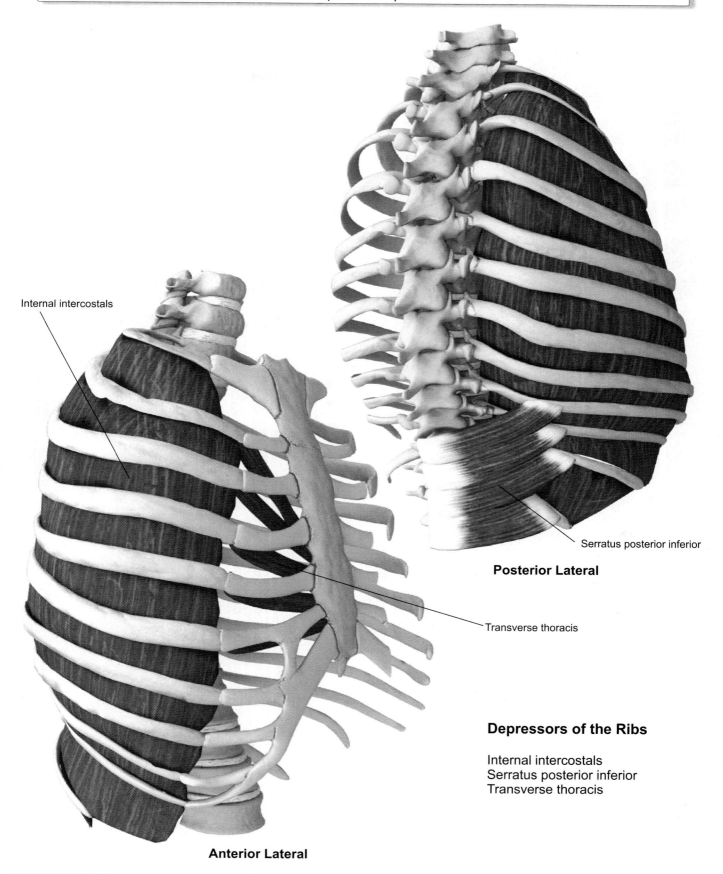

Internal intercostals

Serratus posterior inferior

Posterior Lateral

Transverse thoracis

Depressors of the Ribs

Internal intercostals
Serratus posterior inferior
Transverse thoracis

Anterior Lateral

Stabilizers of the Ribs

External intercostals
Quadratus lumborum

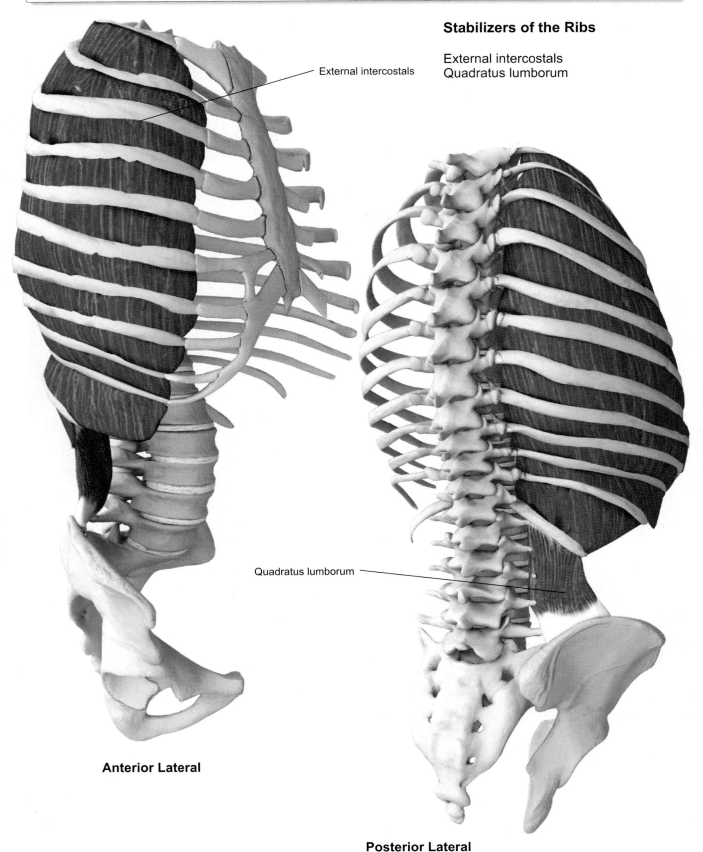

External intercostals

Quadratus lumborum

Anterior Lateral

Posterior Lateral

Unit 4 Muscle Group Movements

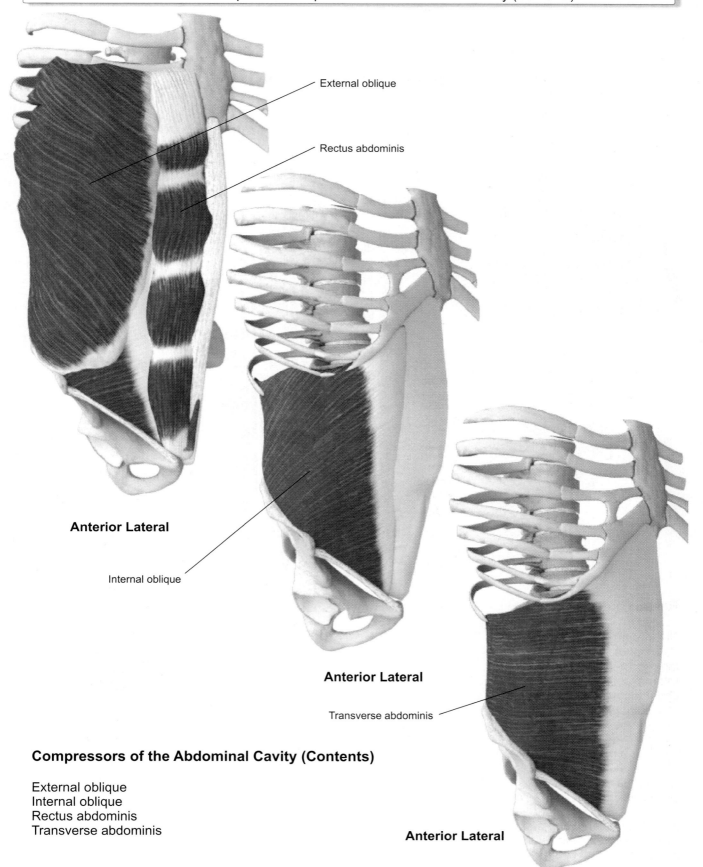

External oblique

Rectus abdominis

Anterior Lateral

Internal oblique

Anterior Lateral

Transverse abdominis

Anterior Lateral

Compressors of the Abdominal Cavity (Contents)

External oblique
Internal oblique
Rectus abdominis
Transverse abdominis

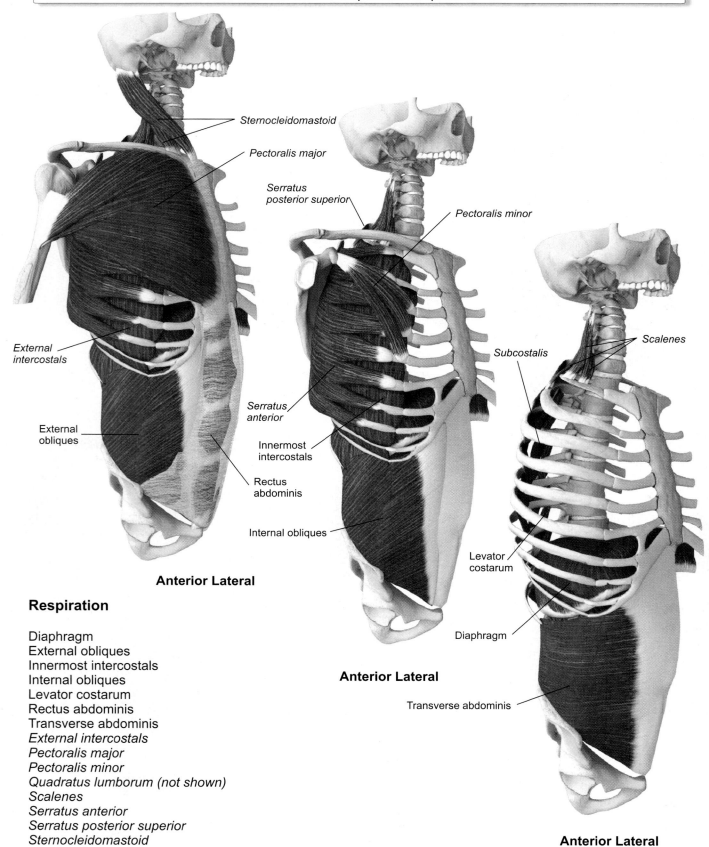

Sternocleidomastoid

Pectoralis major

Serratus
posterior superior

Pectoralis minor

External
intercostals

Scalenes

Subcostalis

External
obliques

Serratus
anterior

Innermost
intercostals

Rectus
abdominis

Internal obliques

Levator
costarum

Diaphragm

Anterior Lateral

Anterior Lateral

Transverse abdominis

Anterior Lateral

Respiration

Diaphragm
External obliques
Innermost intercostals
Internal obliques
Levator costarum
Rectus abdominis
Transverse abdominis
External intercostals
Pectoralis major
Pectoralis minor
Quadratus lumborum (not shown)
Scalenes
Serratus anterior
Serratus posterior superior
Sternocleidomastoid
Subcostalis

Unit 4 Muscle Group Movements

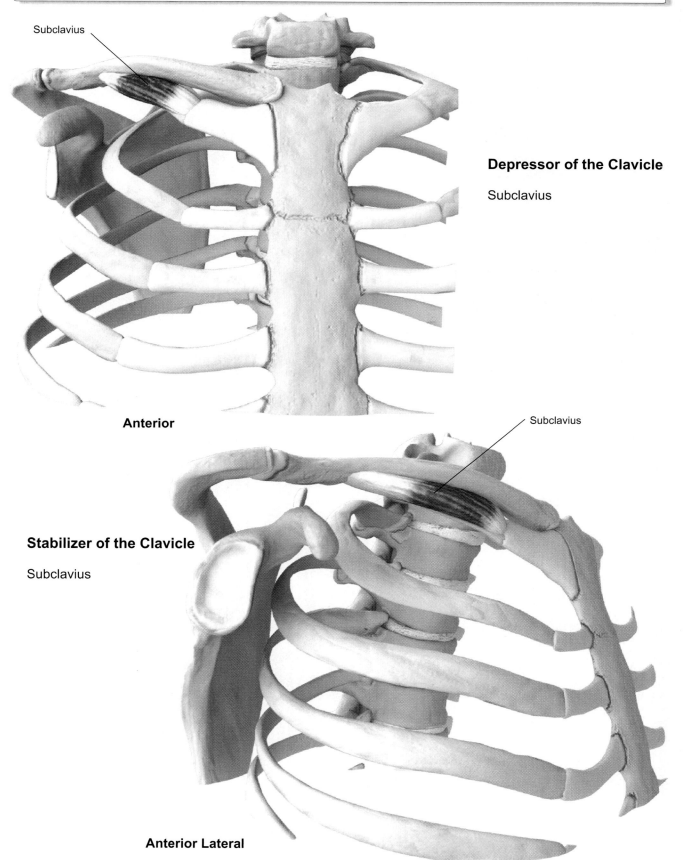

Subclavius

Depressor of the Clavicle

Subclavius

Anterior

Subclavius

Stabilizer of the Clavicle

Subclavius

Anterior Lateral

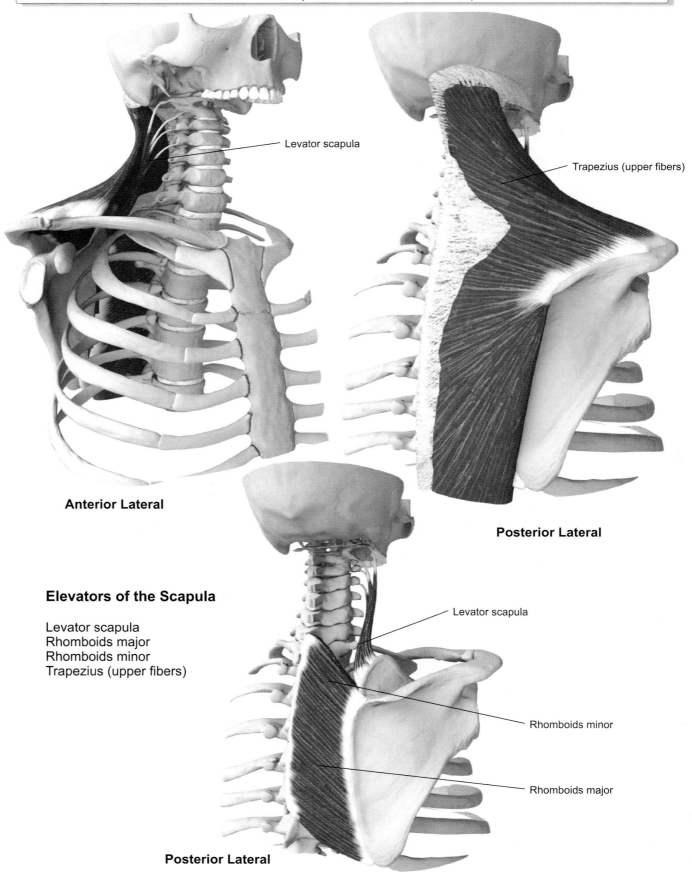

Levator scapula

Trapezius (upper fibers)

Anterior Lateral

Posterior Lateral

Elevators of the Scapula

Levator scapula
Rhomboids major
Rhomboids minor
Trapezius (upper fibers)

Levator scapula

Rhomboids minor

Rhomboids major

Posterior Lateral

Unit 4 Muscle Group Movements

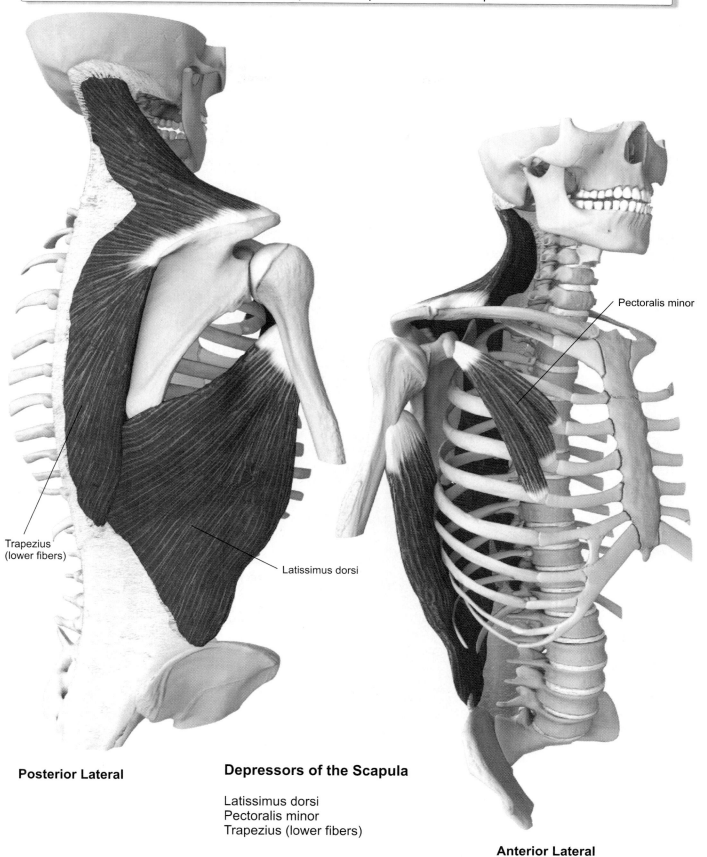

Trapezius
(lower fibers)

Latissimus dorsi

Pectoralis minor

Posterior Lateral

Depressors of the Scapula

Latissimus dorsi
Pectoralis minor
Trapezius (lower fibers)

Anterior Lateral

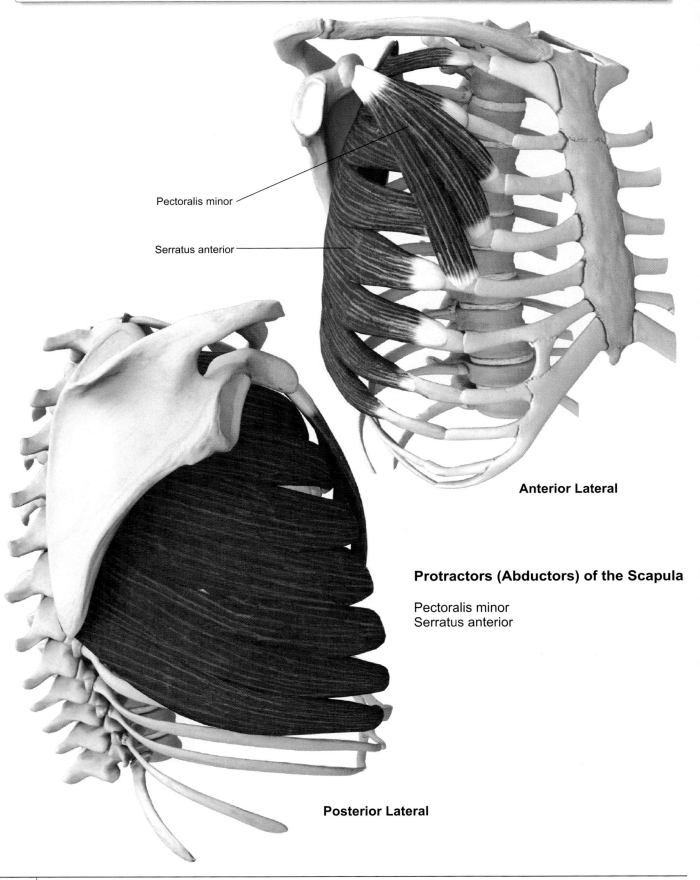

Pectoralis minor

Serratus anterior

Anterior Lateral

Protractors (Abductors) of the Scapula

Pectoralis minor
Serratus anterior

Posterior Lateral

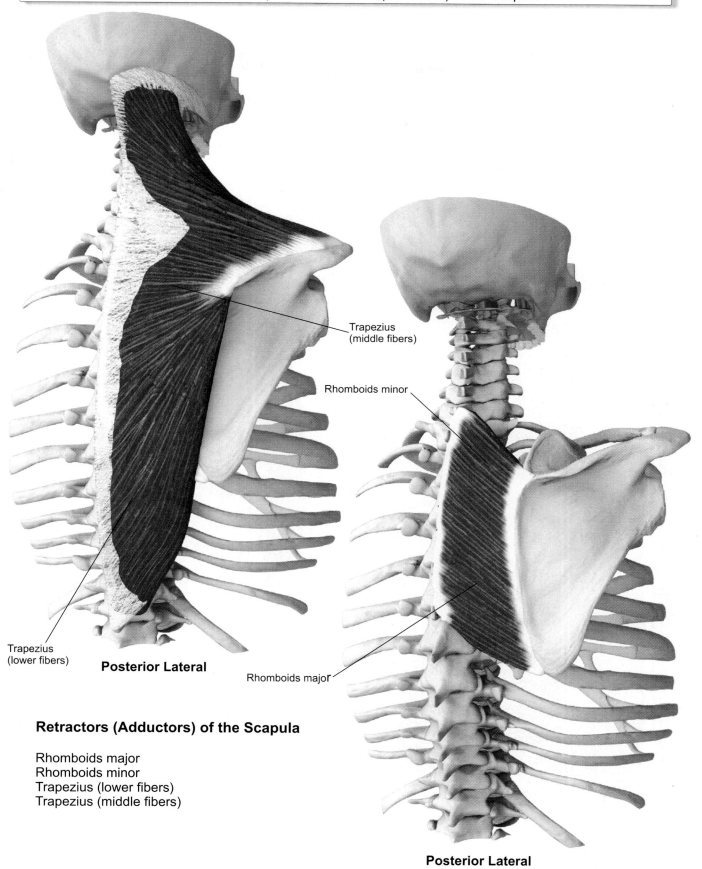

Trapezius
(middle fibers)

Rhomboids minor

Rhomboids major

Trapezius
(lower fibers)

Posterior Lateral

Posterior Lateral

Retractors (Adductors) of the Scapula

Rhomboids major
Rhomboids minor
Trapezius (lower fibers)
Trapezius (middle fibers)

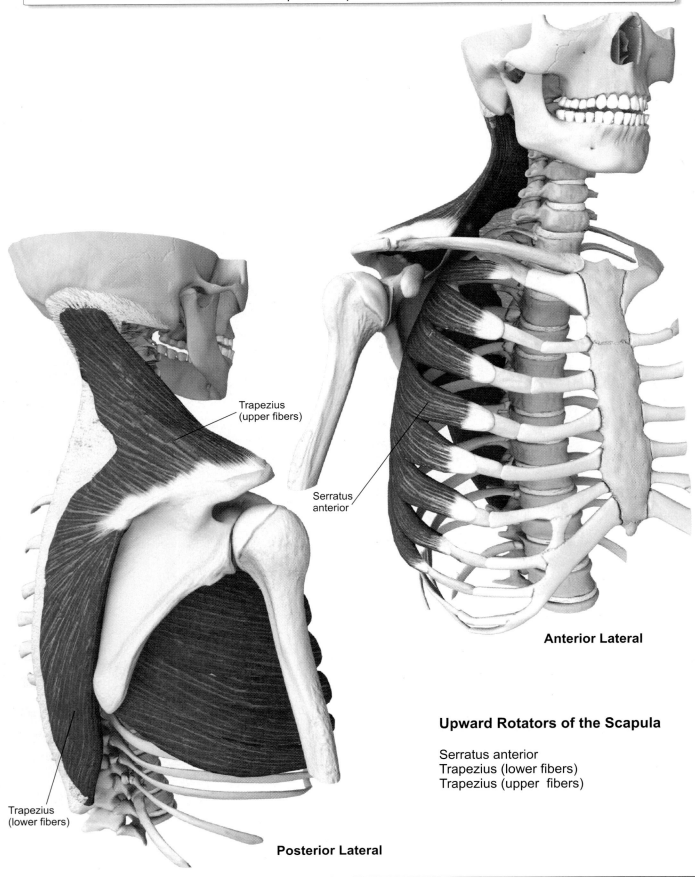

Trapezius
(upper fibers)

Serratus
anterior

Trapezius
(lower fibers)

Posterior Lateral

Anterior Lateral

Upward Rotators of the Scapula

Serratus anterior
Trapezius (lower fibers)
Trapezius (upper fibers)

Unit 4 Muscle Group Movements

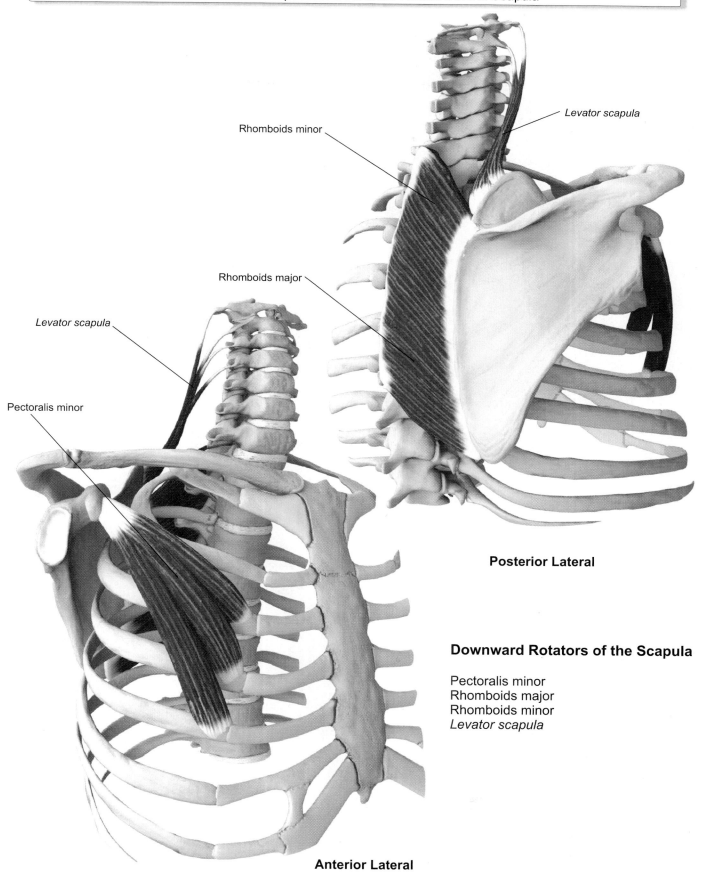

Rhomboids minor

Levator scapula

Rhomboids major

Levator scapula

Pectoralis minor

Posterior Lateral

Downward Rotators of the Scapula

Pectoralis minor
Rhomboids major
Rhomboids minor
Levator scapula

Anterior Lateral

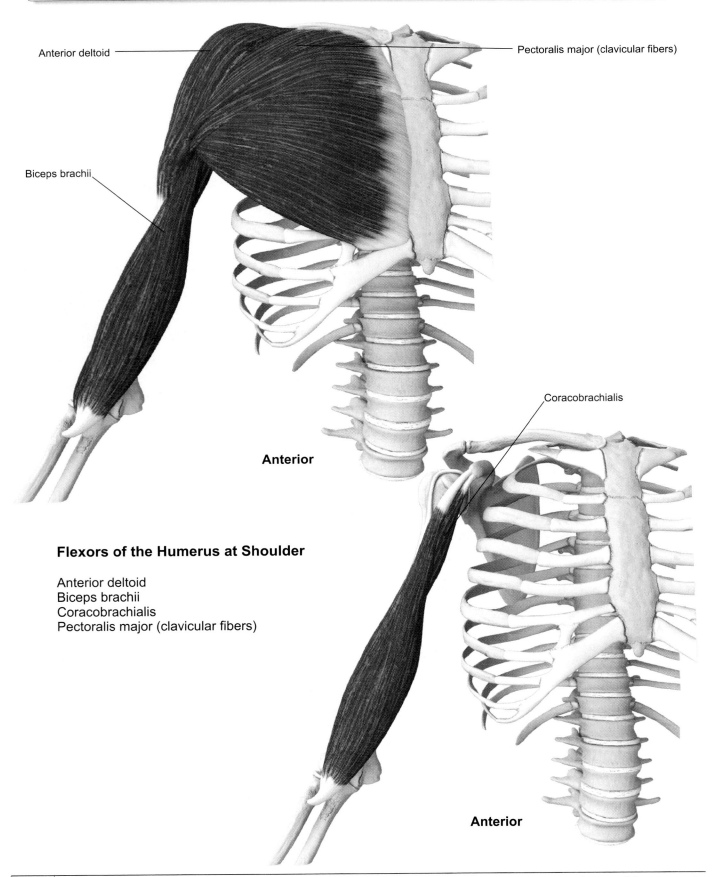

Anterior deltoid

Pectoralis major (clavicular fibers)

Biceps brachii

Anterior

Coracobrachialis

Anterior

Flexors of the Humerus at Shoulder

Anterior deltoid
Biceps brachii
Coracobrachialis
Pectoralis major (clavicular fibers)

Unit 4 Muscle Group Movements

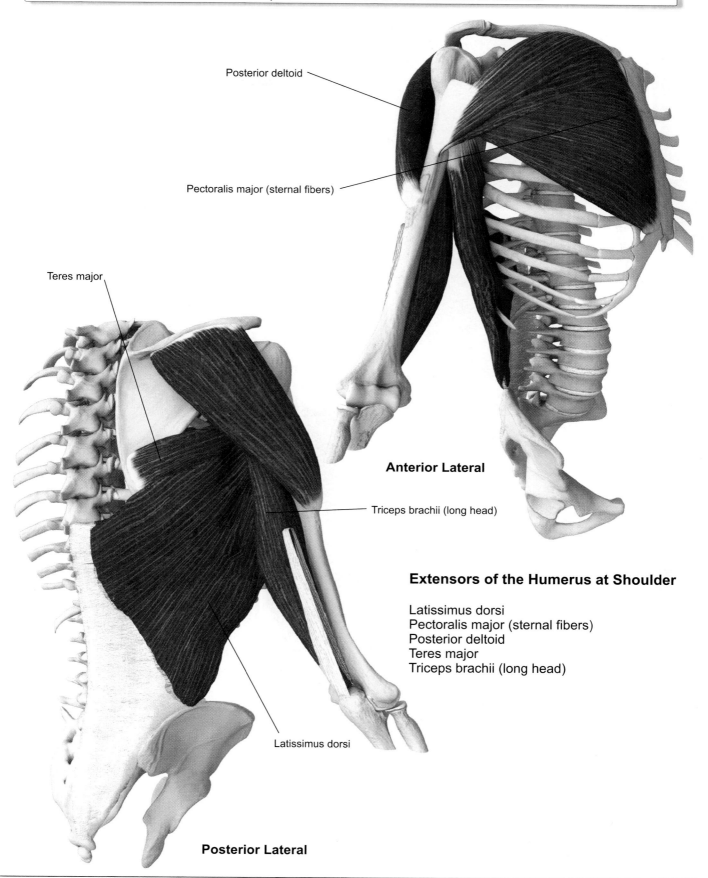

Posterior deltoid

Pectoralis major (sternal fibers)

Teres major

Anterior Lateral

Triceps brachii (long head)

Extensors of the Humerus at Shoulder

Latissimus dorsi
Pectoralis major (sternal fibers)
Posterior deltoid
Teres major
Triceps brachii (long head)

Latissimus dorsi

Posterior Lateral

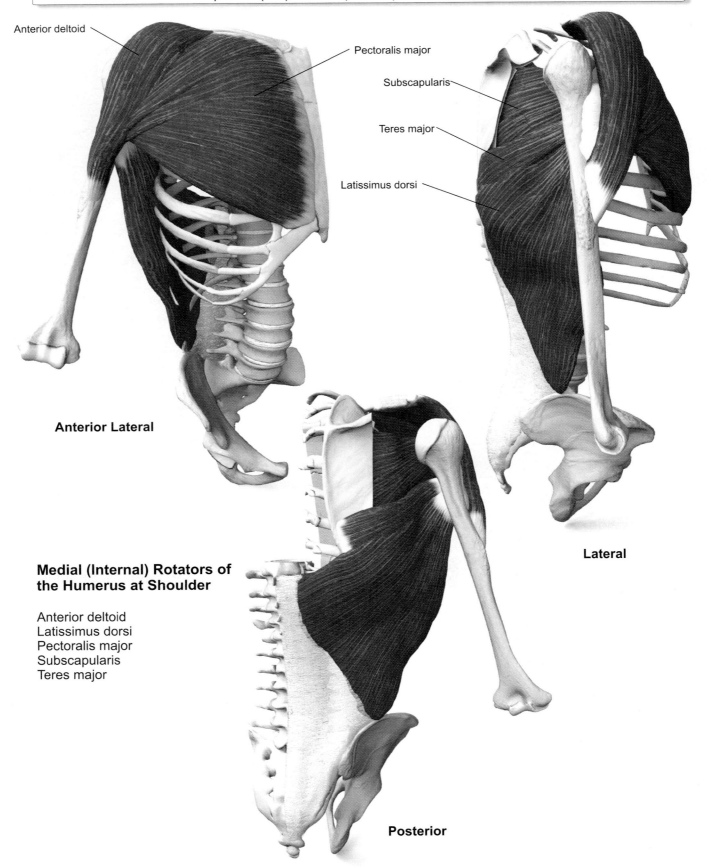

Anterior deltoid

Pectoralis major

Subscapularis

Teres major

Latissimus dorsi

Anterior Lateral

Lateral

Medial (Internal) Rotators of the Humerus at Shoulder

Anterior deltoid
Latissimus dorsi
Pectoralis major
Subscapularis
Teres major

Posterior

Unit 4 Muscle Group Movements

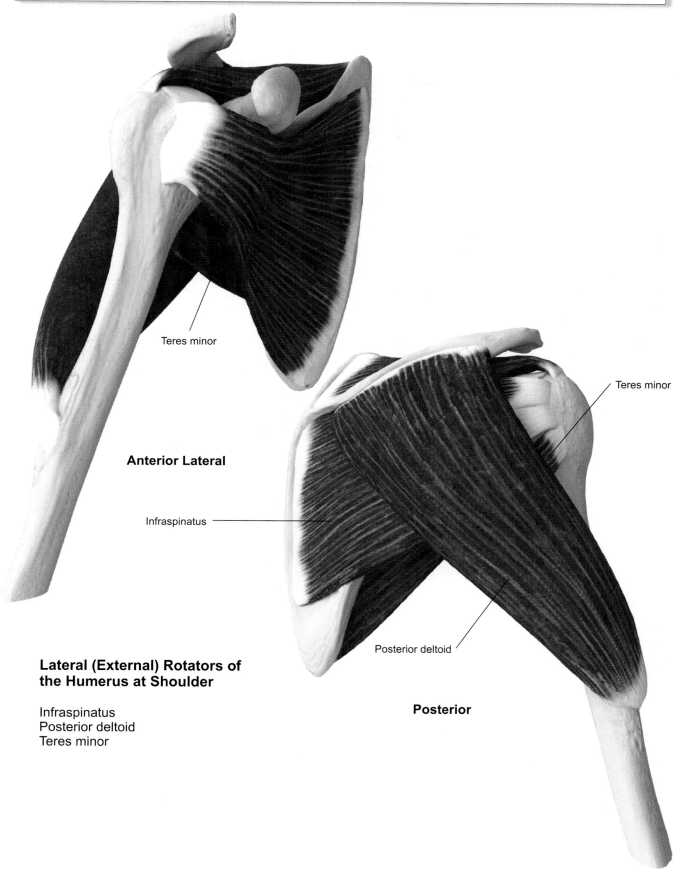

Teres minor

Anterior Lateral

Teres minor

Infraspinatus

Lateral (External) Rotators of the Humerus at Shoulder

Infraspinatus
Posterior deltoid
Teres minor

Posterior deltoid

Posterior

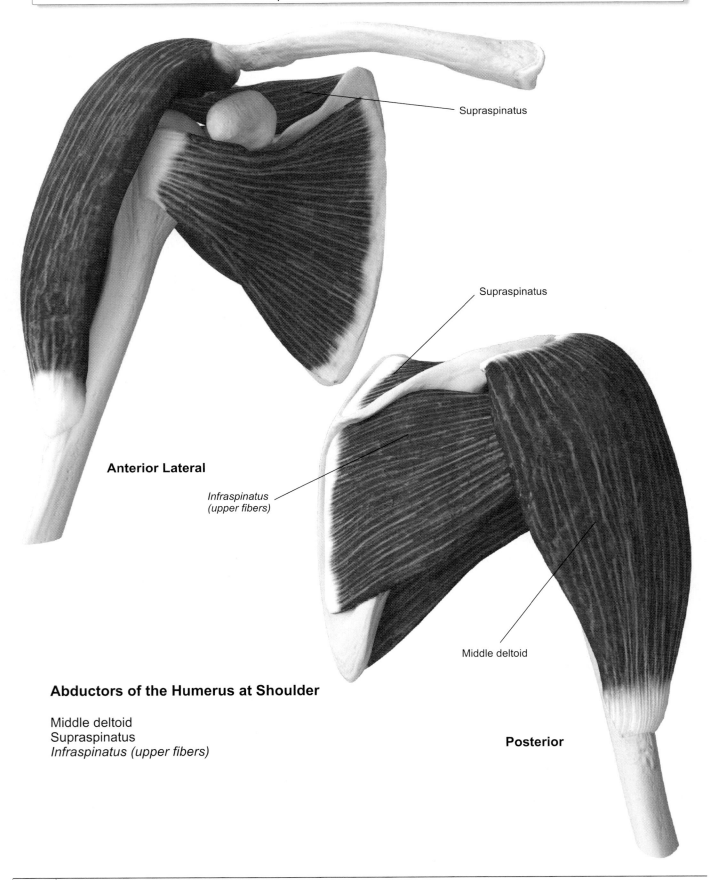

Supraspinatus

Supraspinatus

Anterior Lateral

Infraspinatus (upper fibers)

Middle deltoid

Posterior

Abductors of the Humerus at Shoulder

Middle deltoid
Supraspinatus
Infraspinatus (upper fibers)

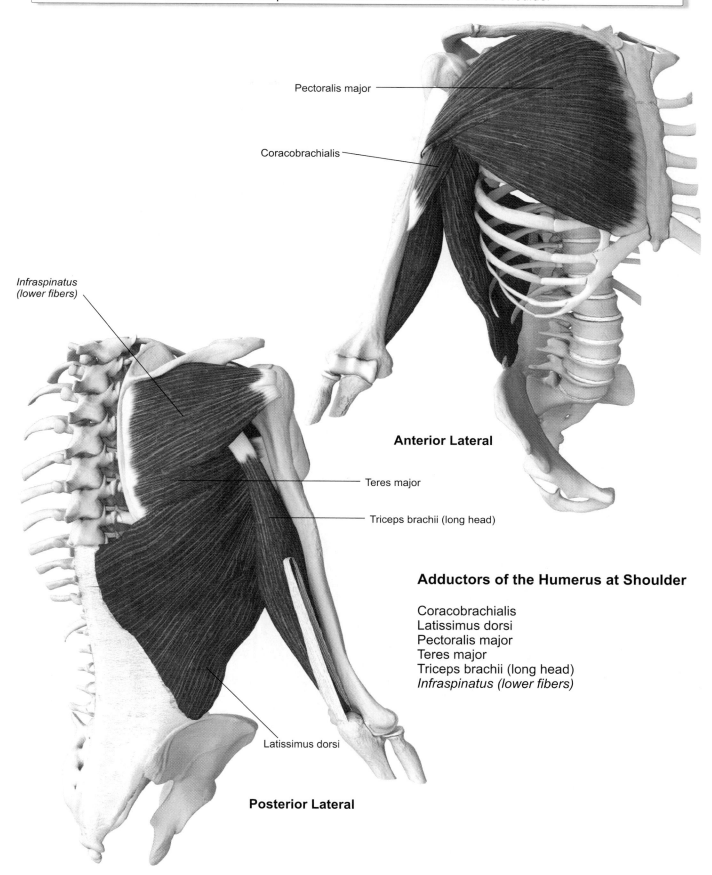

Pectoralis major

Coracobrachialis

Anterior Lateral

Infraspinatus (lower fibers)

Teres major

Triceps brachii (long head)

Latissimus dorsi

Posterior Lateral

Adductors of the Humerus at Shoulder

Coracobrachialis
Latissimus dorsi
Pectoralis major
Teres major
Triceps brachii (long head)
Infraspinatus (lower fibers)

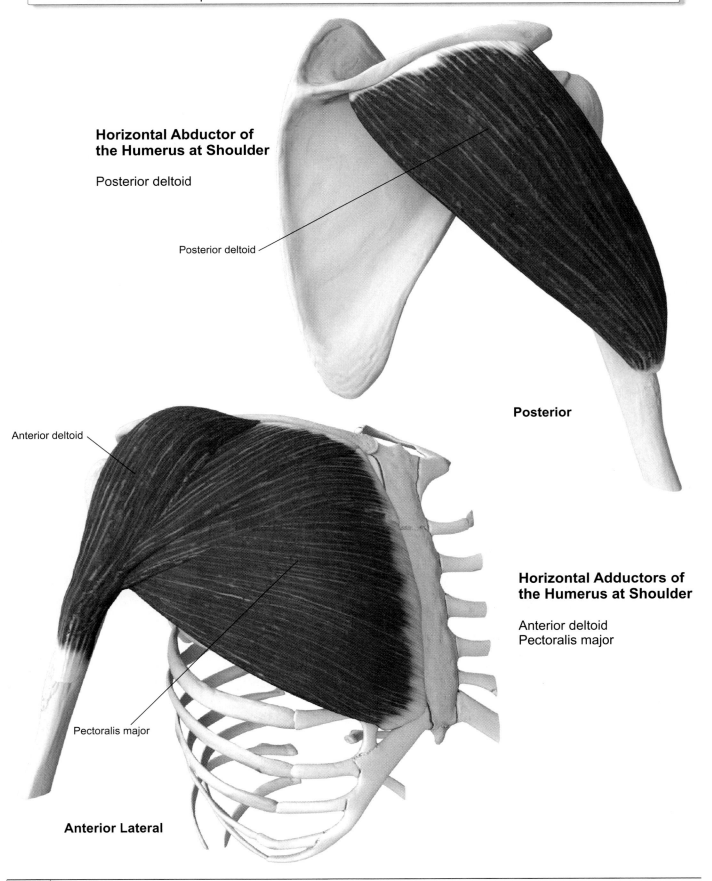

Horizontal Abductor of the Humerus at Shoulder

Posterior deltoid

Posterior deltoid

Posterior

Anterior deltoid

Horizontal Adductors of the Humerus at Shoulder

Anterior deltoid
Pectoralis major

Pectoralis major

Anterior Lateral

Unit 4 Muscle Group Movements

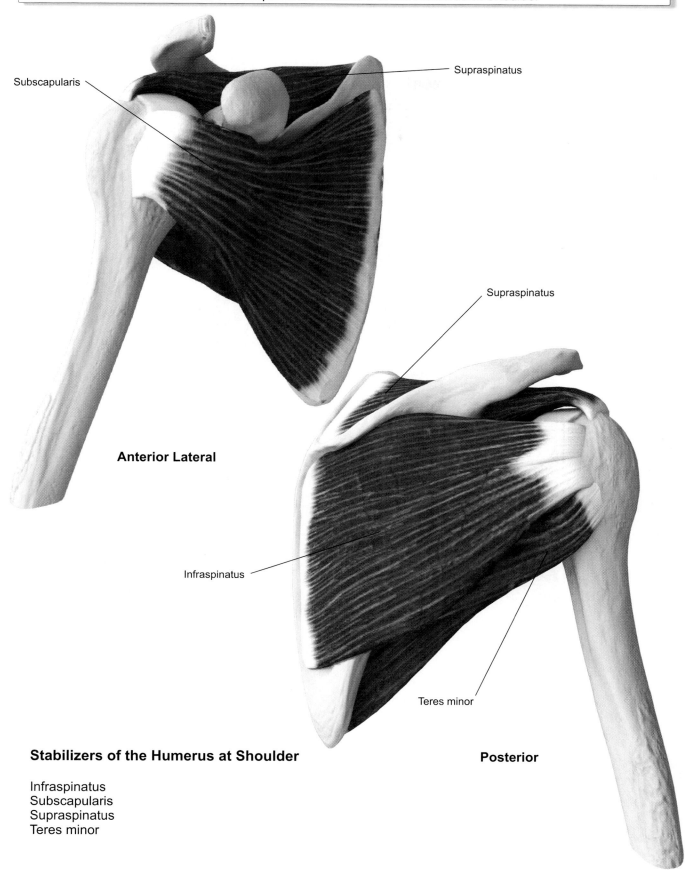

Subscapularis

Supraspinatus

Supraspinatus

Anterior Lateral

Infraspinatus

Teres minor

Stabilizers of the Humerus at Shoulder

Posterior

Infraspinatus
Subscapularis
Supraspinatus
Teres minor

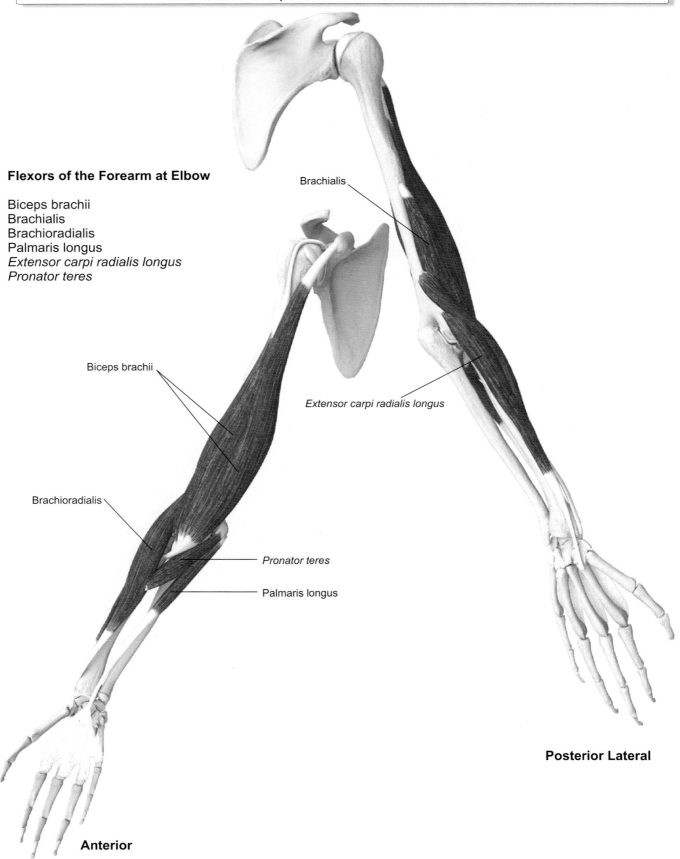

Flexors of the Forearm at Elbow

Biceps brachii
Brachialis
Brachioradialis
Palmaris longus
Extensor carpi radialis longus
Pronator teres

Brachialis

Biceps brachii

Extensor carpi radialis longus

Brachioradialis

Pronator teres

Palmaris longus

Posterior Lateral

Anterior

Unit 4 Muscle Group Movements

Extensors of the Forearm at Elbow

Anconeus
Triceps brachii

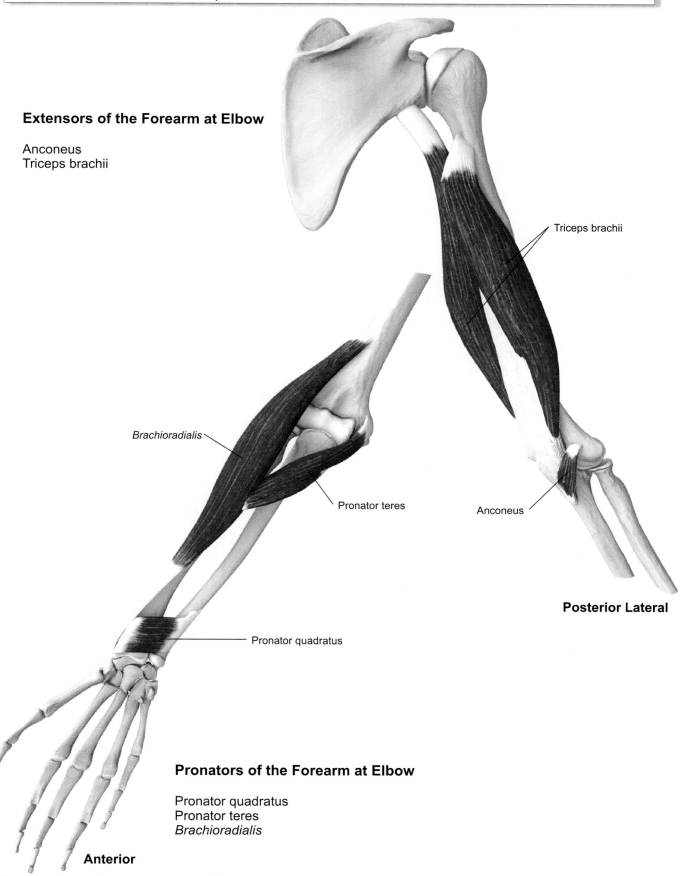

Triceps brachii

Brachioradialis

Pronator teres

Anconeus

Posterior Lateral

Pronator quadratus

Pronators of the Forearm at Elbow

Pronator quadratus
Pronator teres
Brachioradialis

Anterior

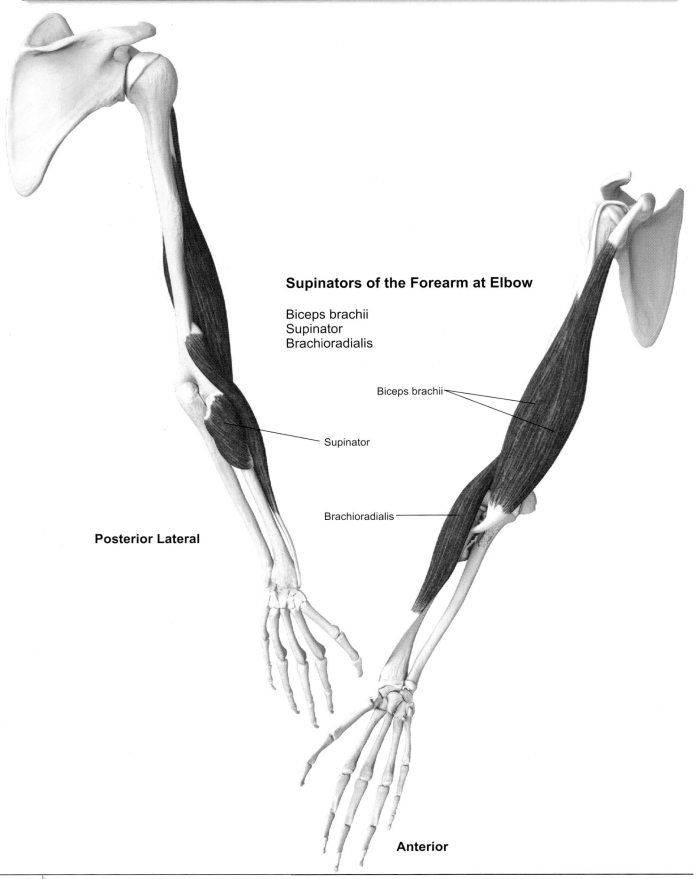

Supinators of the Forearm at Elbow

Biceps brachii
Supinator
Brachioradialis

Biceps brachii

Supinator

Brachioradialis

Posterior Lateral

Anterior

Unit 4 Muscle Group Movements

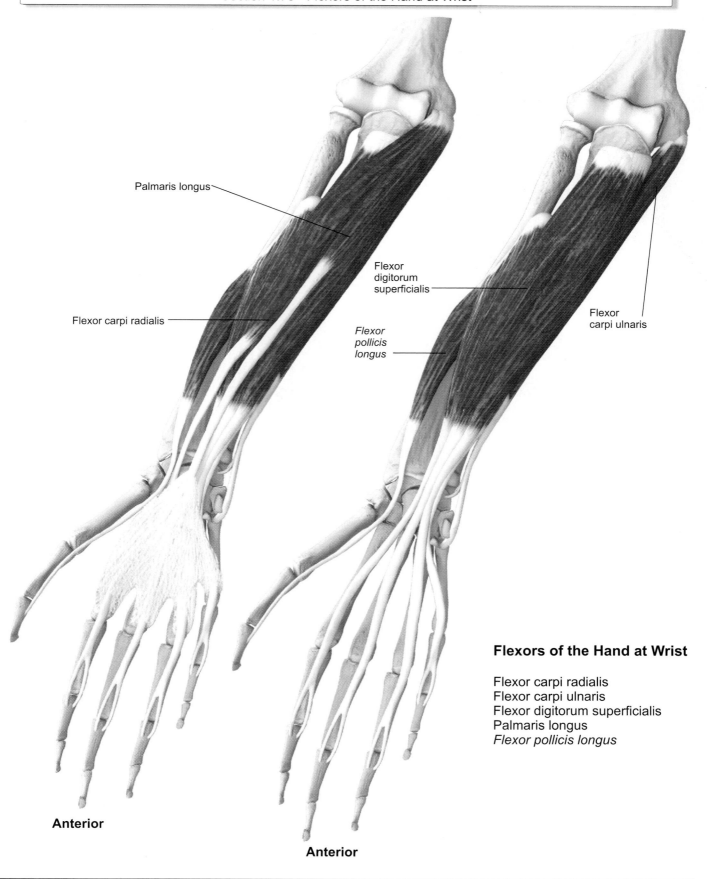

Palmaris longus

Flexor digitorum superficialis

Flexor carpi radialis

Flexor pollicis longus

Flexor carpi ulnaris

Anterior

Anterior

Flexors of the Hand at Wrist

Flexor carpi radialis
Flexor carpi ulnaris
Flexor digitorum superficialis
Palmaris longus
Flexor pollicis longus

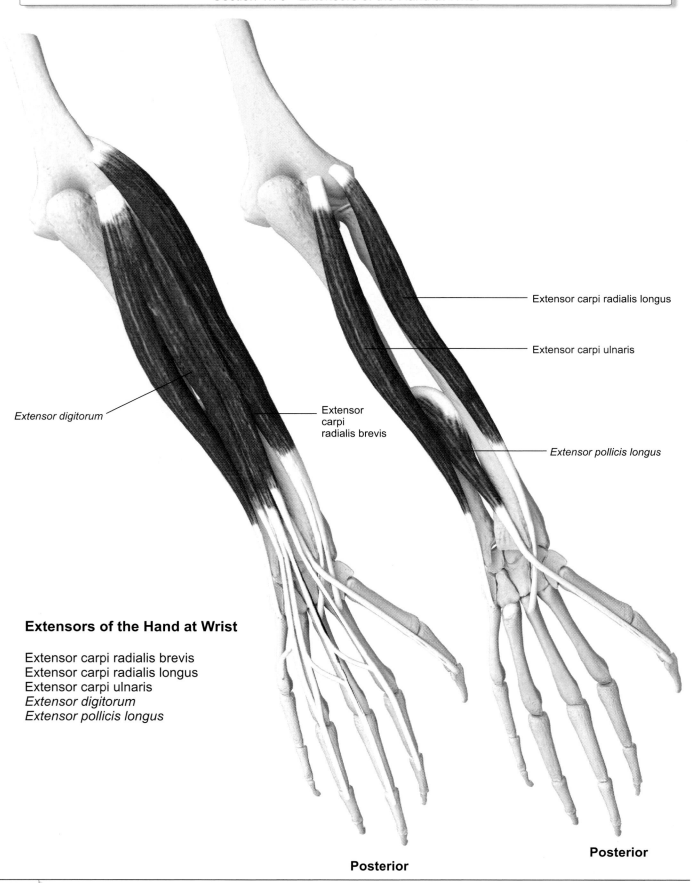

Extensor carpi radialis longus

Extensor carpi ulnaris

Extensor digitorum

Extensor carpi radialis brevis

Extensor pollicis longus

Extensors of the Hand at Wrist

Extensor carpi radialis brevis
Extensor carpi radialis longus
Extensor carpi ulnaris
Extensor digitorum
Extensor pollicis longus

Posterior

Posterior

Unit 4 Muscle Group Movements

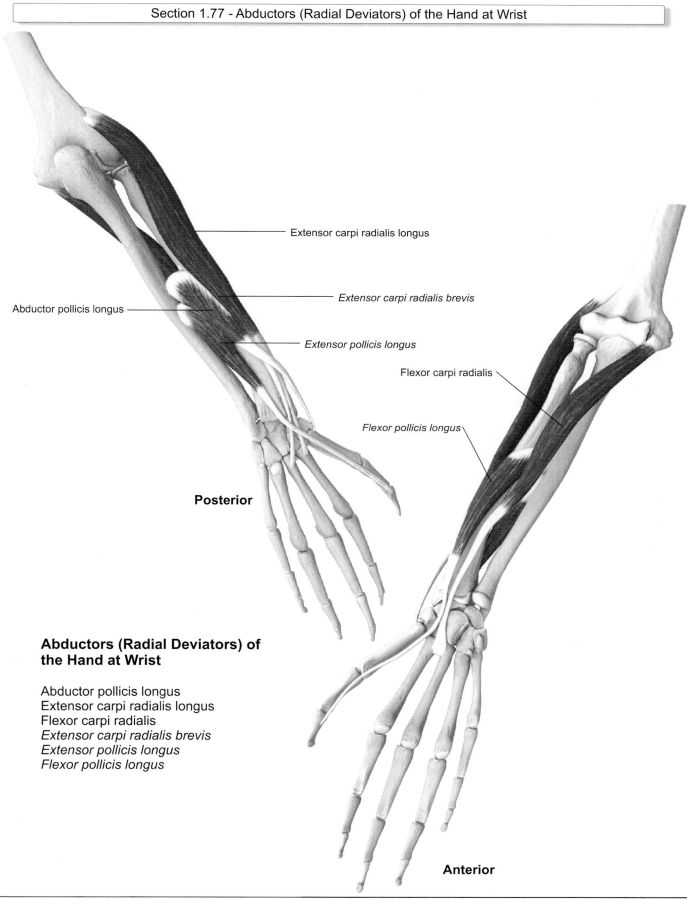

Extensor carpi radialis longus

Extensor carpi radialis brevis

Abductor pollicis longus

Extensor pollicis longus

Flexor carpi radialis

Flexor pollicis longus

Posterior

Anterior

Abductors (Radial Deviators) of the Hand at Wrist

Abductor pollicis longus
Extensor carpi radialis longus
Flexor carpi radialis
Extensor carpi radialis brevis
Extensor pollicis longus
Flexor pollicis longus

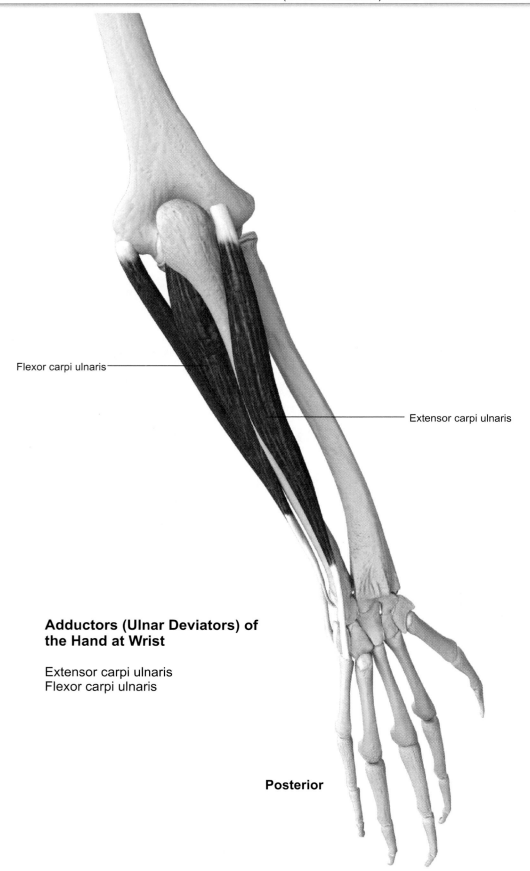

Flexor carpi ulnaris

Extensor carpi ulnaris

**Adductors (Ulnar Deviators) of
the Hand at Wrist**

Extensor carpi ulnaris
Flexor carpi ulnaris

Posterior

Flexors of the Thumb and/or Digits

Flexor digiti minimi
Flexor digitorum profundus
Flexor digitorum superficialis
Flexor pollicis brevis
Flexor pollicis longus
Lumbricals
Adductor pollicis
Dorsal interossei
Palmar interossei

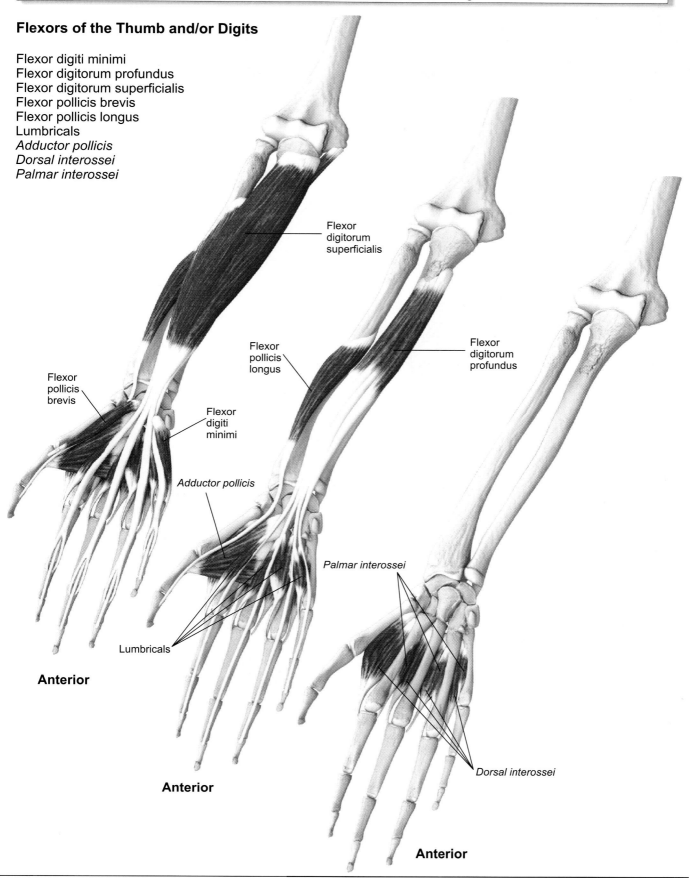

Flexor
digitorum
superficialis

Flexor
pollicis
longus

Flexor
digitorum
profundus

Flexor
pollicis
brevis

Flexor
digiti
minimi

Adductor pollicis

Palmar interossei

Lumbricals

Anterior

Anterior

Dorsal interossei

Anterior

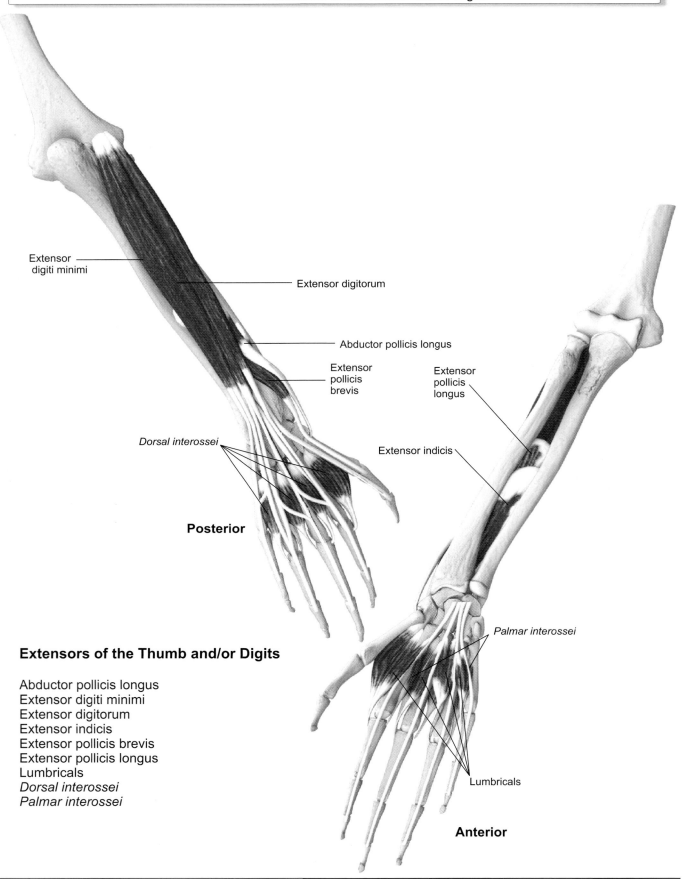

Extensor digiti minimi

Extensor digitorum

Abductor pollicis longus

Extensor pollicis brevis

Dorsal interossei

Posterior

Extensor pollicis longus

Extensor indicis

Palmar interossei

Lumbricals

Anterior

Extensors of the Thumb and/or Digits

Abductor pollicis longus
Extensor digiti minimi
Extensor digitorum
Extensor indicis
Extensor pollicis brevis
Extensor pollicis longus
Lumbricals
Dorsal interossei
Palmar interossei

Unit 4 Muscle Group Movements

Adductors of the Thumb and/or Digits

Adductor pollicis
Palmar interossei
Dorsal interossei

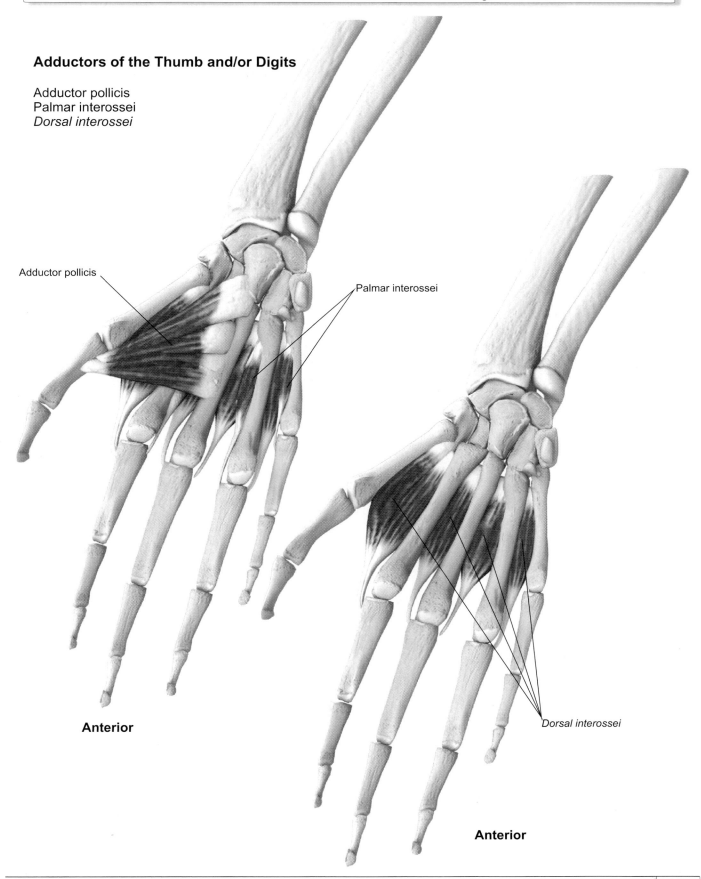

Adductor pollicis

Palmar interossei

Dorsal interossei

Anterior

Anterior

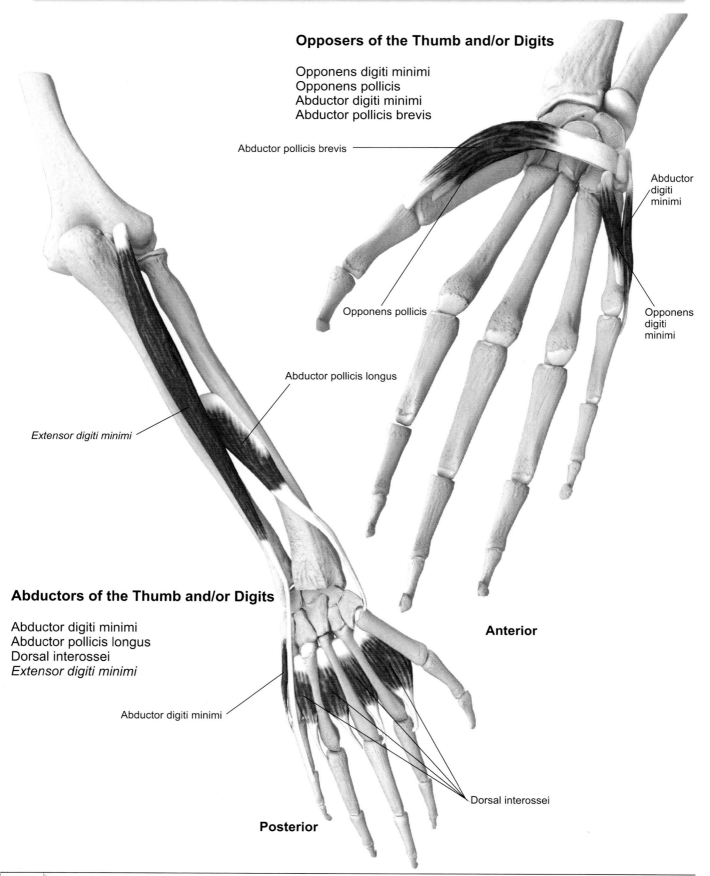

Opposers of the Thumb and/or Digits

Opponens digiti minimi
Opponens pollicis
Abductor digiti minimi
Abductor pollicis brevis

Abductor pollicis brevis

Abductor digiti minimi

Opponens pollicis

Opponens digiti minimi

Abductor pollicis longus

Extensor digiti minimi

Anterior

Abductors of the Thumb and/or Digits

Abductor digiti minimi
Abductor pollicis longus
Dorsal interossei
Extensor digiti minimi

Abductor digiti minimi

Dorsal interossei

Posterior

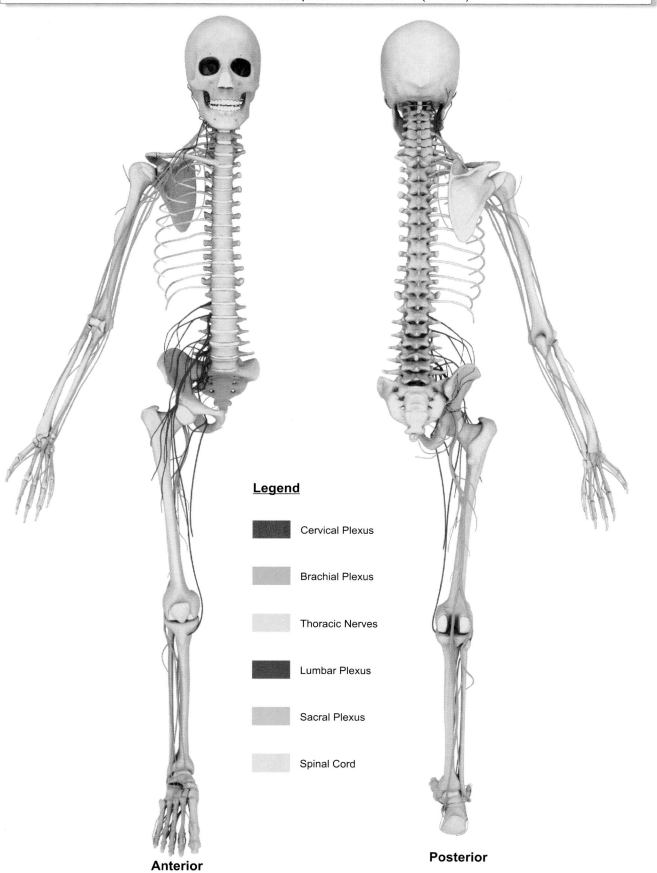

Legend

Cervical Plexus

Brachial Plexus

Thoracic Nerves

Lumbar Plexus

Sacral Plexus

Spinal Cord

Anterior

Posterior

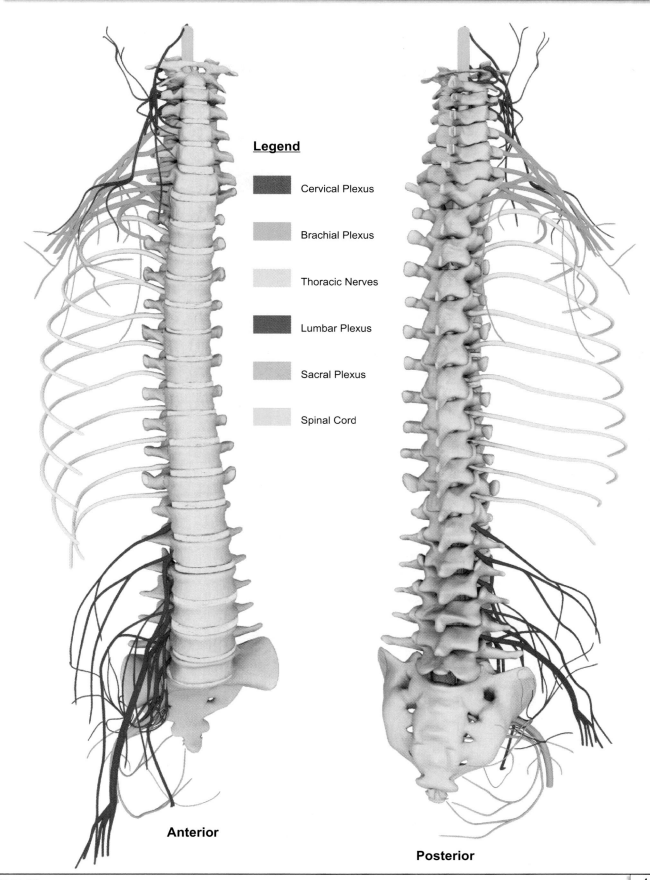

Legend

Cervical Plexus

Brachial Plexus

Thoracic Nerves

Lumbar Plexus

Sacral Plexus

Spinal Cord

Anterior

Posterior

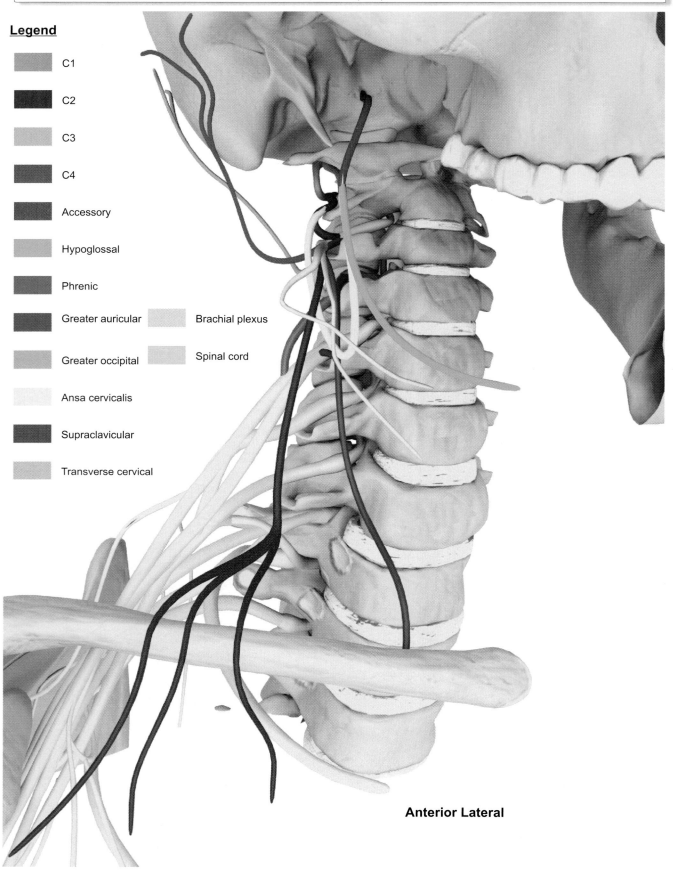

Legend

- C1
- C2
- C3
- C4
- Accessory
- Hypoglossal
- Phrenic
- Greater auricular
- Greater occipital
- Ansa cervicalis
- Supraclavicular
- Transverse cervical
- Brachial plexus
- Spinal cord

Anterior Lateral

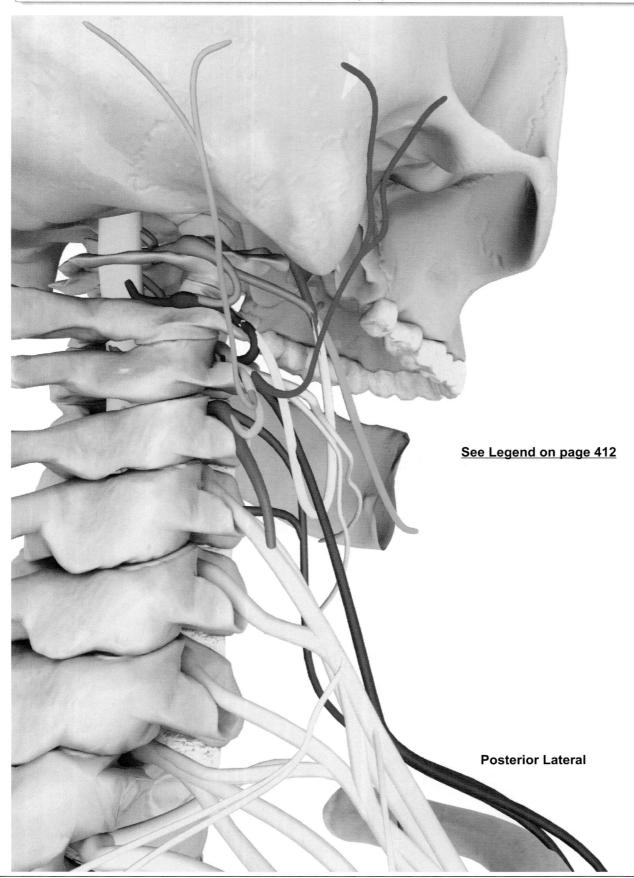

See Legend on page 412

Posterior Lateral

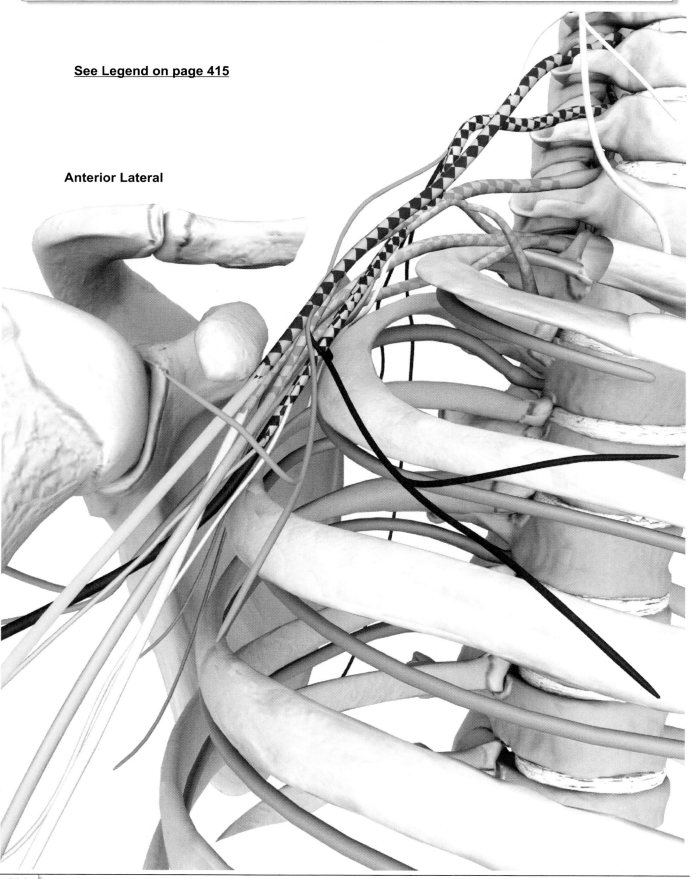

See Legend on page 415

Anterior Lateral

Unit 5 Nerves

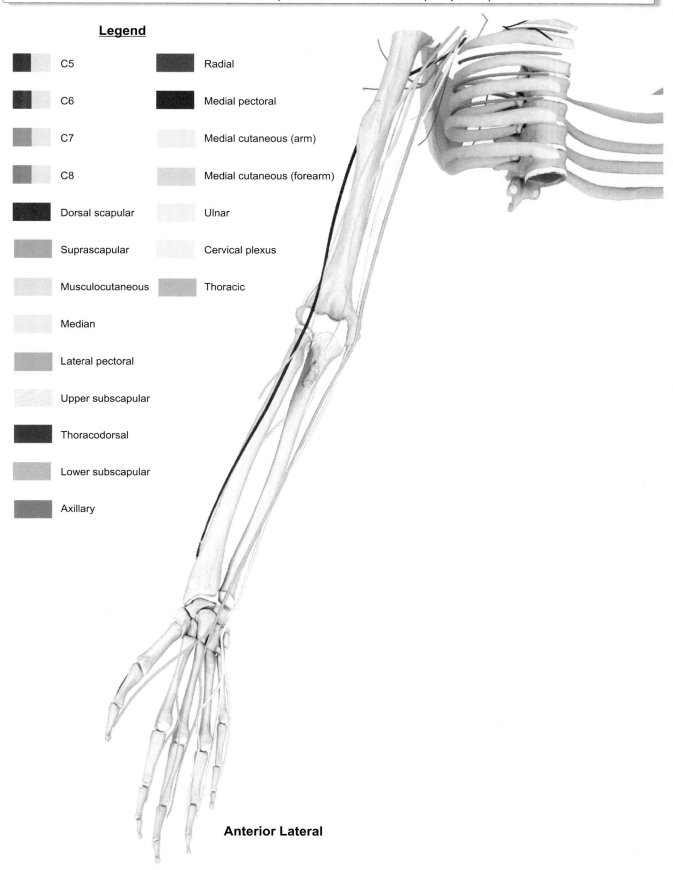

Legend

C5	Radial
C6	Medial pectoral
C7	Medial cutaneous (arm)
C8	Medial cutaneous (forearm)
Dorsal scapular	Ulnar
Suprascapular	Cervical plexus
Musculocutaneous	Thoracic
Median	
Lateral pectoral	
Upper subscapular	
Thoracodorsal	
Lower subscapular	
Axillary	

Anterior Lateral

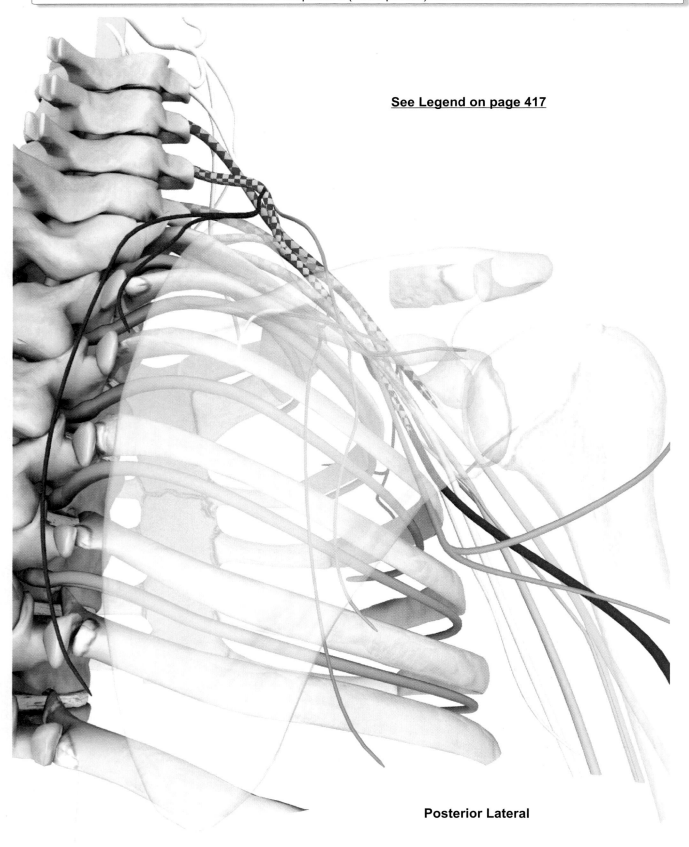

See Legend on page 417

Posterior Lateral

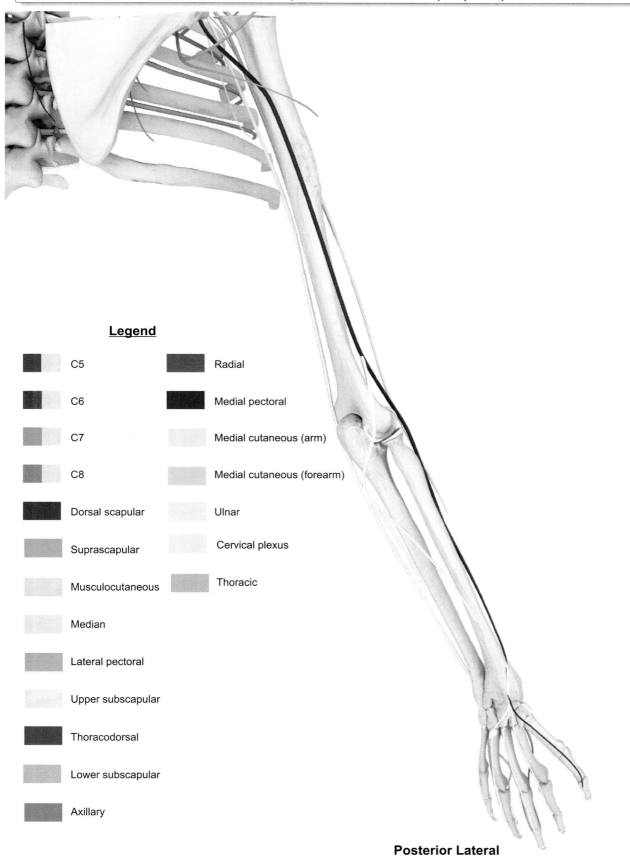

Legend

C5	Radial
C6	Medial pectoral
C7	Medial cutaneous (arm)
C8	Medial cutaneous (forearm)
Dorsal scapular	Ulnar
Suprascapular	Cervical plexus
Musculocutaneous	Thoracic
Median	
Lateral pectoral	
Upper subscapular	
Thoracodorsal	
Lower subscapular	
Axillary	

Posterior Lateral

See Legend on page 419

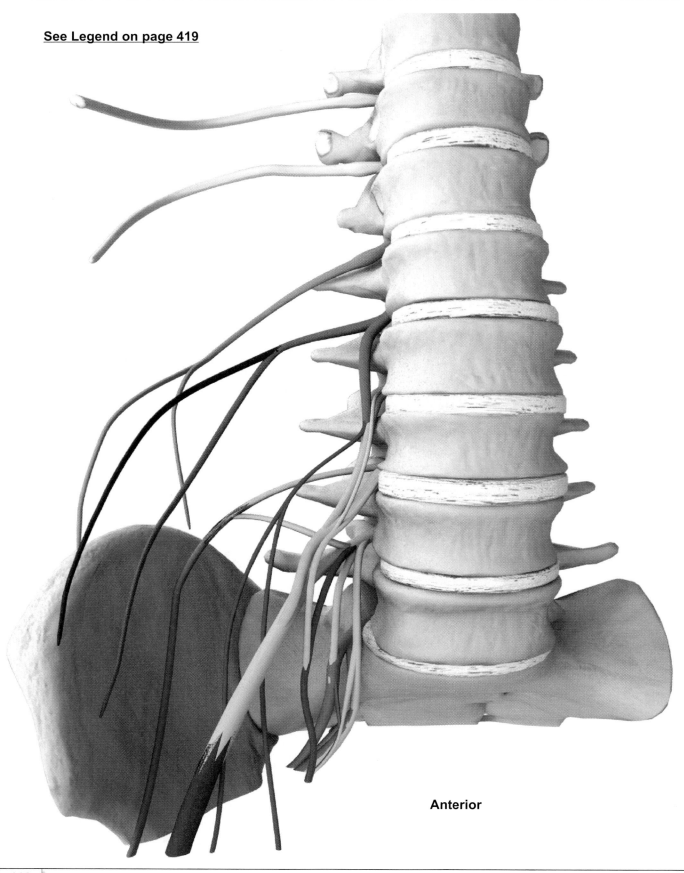

Anterior

Legend

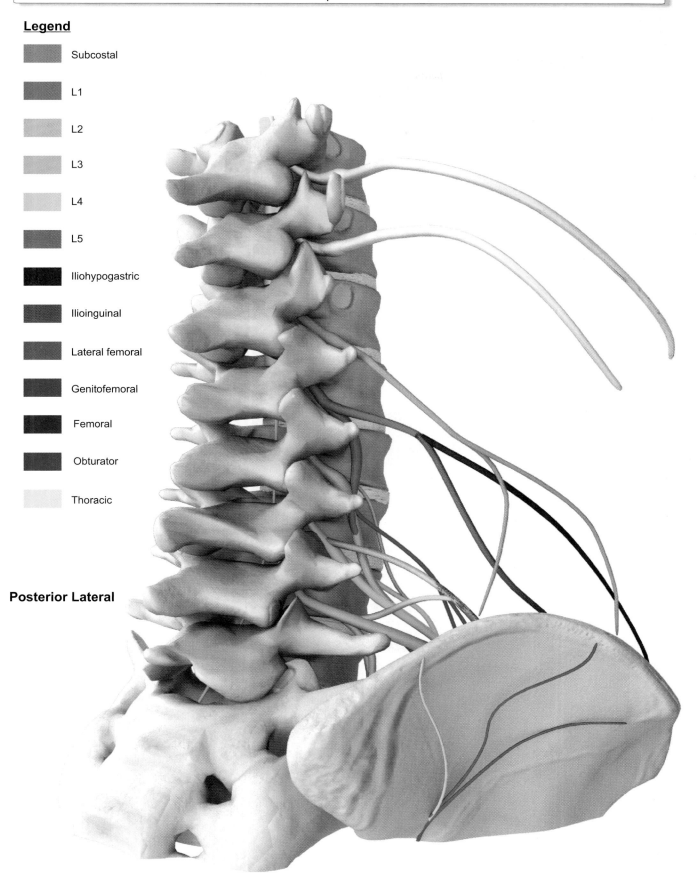

Subcostal

L1

L2

L3

L4

L5

Iliohypogastric

Ilioinguinal

Lateral femoral

Genitofemoral

Femoral

Obturator

Thoracic

Posterior Lateral

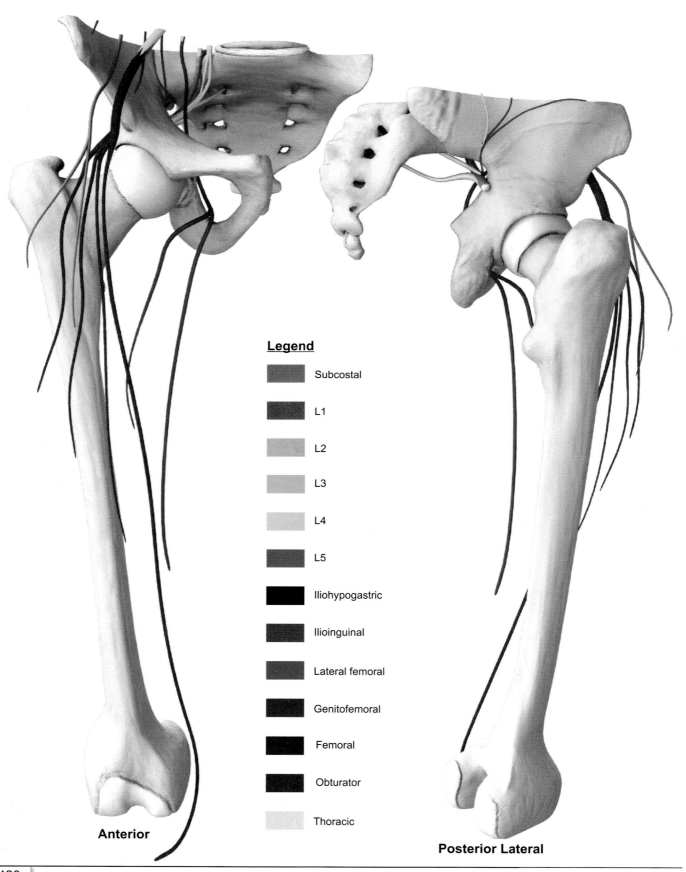

Legend

Subcostal

L1

L2

L3

L4

L5

Iliohypogastric

Ilioinguinal

Lateral femoral

Genitofemoral

Femoral

Obturator

Thoracic

Anterior

Posterior Lateral

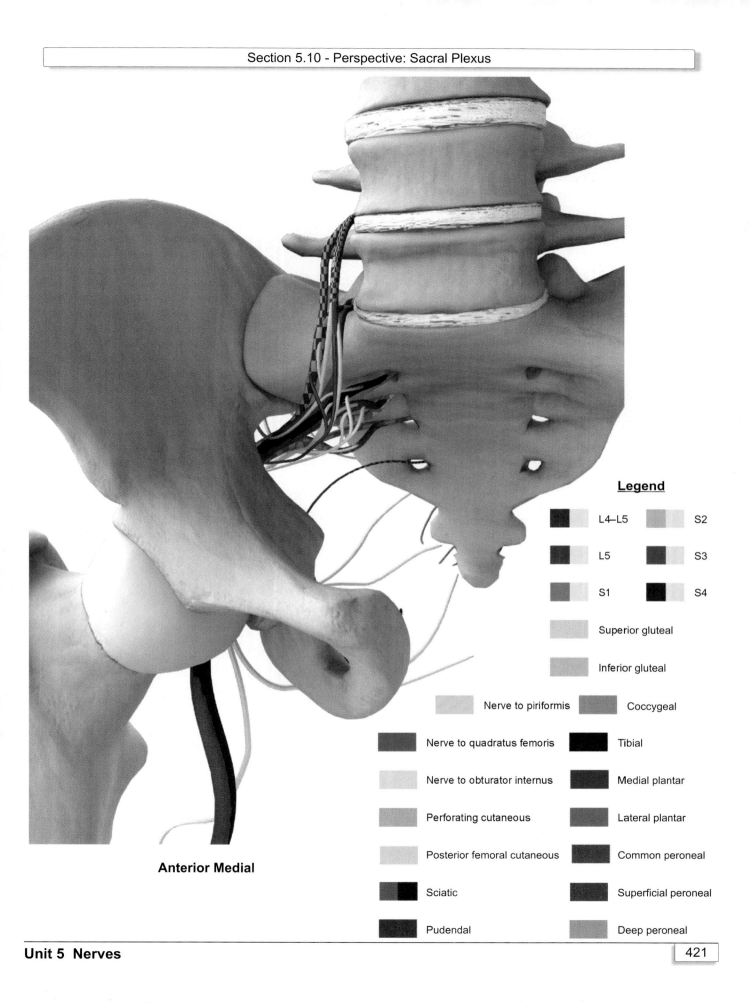

Anterior Medial

Legend

L4–L5	S2
L5	S3
S1	S4

Superior gluteal

Inferior gluteal

Nerve to piriformis   Coccygeal

Nerve to quadratus femoris   Tibial

Nerve to obturator internus   Medial plantar

Perforating cutaneous   Lateral plantar

Posterior femoral cutaneous   Common peroneal

Sciatic   Superficial peroneal

Pudendal   Deep peroneal

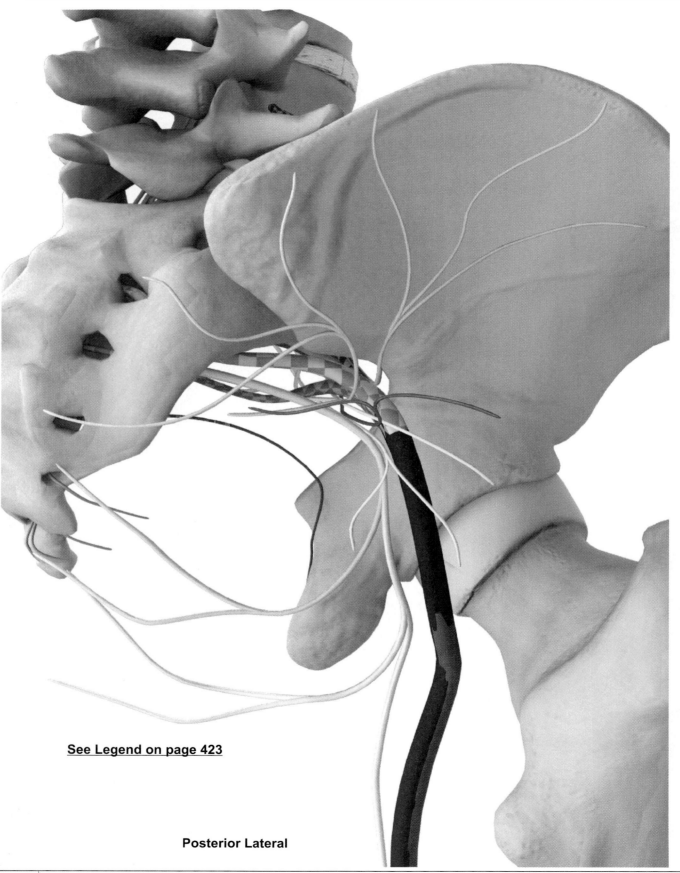

See Legend on page 423

Posterior Lateral

Unit 5 Nerves

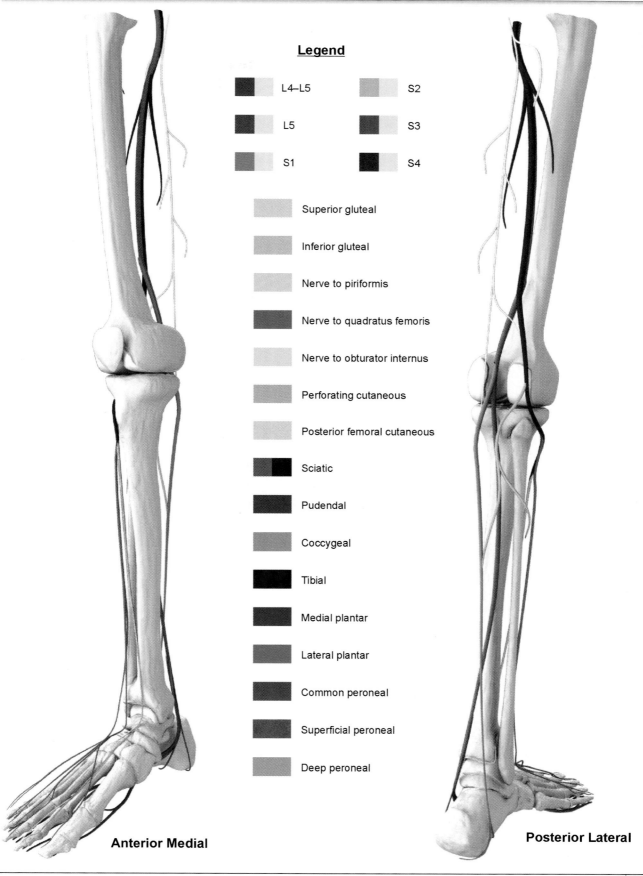

Legend

L4–L5		S2	
L5		S3	
S1		S4	

Superior gluteal

Inferior gluteal

Nerve to piriformis

Nerve to quadratus femoris

Nerve to obturator internus

Perforating cutaneous

Posterior femoral cutaneous

Sciatic

Pudendal

Coccygeal

Tibial

Medial plantar

Lateral plantar

Common peroneal

Superficial peroneal

Deep peroneal

Anterior Medial

Posterior Lateral

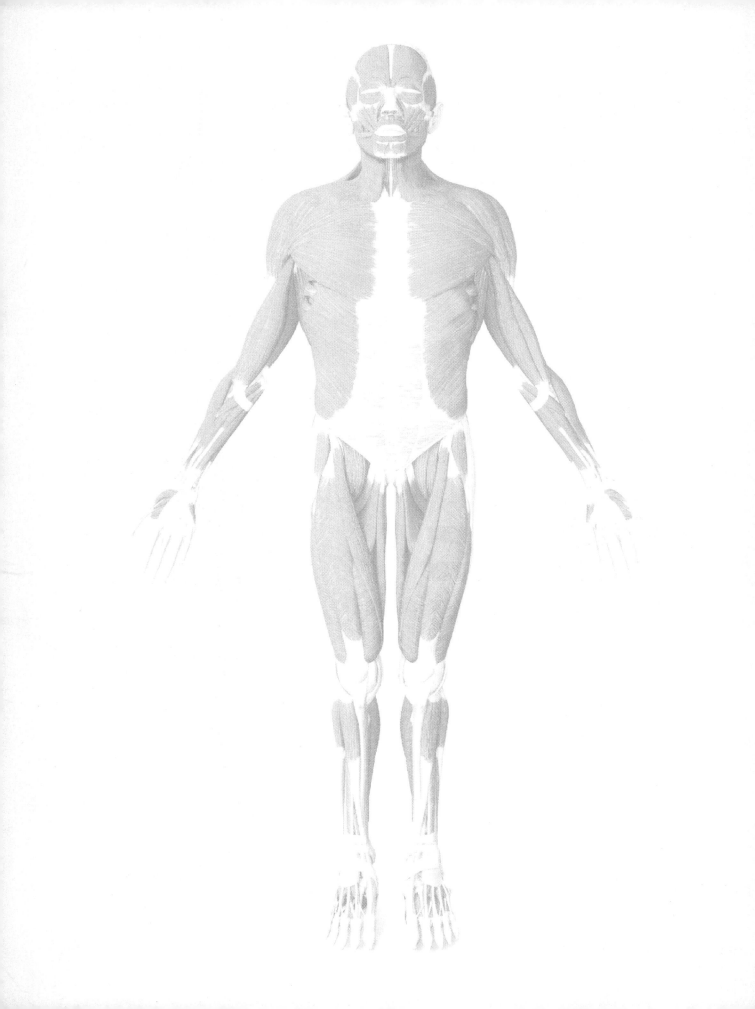

Glossary of Terms/Relative Terminology

A

Abduction - The movement of a body part away from the axis or midline of the body; movement of a digit away from the axis of the limb; opposite of *adduction*.

Acetabulum - A cup-shaped socket in the lateral surface of the hipbone (os coxa) with which the head of the femur articulates.

Adduction - The movement of a body part toward the axis or midline of the body; movement of a digit toward the axis of the limb; retraction; opposite of *abduction*.

Ankle - The area of the joint between the leg and foot; the tarsus.

Anterior (ventral) - Situated or directed toward the front; the opposite of *posterior*.

Annulous fibrosis - 1. A small ring or a circular structure. 2. Fibrous ring of intervertebral disk.

Aperture - An opening or orifice.

Aponeurosis - A fibrous or membranous sheet like tendinous expansion, serving to connect a muscle with the parts it moves.

Articular - Pertaining to a joint.

Articulation - A joint; the place of union or junction between two or more bones of the skeleton.

Atlas - The first cervical vertebra.

Auricle - Flap of elastic cartilage covered by thick skin, attached to the head by ligaments and muscles (forming the external ear).

Axillary - Pertaining to the depressed hollow between the upper arm and lateral chest, commonly called the "armpit."

Axis - The second cervical vertebra.

B

Bilateral - Pertaining to two sides.

Body - Any mass or collection of material.

Bone - Solid, rigid ossified connective tissue that collectively forms the skeletal system.

Brachium - Pertaining to the arm, particularly the arm from shoulder to elbow.

Bursa - A saclike structure filled with synovial fluid. Bursae are located at friction points, such as around joints, over which tendons can slide without contacting bone.

C

Canal - A narrow tube, channel, or passageway.

Capsule - A cartilaginous, fatty, fibrous, membranous structure enveloping another structure, organ, or part.

Carpal - Pertaining to the carpus; referring to the wrist.

Carpus - The proximal portion of the hand that contains the eight carpal bones; the wrist.

Cartilage - A specialized type of fibrous, elastic, connective tissue present in adults and forming the temporary skeleton in the embryo.

Cauda - A tail or tail-like appendage.

Caudal - 1. Pertaining to a cauda. 2. Situated more toward the cauda or tail, than some specified reference point; toward the inferior.

Cervical - Pertaining to the neck, or narrowed portion of a body part.

Cervix - Neck.

Circumduction - Movement at a synovial joint in which the distal end of a bone moves in a circle while the proximal end remains reasonably stable.

Coccyx - The tailbone; the small bone that forms the caudal extremity of the vertebral column.

Coccygeal - Pertaining to the region of the vertebral column that is most inferior.

Collateral - Running side by side; parallel.

Condyle - A rounded process at the end of a long bone, usually for articulation with another bone.

Contralateral - Pertaining to, situated on, or affecting the opposite side; opposite of *ipsilateral*.

Corrugate - To shape into folds or alternate furrows; wrinkle.

Costal - Pertaining to the ribs.

Coxa - Pertaining to the hip or hip joint.

Cranium - The bones of the skull that enclose or support the brain and the organs of sight, hearing, and balance.

Crest - A projection or projecting structure or high ridge, especially one surmounting a bone or its border, for the attachment of muscle.

Cruciate - "Shaped like a cross"; a crossed arrangement of structures.

Cubital - Pertaining to the elbow.

D

Demi - A prefix signifying half.

Dens - A tooth or toothlike structure.

Depression - Movement in which a part of the body moves downward; opposite of *elevation*.

Digit - A finger or toe.

Disc (disk) - A circular or rounded flat plate.

DIP - Distal interphalangeal joint.

Distal - Away from the midline or origin; the opposite of *proximal*.

Dorsal - Pertaining to the back or dorsum.
Dorsiflexion - Movement at the ankle as the foot or toes are raised upward; opposite of *plantarflexion*.
Dorsum - The back.

E

Elevation - Movement in which a part of the body moves upward.
Eminence - A projection.
Epicondyle - A protuberance directly above a condyle to which tendons or ligaments attach.
Eversion - A turning outward; opposite of *inversion*.
Extension - 1. A movement that increases the angle between two bones. 2. Restoring a body part to its anatomical position after flexion; opposite of *flexion*.
Extensor - Any muscle that increases the angle between two bones as it contracts.
External - Situated toward or near the outside; lateral.

F

Facet - A small, smooth area on a bone where articulation occurs.
Fascia - A sheet or band of loose or dense fibrous connective tissue.
Femoral - Pertains to the thigh or the femur.
Fissure - A groove or narrow cleft.
Flexion - A movement that decreases the angle between two bones; opposite of *extension*.
Flexor - A muscle that decreases the angle between two bones as it contracts.
Foot -The distal portion of the leg.
Foramen - A hole or opening in a bone for passage of vessels or nerves.
Forearm - The portion of the upper limb between the wrist and elbow joints.
Fossa - A hollow or shallow depression.
Fovea - A small pit or depression.
Frontal - Pertaining to the region of the forehead; constituting the anterior part of the skull.

G

Glabella - The area on the frontal bone above the nasion (the middle point of the frontonasal suture) and between the eyebrows.
Gluteal - Pertaining to the buttocks.
Groove for radial nerve - A narrow linear hollow, synonymous with spiral groove.

H

Hallux - Pertaining to the big or "great" toe.
Hand - The distal portion of the arm.

Head - A rounded projection beyond a constricted part of a bone. The proximal extremity of a structure.
Horizontal - A directional plane that runs parallel to the ground differentiating between superior and inferior or proximal and distal portions. Also called a transverse plane.

I

Inferior - Below; away from the head or toward the lower part of a structure.
Inguinal - Pertaining to the groin region.
Innervation - The nerve supply to a body structure or area.
Insertion - The site of attachment, as of a muscle to the bone it moves. The opposite of *origin*.
Internal - Located toward the center, away from the surface of the body.
Inversion - A turning inward; opposite of *eversion*.
IP - Interphalangeal joint.
Ipsilateral - Situated on or affecting the same side; opposite of *contralateral*.

J

Joint - The site of junction or union between two or more bones.

L

Lacrimal - Pertaining to tears.
Lacuna - A small pit or hollow cavity, such as that found in bones.
Lambdoid suture - The line of union in the cranium between the occipital bone and the parietal bones.
Lamina - A thin, flat plate or layer that extends superiorly from the body of a vertebra to form either side of the arch of a vertebra.
Lateral - Pertaining to the side; farther away from the midline of the body; opposite of *medial*.
Leg - The portion of the lower limb between the knee and the ankle.
Ligament - A tough cord or fibrous band of dense connective tissue that attaches bone to bone to strengthen and provide flexibility to a joint.
Ligamentum flavum - One of a series of bands of elastic tissue attached to and extending between the anterior portions of the laminae of two adjacent vertebrae from the joint of the axis and the third cervical vertebra to the joint of the fifth lumbar vertebra and the sacral bone. They support the erect position and serve to close in the gaps between the arches.
Line - A ridge of bone less prominent than a crest.

Glossary of Terms/Relative Terminology

Linea aspera - A rough, longitudinal line on the back of the femur for muscle attachments.

Lumbar - Region of the back and side between the ribs and pelvis; pertaining to the loin.

M

Malleolus - A large process at the distal end of the tibia and the fibula.

Margin - An edge or border.

Mass - A lump or collection of cohering particles.

MCP - Metacarpal phalangeal joint.

Meatus - A passage or opening.

Medial - Toward or nearer the midline of the body or structure; opposite of *lateral*.

Membrane - A thin, flexible layer of tissue that covers a surface.

Meniscus - Crescent-shaped fibrocartilages in specific synovial joints.

Mental - Pertaining to the chin.

Metacarpal - Pertaining to the metacarpus.

Metacarpus - The part of the hand between the wrist and the phalanges, including the five metacarpal bones that support the palm of the hand. These are numbered one to five beginning at thumb side.

Metatarsal - Pertaining to the metatarsus. These bones are numbered one to five starting at the great toe.

Metatarsus - The part of the foot between the ankle and the phalanges that includes the five metatarsal bones.

MTP - Metatarsal phalangeal joint.

Muscle - A main type of tissue with contractibility that produces voluntary or involuntary movements of body parts. The three types of muscle are skeletal, smooth, and visceral.

N

Nares - The nostrils.

Nasal - Pertaining to the nose.

Neck - A constricted portion.

Nerve - A bundle of nerve fibers and associated connective tissue, outside the central nervous system, that transmits impulses between a part of the central nervous system and another part of the body.

Notch - An indentation on the edge of a bone.

Nuchal - Pertaining to the nape or back of the neck.

Nucleus pulposus - A soft, pulpy, elastic mass forming the center of an intervertebral disk.

O

Occipital - The bone that makes up the back and part of the base of the skull.

Opposition - Movement of the thumb toward one or more of the fingers; opposite of *reposition*.

Orbit - The bony cavity of the skull that holds the eyeball and its related muscles, vessels, and nerves.

Orifice - An opening or outlet of a body cavity or tube.

Origin - The more stationary end or attachment of a muscle; opposite of *insertion*.

Os coxa - A large flat bone formed by the fusion of the ilium, ischium, and pubis (in the adult), which constitutes the lateral half of the pelvis.

P

Palate - The roof of the mouth, horizontally separating the oral and nasal cavities.

Palmar - Pertaining to the palm of the hand.

Parietal - 1. The bone between the frontal and occipital bones that forms the superior and lateral parts of the skull. 2. Pertaining to a wall or organ of a cavity.

Pectoral - Pertaining to the chest or breast.

Pedicle - 1. The portion of the vertebra that connects and attaches the lamina to the body. 2. A footlike structure.

Pelvis - A basinlike bony structure formed by the two hip bones, the sacrum, and the coccyx.

Phalanx - (*Plural*, phalanges) Any bone of a finger or toe. The fingers are numbered one to five beginning with the thumb. Toes are numbered one through five starting with the great toe.

PIP - Proximal interphalangeal joint.

Plantar - Pertaining to the sole of the foot.

Plantarflexion - Movement at the ankle as the foot bends in the direction of the plantar surface.

Plate - A flat structure or layer, as a thin layer of bone.

Plexus - A network; primarily of nerves or vessels.

Pollicis - Pertaining to the thumb.

Popliteal - Pertaining to the concave area on the posterior aspect of the knee.

Posterior - Toward or situated at the back; also called dorsal; opposite of *anterior*.

Process - A prominence or projection.

Promontory - A projecting eminence or process.

Pronation - The rotational movement of turning downward; opposite of *supination*.

Protraction - The forward movement of a body part on a plane parallel to the ground; opposite of *retraction*.

Protuberance - A projecting or elevated part.

Proximal - Closer to the midline of the body or to the origin of an appendage; the opposite of *distal*.

R

Radiate - Radiating from a central point or part.

Ramus - A branch of bone, artery, or nerve.

Raphe - The line of union of the halves of various symmetrical parts.

Rectus - Pertains to something that is straight.

Reposition - Returning the thumb to a parallel position with the fingers; opposite of *opposition*.

Retinaculum - A structure that holds an organ or tissue in place.

Retraction - The backward movement of a body part; on a plane parallel with the ground; adduction; opposite of *protraction*.

Ribs - Arches of bone that form the chief part of the thoracic walls. They articulate with the vertebrae and occur in pairs, 12 on each side. The first 7 are called **true ribs**. The remaining 5 are **false ribs** of which the last 2 are termed **floating ribs**.

Ridge - A linear projection or projecting structure.

Rotation - The movement of a bone around its own longitudinal axis, with no other movement.

S

Sacral - Pertaining to the sacrum.

Sacroiliac joint - The joint between the sacrum and adjacent surface of the ilium.

Sacrum - Wedge-shaped bone formed by fusion of 5 vertebrae, making up posterior wall of pelvis.

Septum - A dividing wall or partition.

Shaft - An elongated slender part, as the segment of a long bone between the wider ends.

Shoulder - A synovial joint where the humerus articulates with the scapula.

Skull - The cranium; the skeleton of the head consisting of the cranial and facial bones.

Spine - 1. A slender, sharp projection. 2. The vertebral column.

Spiral groove - Groove for radial nerve.

Styloid - A long and tapered bony prominence for muscle attachment.

Sulcus - Open, ditchlike groove.

Superficial - Situated on or near the surface of the body.

Superior - Toward the upper part of a structure or the head (also called *cephalic*).

Supination - The rotational movement of turning upward (opposite of *pronation*).

Suture - A fibrous joint between bones of the skull.

Symphysis - A joint distinguished by a fibrocartilaginous pad between the articulating bones that provides slight movement.

T

Tarsal - Pertaining to the tarsus.

Tarsus - A collective term for the seven bones of the ankle.

Tendon - A white, fibrous cord of dense, connective tissue that attaches muscle to bone.

Thigh - The portion of the lower extremity above the knee and beneath the hip; femur.

Thoracic - Pertaining to the chest.

Thorax - The chest.

Trochanter - Broad, flat process.

Trochlea - A pulleylike structure.

Trunk - The main part of the body to which the head and extremities are attached.

Tubercle - A small rounded eminence.

Tuberosity - A protuberance on a bone.

U

Unilateral - Pertaining to one side.

Upper extremity - The appendage connected to the shoulder girdle consisting of the arm, forearm, wrist, hand, and fingers.

V

Ventral - Toward the anterior or front side of the body (opposite of *dorsal*).

Vertebrae - Any of the bones of the vertebral column (26 in an adult, 33 in an infant).

Vertebral column - The 26 vertebrae that collectively enclose and protect the spinal cord. It serves as a point of attachment for the ribs and back muscles. Also called the spine, spinal column, or backbone.

X

Xiphoid - Sword-shaped.

Glossary of Terms/Relative Terminology

References

Austrin, Miriam G. & Austrin, Harvey R., *Learning Medical Terminology*, 8th edition. St. Louis, MO: Mosby Life Line, 1995.

Birn, Jeremy, *Lighting and Rendering* (digital). Indianapolis, IN: New Riders, 2000.

Bowden, Bradley & Bowden, Joan, *An Illustrated Atlas of the Skeletal Muscles*. Englewood, CO: Morton Publishing Company, 2002.

Calais Germain, Blandine, *Anatomy of Movement*. Seattle: Eastland Press, 1993.

Chaitow, Leon, *Palpatory Skills*. New York: Churchill Livingstone, 1997.

Clemente, Carmine, *Gray's Anatomy*, 30th edition. Philadelphia: Lea & Febiger, 1985.

Cyriax J. & Cyriax P., *Illustrated Manual of Orthopaedic Medicine*. Boston: Butterworths, 1983.

Dorland's Illustrated Medical Dictionary, 25th edition. Philadelphia, W. B. Saunders Co., 1995.

Hay, James G. & Reid, J. Gavin, *Anatomy, Mechanics and Human Motion*, 2nd edition. Englewood Cliffs, NJ: Prentice Hall, 1988.

Hole, John, *Essentials of Human Anatomy and Physiology*, 4th edition. Dubuque, IA: Wm. C. Brown Publishers, 1992.

Kendall, F. P., McCreary, E. K., Provance P. G., *Muscles, Testing and Function*, 4th edition. Baltimore: Williams and Wilkins, 1993.

Magee, David, *Orthopedic Physical Assessment*, 2nd edition. Philadelphia: W. B. Saunders, 1992.

Netter, Frank H., *Atlas of Human Anatomy*, 3rd edition. Teterboro, NJ: Icon Learning Systems, 2003.

Nordin, Margareta & Frankel, Victor H., *Basic Biomechanics of the Musculoskeletal System*, 2nd edition. Philadelphia: Lea & Febiger, 1989.

Rohen, Johannes & Yokochi, Chihiro, *Atlas of Color Anatomy*, 3rd. Edition. New York: Igaku Shoin Publishers, 1993.

Seig, Kay & Adams, Sandra, *Illustrated Essentials of Musculoskeletal Anatomy*, 3rd edition. Gainsville, FL: Megabooks, 1996.

Taber's Cyclopedic Medical Dictionary, 17th edition. Philadelphia: F. A. Davis, 1993.

Tortora, G. J. & Grabowski, S. R., *Principles of Anatomy and Physiology*, 7th edition. New York: HarperCollins College Publishers, 1993.

Travell, Janet & Simons, David, *Myofascial Pain and Dysfunction: Trigger Point Manual*, Volume 1. Baltimore: Williams and Wilkins, 1983.

Travell, Janet & Simons, David, *Myofascial Pain and Dysfunction: Trigger Point Manual*, Volume 2. Baltimore: Williams and Wilkins, 1992.

Websites

http://anatomy.uams.edu/HTMLpages/anatomyhtml/muscles_alpha.html

http://medical-dictionary.com/

http://www.geocities.com/medinotes/main_anatomy_index.htm

http://www.gpnotebook.co.uk/homePage.cfm

http://www.med.umich.edu/lrc/coursepages/M1/anatomy/html/anatomytables/muscles.html

http://www.meddean.luc.edu/lumen/MedEd/GrossAnatomy/dissector/mml/index.htm

http://www.ortho-u.net/Welcome.html

http://www.pccclass041.org/classes/tri2/gross2/unit1muscles.htm

http://www.ptcentral.com/muscles/

http://www.rad.washington.edu/atlas/

http://www.rad.washington.edu/atlas2/

http://www.recnet.ca/anatomy101/

http://www.tedmontgomery.com/the_eye/eom.html

http://www.vh.org/adult/provider/anatomy/AnatomicVariants/MuscularSystem/

Index